ADVANCES IN
HUMAN GENETICS 15

CONTRIBUTORS TO THIS VOLUME

Charles Auffray
Institut d'Embryologie du CNRS et du
* Collège de France*
Nogent sur Marne, France

Arthur L. Beaudet
Departments of Pediatrics and Cell Biology
Baylor College of Medicine
Houston, Texas

Hans-Georg O. Bock
Department of Pediatrics
Baylor College of Medicine
Houston, Texas

Svend O. Freytag
Department of Pediatrics
Baylor College of Medicine
Houston, Texas

Michelle M. Le Beau
Department of Medicine
Section of Hematology/Oncology
University of Chicago
Chicago, Illinois

James V. Neel
Department of Human Genetics
University of Michigan Medical School
Ann Arbor, Michigan

William E. O'Brien
Departments of Pediatrics and Bioche
Baylor College of Medicine
Houston, Texas

Janet D. Rowley
Department of Medicine
Section of Hematology/Oncology
University of Chicago
Chicago, Illinois

Michael M. Skolnick
Department of Human Genetics
University of Michigan Medical Schoo
Ann Arbor, Michigan

Moyra Smith
Department of Pediatrics
University of California at Irvine
Irvine, California

Jack L. Strominger
Department of Biochemistry and
* Molecular Biology*
Harvard University
Cambridge, Massachusetts

Tsung-Sheng Su
Department of Pediatrics
Baylor College of Medicine
Houston, Texas

A Continuation Order Plan is available for this series. A continuation order will bring delivery of
each new volume immediately upon publication. Volumes are billed only upon actual shipment.
For further information please contact the publisher.

ADVANCES IN HUMAN GENETICS 15

Edited by

Harry Harris

Harnwell Professor of Human Genetics
University of Pennsylvania, Philadelphia

and

Kurt Hirschhorn

Herbert H. Lehman Professor and Chairman of Pediatrics
Mount Sinai School of Medicine of The City University of New York

PLENUM PRESS • NEW YORK AND LONDON

The Library of Congress catalogued the first volume of this title as follows:

Advances in human genetics. 1—
  New York, Plenum Press, 1970—
    (1) v. illus. 24-cm.
    Editors: V. 1—   H. Harris and K. Hirschhorn.
  1. Human genetics—Collected works. I. Harris, Harry, ed. II. Hirschhorn, Kurt, 1926—
  joint ed.
QH431.A1A32   573.2′1   77-84583

ISBN-13: 978-1-4615-8358-5   e-ISBN-13: 978-1-4615-8356-1
DOI: 10.1007/978-1-4615-8356-1

ARTICLES PLANNED FOR FUTURE VOLUMES

CONTENTS OF EARLIER VOLUMES

Preface to Volume 1

During the last few years the science of human genetics has been expanding almost explosively. Original papers dealing with different aspects of the subject are appearing at an increasing rapid rate in a very wide range of journals, and it becomes more and more difficult for the geneticist and virtually impossible for the nongeneticist to keep track of the developments. Furthermore, new observations and discoveries relevant to an overall understanding of the subject result from investigations using very diverse techniques and methodologies and originating in a variety of different disciplines. Thus, investigations in such various fields as enzymology, immunology, protein chemistry, cytology, pediatrics, neurology, internal medicine, anthropology, and mathematical and statistical genetics, to name but a few, have each contributed results and ideas of general significance to the study of human genetics. Not surprisingly it is often difficult for workers in one branch of the subject to assess and assimilate findings made in another. This can be a serious limiting factor on the rate of progress.

Thus, there appears to be a real need for critical review which summarizes the positions reached in different areas, and it is hoped that *Advances in Human Genetics* will help to meet this requirement.

Each of the contributors has been asked to write an account of the position that has been reached in the investigations of a specific topic in one of the branches of human genetics. The reviews are intended to be critical and to deal with the topic in depth from the writer's own point of view. It is hoped that the articles will provide workers in other branches of the subject, and in related disciplines, with a detailed account of the results so far obtained in the particular area, and help them to assess the relevance of these discoveries to aspects of their own work, as well as to the science as a whole. The reviews are also intended to give the reader some idea of the nature of the technical and methodological problems involved, and to indicate new directions stemming from recent advances.

The contributors have not been restricted in the arrangement or organization of their material or in the manner of its presentation, so that the reader should be able to appreciate something of the individuality of approach which goes to make up the subject of human genetics, and which, indeed, gives it much of its fascination.

HARRY HARRIS
The Galton Laboratory
University College London

KURT HIRSCHHORN
Division of Medical Genetics
Department of Pediatrics
Mount Sinai School of Medicine

Preface to Volume 10

This is the tenth volume of *Advances in Human Genetics* and some fifty different reviews covering a very wide range of topics have now appeared. Many of the earlier articles still stand as valuable sources of reference. But the subject continues to move forward at an increasing speed and its vitality is indicated by its remarkable recruitment of young investigators. New areas of research which could hardly have been envisaged only a few years ago have emerged, and quite unexpectedly dicoveries have been made in parts of the subject which only recently had come to be thought as full explored. So there continues to be a need for authoritative and critical reviews intended to keep workers in the various branches of this seemingly ever-expanding subject fully informed about the progress that is being made and also, of course, to provide a ready and accessible account of new developments in human genetics for those whose primary interests are in other fields of biological and medical research.

We see no reason to alter the general policy which was outlined in the preface to the first volume. We believe that it has served our readers well. The subject seems to us to be just as exciting and intellectually stimulating and rewarding as it did when this series was first started. We expect the next decade of research in human genetics to be as innovative and productive as the last and our aim is to record its progress in *Advances in Human Genetics*.

HARRY HARRIS
University of Pennsylvania, Philadelphia

KURT HIRSCHHORN
*Mount Sinai School of Medicine
of the City University of New York*

NOTE ABOUT ADDENDUM

To make the volume as up-to-date as possible, each author was given the opportunity to write a short Addendum at the time he or she received the page proofs of that particular chapter. This allows for any important new material to be presented at the latest possible time in the publication process. The Addendum is presented at the end of the book, beginning on page 291.

Contents

Chapter 1
**Chromosomal Abnormalities in Leukemia and Lymphoma:
Clinical and Biological Significance**

Michelle M. Le Beau and Janet D. Rowley

Chapter 2

**An Algorithm for Comparing Two-Dimensional Electrophoretic Gels,
with Particular Reference to the Study of Mutation**

Michael M. Skolnick and James V. Neel

Chapter 3

The Human Argininosuccinate Synthetase Locus and Citrullinemia

Arthur L. Beaudet, William E. O'Brien, Hans-Georg O. Bock,
Svend O. Freytag, and Tsung-Sheng Su

Chapter 4

Molecular Genetics of the Human Major Histocompatibility Complex

Charles Auffray and Jack L. Strominger

Chapter 5

Genetics of Human Alcohol and Aldehyde Dehydrogenases

Moyra Smith

Chromosomal Abnormalities in Leukemia and Lymphoma: Clinical and Biological Significance

Michelle M. Le Beau and Janet D. Rowley

Department of Medicine
Section of Hematology/Oncology
University of Chicago
Chicago, Illinois 60637

INTRODUCTION

Cytogenetic analysis of human tumors is one of the most rapidly progressing and exciting areas of cancer research. Major advances in our understanding of the specificity of some of the abnormalities observed have occurred within the last 10 years with the application of both chromosome banding techniques and improved methods of cell culture. Thus, the hypothesis put forward by Boveri at the turn of the century, that an abnormal chromosome pattern was intimately associated with the malignant phenotype of the tumor cell, can now be tested with the substantial hope of obtaining a valid answer (Boveri, 1914).

The study of the chromosome pattern in human leukemias can be divided into two periods, each one covering 10 years. The first lasted from 1960 to 1970, and the second from 1970 to 1980. During the first period, the chromosome abnormalities seen in leukemic cells were identified without banding, and therefore they include only structural rearrangements that resulted in a change in morphology and abnormal modal chromosome numbers. The most significant observation during this initial period was the identification of the Philadelphia (Ph[1]) chromosome in leukemic cells from patients with chronic myelogenous leukemia (CML)

1

(Nowell and Hungerford, 1960). In 1960, when this abnormality was discovered by Nowell and Hungerford, it appeared to represent a deletion of about half of the long arm of one G-group chromosome; whether pair 21 or 22 was affected was not determined. This observation led to a search for similar abnormalities closely associated with other types of malignant hematologic diseases. The results were quite disappointing, in that although the abnormalities seemed to be consistent in any particular patient, the patterns varied greatly from one patient to another. Moreover, about half of the patients with acute leukemia of both the myeloid and lymphoid types appeared to have a normal karyotype in their leukemic cells (Rowley, 1980a, 1983a; Sandberg, 1980). Thus the accepted notion was that the Ph[1] was a unique example of a consistent karyotypic abnormality, and that the general rule was one of marked variability in karyotype. This in turn led most investigators to assume that chromosome changes were a secondary phenomenon not fundamentally involved with the process of malignant transformation.

The evidence obtained during the second period showed that these assumptions were probably not correct. With the use of banding techniques, other specific structural abnormalities were found to be associated with certain leukemias and lymphomas (Rowley, 1980a). Moreover, banding techniques revealed that the gains and losses of chromosomes were also distinctly nonrandom. These major advances in our understanding of the specificity of cancer chromosomal abnormalities were in large part the result of collaborative efforts among cytogeneticists, clinicians, and morphologists. Using the newly proposed French–American–British (FAB) Cooperative Group criteria for the morphological classification of acute leukemias (Bennett et al., 1976) (Table I, Fig. 1), investigators during this second period recognized that the specific chromosomal abnormalities often correlated with subtypes of leukemia that had chracteristic morphological and clinical features, such as response to therapy (First International Workshop on Chromosomes in Leukemia, 1978; Second International Workshop on Chromosomes in Leukemia, 1980).

Cancer cytogenetists have now embarked upon a third period of analysis, characterized by substantial improvements in the quality of the chromosome preparations available for analysis. Many of the studies prior to 1980 used chromosomes that were relatively contracted, and the banding pattern was often fuzzy and poorly defined. For this reason, subtle abnormalities, such as a deletion or a duplication of one-third of a chromosome band, involving about 3×10^6 nucleotide pairs, would be un-

TABLE I. French–American–British (FAB) Classification of Acute Leukemia[a]

FAB subtype		Percent of patients[b]
	Lymphoblastic (ALL)	
L1	Small cells; homogeneous morphology	41
L2	Large cells; heterogeneous morphology	52
L3	Large cells; homogeneous morphology (Burkitt type)	7
	Myeloid (ANLL)	
M1	Acute myeloblastic leukemia without maturation (AML)	15
M2	Acute myeloblastic leukemia with maturation	34
M3	Acute promyelocytic leukemia, hypergranular (APL)	9.5
M3V	Acute promyelocytic leukemia, microgranular	
M4	Acute myelomonocytic leukemia (AMMoL)	23
M5a	Acute monocytic leukemia, poorly differentiated (AMoL)	14.0
M5b	Acute monocytic leukemia, well differentiated	
M6	Erythroleukemia (EL)	4.5

[a] Bennett et al. (1976).
[b] Third International Workshop on Chromosomes in Leukemia (1981); Fourth International Workshop on Chromosomes in Leukemia (1984).

detectable. It is noteworthy that the chromosomal abnormalities described in the past few years [i.e., inv(16)(p13q22), t(9;11)(p22;q23), and t(6;9)(p23;q34)] represent subtle rearrangements that in all likelihood were previously overlooked. With improvements in the quality of preparations' we anticipate that the proportion of leukemic patients in whom abnormalities are detected should increase over the 50% figure determined by earlier investigations. In fact, Yunis et al. (1981) reported that by using cell synchronization and high-resolution banding techniques to study patients with acute nonlymphocytic leukemia (ANLL), they identified karyotypic abnormalities in each of 24 patients examined. The data obtained prior to 1970 have been reviewed in a number of reports and they will not be considered here (Sandberg, 1980). The data presented here have been gathered primarily during the period 1974–1983 [for review, see Mitelman and Levan (1978), Sandberg (1980), Rowley (1980a,b, 1983), Rowley and Testa (1982), Yunis (1983)].

Several major types of chromosome abnormalities have been identified in human leukemias and other malignant diseases (Table II) (Yunis, 1983). These include gain of a whole chromosome or a portion thereof, loss of part or all of a chromosome, consistent translocations, and other structural rearrangements. This diversity of abnormalities implies an

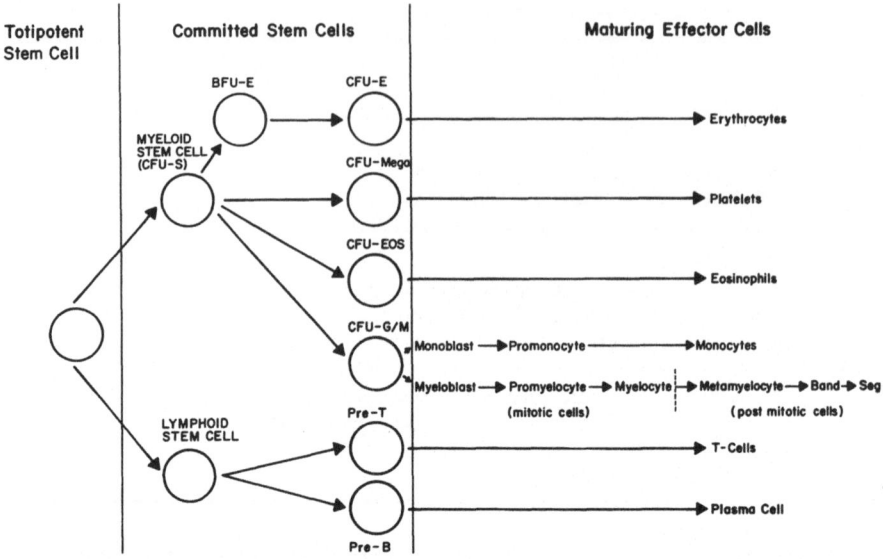

Fig. 1. A schematic outline of hematopoiesis. Lymphoid and myeloid stem cells are derived from totipotent stem cells. Committed stem cells give rise to mature circulating blood cells following division and terminal differentiation. CFU-S, colony-forming unit-spleen; BFU-E, burst-forming unit-erythroid; CFU-E, colony-forming unit-erythroid; CFU-Mega, colony-forming unit-megakaryocyte; CFU-Eos, colony-forming unit-eosinophil; CFU-G/M, colony-forming unit-granulocyte/monocyte. In a pathological situation, cell differentiation is blocked, and a progressive clonal expansion of a population of immature cells occurs.

equal diversity in the mechanisms of genetic changes that can be associated with malignant transformation. For example, a gain of all or part of a chromosome implies amplification of a gene, suggesting that an increase in a gene product is an important factor in the malignant process. Deletion of part or all of a chromosome suggests that loss of certain elements regulating cell growth may be significant. Consistent translocations, on the other hand, imply that a more complex process is involved, because two chromosomes and presumably two genes are affected by this rearrangement. It should be emphasized that for each type of abberation certain chromosomes are preferentially affected. Thus, a gain of chromosome 8 is the most frequent aberration in a variety of myeloid disorders (Mitelman and Levan, 1978; Sandberg, 1980; Rowley and Testa, 1982). When a chromosome is lost, chromosome 7 is most commonly affected. The consistent translocations in myeloid disorders are t(9;22) in CML (Rowley, 1973a), t(8;21) in acute myelogenous leukemia with maturation

TABLE II. Consistent Chromosomal Abnormalities in Hematologic Malignancies

Malignancy	Chromosomal abnormality	Percent of patients
CML		
Chronic phase	t(9;22)(q34;q11)	85–100
Blast crisis	t(9;22)(q34;q11), +8, +Ph[1], i(17q)	—
ANLL	+8	25
	−7	12
AML (M2)	t(8;21)(q22;q22)	10
APL (M3)	t(15;17)(q22;q21)	70
AMMoL (M4)	inv(16)(p13q22), del(16)(q22)	25
AMoL (M5) or AMMoL (M4)	t(9;11)(p21 or p22;q23), t(11q), del(11q)	10
ALL	t(9;22)(q34;q11)	12
	t(4;11)(q21;q23)	5
	t(8;14)(q24;q32)	5
	Hyperdiploidy (50–60 chromosomes)	9
B-Cell ALL	14q+	100
Burkitt lymphoma	t(8;14)(q24;q32)	80
Non-Hodgkin lymphoma	t(14;18)(q32;q21)	20
	t(11;14)(q13;q32)	10
	del(6q)	20
	+12	19
	+18	13
	+7	12
	+21	10

(AML-M2) (Rowley, 1973*b*), and t(15;17) in acute promyelocytic leukemia (APL-M3) (Rowley *et al.*, 1977). More recently, translocations or deletions involving chromosome 11 have been observed primarily in acute monocytic leukemia (AMoL-M5) (Berger *et al.*, 1982), and an inversion of chromosome 16 has been described in acute myelomonocytic leukemia (AMMoL-M4) (Le Beau *et al.*, 1983). Different chromosomes are involved in lymphoid disorders, e.g., t(8;14), t(2;8), t(8;22), and t(14;18) (Mitelman and Levan, 1978; Sandberg, 1980; Rowley and Testa, 1982).

METHODS

Cytogenetic analyses in malignant disease must be based upon the study of the tumor cells themselves. In leukemia, the specimen is usually a bone marrow aspirate either processed immediately (direct preparation) or cultured for 24–48 hr. When a bone marrow aspirate cannot be obtained, a bone marrow biopsy (bone core specimen) can often be successfully processed. Alternatively, in patients with a white blood cell count higher than 15,000 with about 10% immature myeloid or lymphoid cells, a sample of peripheral blood can be cultured without adding phytohemagglutinin (PHA). The karyotype of the dividing cells will be similar to that obtained from the bone marrow. Mitogens such as PHA are not routinely added to peripheral blood cultures in acute leukemia since stimulation of division of normal lymphoid cells may interfere with the analysis of spontaneously dividing malignant cells. The use of amethopterin or fluorodeoxyuridine to synchronize dividing cells enables one to obtain elongated chromosomes that have an increased number of bands.

Chromosomal abnormalities are described according to the International System for Human Cytogenetic Nomenclature (1978), and the criteria initially suggested by Rowley and Potter (1976) and accepted at the First International Workshop on Chromosomes in Leukemia (1978) are used for the identification of abnormal clones. Following these criteria, the observation of at least two "pseudodiploid" (e.g., translocations, deletions, inversions) or hyperdiploid cells, or three hypodiploid or monosomic cells, each showing the same abnormality, is considered evidence for the presence of an abnormal clone. However, one cell with a normal karyotype is considered evidence for the presence of a normal cell line. Patients whose cells show no alteration, or in whom the alterations involve different chromosomes in different cells, are considered normal. Isolated changes such as chromosome loss may be due to technical artifacts or to random mitotic errors. The presence of a single cell showing an abnormality that is a recognized nonrandom rearrangement must be interpreted with care, however, and it may be necessary to analyze additional cells or to request a second sample to establish the presence of an abnormal clone. In some of the lymphoproliferative diseases charactized by a low mitotic rate, such as multiple myeloma, chronic lymphocytic leukemia, or Hodgkin disease, a single abnormal cell may represent the only dividing malignant cell noted in a particular sample.

CHRONIC MYELOGENOUS LEUKEMIA (CML)

Chronic Phase of CML

Chronic myelogenous leukemia is a particularly important subtype of leukemia because it was in this disease that the first consistent chromosomal abnormality in a malignant disease was noted. This abnormality, the Philadelphia or Ph[1] chromosome, was first described by Nowell and Hungerford (1960) as a deletion of part of the long arm of a G-group chromosome, and later with the use of quinacrine fluorescence banding techniques as a 22q − (Caspersson et al., 1970; O'Riordan et al., 1971). The nature of the chromosome aberration was clarified by Rowley who reported that the Ph[1] chromosome resulted from a translocation rather than a deletion as many investigators had previously assumed (Rowley, 1973a). In each of nine patients examined by Rowley, additional pale fluorescent material was present at the end of the long arm of chromosome 9. This additional material was approximately equal in length to that missing from the Ph[1] chromosome, and it had staining characteristics similar to those of the distal portion of the long arm of chromosome 22. It was proposed that the abnormality of CML was an apparently balanced reciprocal translocation t(9;22)(q34;q11) (Fig. 2a). Subsequent measurement of the DNA content of the affected pairs (9 and 22) have shown that the amount of additional DNA present on 9 is equal to that missing from the Ph[1]; thus, there is no detectable loss of DNA in this chromosomal rearrangement (Mayall et al., 1977). The reciprocal nature of this translocation was established only recently, when the Abelson oncogene c-abl, normally located on chromosome 9, was identified on the Ph[1] chromosome (de Klein et al., 1982). Other studies with chromosomal polymorphisms have shown that in a particular patient, the same 9 or 22 is involved in each cell (Gahrton et al., 1974). These observations confirm earlier work based on enzyme markers, indicating that the CML cells originated from a single cell and were therefore clonal in origin (Fialkow, 1974).

Historically, about 85% of patients diagnosed as having CML were found to have the Ph[1] chromosome (Whang-Peng et al., 1968; Rowley, 1980c). Identification of patients as Ph[1]-positive or Ph[1]-negative was found to be clinically significant in that Ph[1]-positive patients had a better prognosis than did those patients with Ph[1]-negative CML (42 vs. 15 months survival). Moreover, patients with a Ph[1] chromosome and additional chromosomal abnormalities do not have a substantially poorer survival than do those patients who have only a Ph[1] chromosome. A change in the karyotype, however, is considered to be a grave prognostic sign indicating impending acute phase; the median survival after such a change is 2–5 months (Whang-Peng et al., 1968). A recent study by Pugh et al. (1983) of patients initially diagnosed as having CML whose cells lacked the Ph[1] chromosome showed that most of the 25 Ph[1]-negative patients did not have CML, but instead had some type of myelodysplasia, most

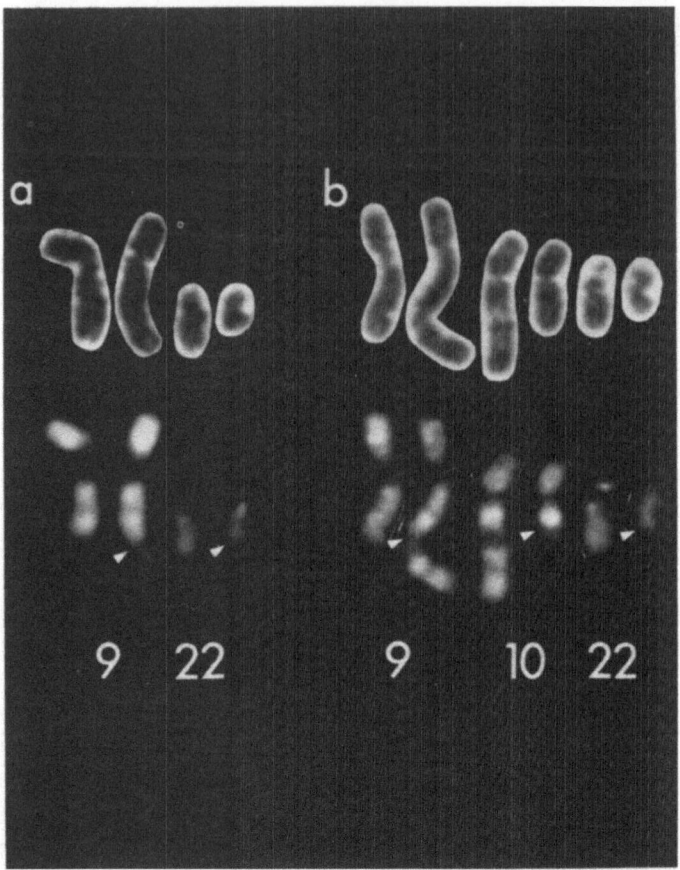

Fig. 2. Partial karyotypes of Giemsa-stained and quinacrine fluorescent-banded metaphase cells obtained from bone marrow of two CML patients. (a) t(9;22)(q34;q11). The Ph[1] and 9q+ chromosomes are on the right of each pair. (b) Variant Ph[1] translocation. Three-way translocation involving chromosomes 9, 10, and 22 [t(9;22;10)(q34;q11;q22)]. Chromosomal material from the long arm of 9 is translocated to 22; the long arm of 10 is translocated to 9q, and material from 22q is present on 10q. Rather than a Ph[1], this cell contains an isochromosome (22q−). The rearranged chromosomes are on the right in each pair. Chromosomal breakpoints are identified with arrowheads.

commonly chronic myelomonocytic leukemia or refractory anemia with excess blasts. This observation raises the question as to whether Ph[1]-negative CML really exists and whether these patients are more appropriately classified within the myelodysplasias. Interestingly, the most common abnormality in these patients was a gain of chromosome 8.

The karyotypes of many Ph[1]-positive patients with CML have been examined with banding techniques by a number of investigators; in a recent review of 1129 Ph[1]-positive patients, the 9;22 translocation was identified in 1036 (92%) (Rowley and Testa, 1982). Variant translocations have been discovered, however, in addition to the typical t(9;22) (Fig. 2b). Until very recently, these were thought to be of two kinds; one appeared to be a simple translocation involving chromosome 22 and some chromosome other than 9 (42 patients; 3.7%), and the other was a complex translocation involving three or more chromosomes, two of which were 9 and 22 (46 patients; 4.1%). Five patients were reported not to have had a translocation; the chromosomal material from 22q was presumed to be missing. Recent data clearly demonstrate that chromosome 9 is affected in the simple as well as the complex translocations, and that its involvement had previously been overlooked (Hagemeijer et al., 1984). Mitelman and Levan (1978) observed that, in the "simple" translocations, the breaks were localized to the ends of the chromosomes other than 22. This phenomenon may account for the failure to detect the involvement of chromosome 9, in that the size and often the staining characteristics of the band on the other involved chromosome were similar to those of the terminal band on 9. Virtually all chromosomes have been involved in these variant translocations, but 17 is affected more often than are other chromosomes. The genetic consequences of the standard t(9;22) or the complex translocation involving at least three chromosomes is to move the c-*abl* gene on 9 next to a gene on 22 whose identity is currently unknown.

Acute Phase of CML

When patients with CML enter the terminal acute phase (blast crisis), about 20% appear to retain the 46,Ph[1]-positive cell line unchanged, whereas 80% of patients show karyotypic evolution (Rowley, 1980c). That is, new chromosomal abnormalities in very distinct patterns are present in addition to the Ph[1] chromosome. In many cases, the change in the karyotype precedes the clinical signs of blast crisis by 2–4 months (Rowley, 1980c). Thus, a change in the karyotype is considered to be a grave prognostic sign; the median survival from the time of change until death was found by Whang-Peng et al. (1968) to be 2–5 months. Similar results were also reported by the same group in a new series of patients (Cannelos et al., 1976). It is now recognized that the blast cells of some patients in the acute phase of CML have lymphoid rather than myeloid character-

TABLE III. Frequent Chromosomal Changes in 303 Ph[1]-Positive
Patients in Acute Phase of Chronic Myelogenous Leukemia[a]

	Number of patients			
Change	Chr 8	Chr 17	Chr 19	Ph[1]
Gain	119	31	45	113
Rearrangement	9	89[b]	2	8[c]

[a] Taken from Rowley and Testa (1982).
[b] Seventy-nine were i(17q).
[c] All were i(Ph[1]).

istics. At present, the data are insufficient to enable us to determine
whether a particular karyotype is associated with the lymphoid or with
the myeloid type of blast crisis (Rowley and Testa, 1982).

Bone marrow chromosomes from 392 patients with Ph[1]-positive
CML, who were in the acute phase, have been analyzed with banding
techniques [see Mitelman and Levan (1978) and Rowley and Testa (1982)
for review and references]. Eightly-nine (22%) showed no change in their
karyotype, whereas 303 patients had additional chromosomal abnormalities. The most frequently observed chromosomal changes observed in
these patients are summarized in Table III. The most common changes,
gain of chromosome 8 or 19 or a second Ph[1] and i(17q), frequently occur
in combination to produce modal chromosome numbers of 47–50. When
patients had only a single new chromosome change, this most commonly
involved the gain of a second Ph[1], an i(17q), or a +8, in descending
order of frequency. When several changes were seen together, those occurring most often were an extra chromosome 8 and i(17q); a +8 and +17
were never seen as the only changes. On the other hand, if the patient's
cells also had an extra Ph[1], then +8, i(17q), +Ph[1] and +8, +17, +Ph[1]
were seen with equal frequency. In nine patients, it was possible to tell
which change occurred first; i(17q) was the initial change in seven of them.
A gain of chromosome 19 seems to be of lesser importance because, unlike
the other three abnormalities, it was never observed as the only new
change in the acute phase. Chromosome loss occurs only rarely; that most
often seen was −7, which occurred in only 3% of patients (Rowley and
Testa, 1982). The relatively limited number of recurring chromosome abnormalities in the acute phase implies that the chromosomes involved
carry genes that provide a proliferative advantage to the Ph[1]-positive mye-

loid or lymphoid cell that has an extra copy of one or a combination of these chromosomes.

The data regarding the prognostic implications of particular karyotypic changes in the acute phase are conflicting. Sonta and Sandberg (1978) stated that the survival of patients who developed additional abnormalities was similar to that of patients without further changes. This view differs from that of Prigogina et al. (1978), who reported a higher remission rate and a longer survival in patients who remained only Ph[1]-positive compared with those whose cells had additional changes. Recently, Alimena et al. (1982) have reviewed the data from 69 patients in blast crisis; no difference in survival was noted in patients whose karyotype did not change. However, they did observe that survival was longer in patients with a lymphoid rather than a myeloid blast crisis.

The Ph[1] Chromosome As a Biological Marker

Our interpretation of the biological implications of the Ph[1] chromosome has been modified as our clinical experience with this marker has widened. Early cases of acute leukemia in which the Ph[1] chromosome was present were classified as chronic myeloid leukemia presenting in blast transformation. More recently, however, the tendency has been to refer to patients who have no prior history suggestive of CML as having Ph[1]-positive acute leukemia (Rowley, 1980c). It is evident that the interrelationships of various forms of Ph[1]-positive leukemia are complex. The difficult distinctions between some forms have often been determined by the arbitrary judgment of the investigator. The increasing availability of special cytochemical markers and of monoclonal antibodies for cell surface determinants will result in more precise, objective identification of the particular cell type that is affected.

The question as to which cells in CML contain a Ph[1] chromosome has not been completely resolved. It was shown relatively early that the Ph[1] chromosome was present in granulocytic, erythroid, and megakaryocytic cells (Sandberg, 1980). It was assumed that the Ph[1] chromosome was not present in lymphoid cells because most peripheral blood cells stimulated to divide by the mitogen phytohemagglutinin lacked a Ph[1] chromosome. As techniques of cell separation improved and immunologic markers were developed, it was established that some B cells were also Ph[1]-positive. At present, there are no data definitively showing that T cells are Ph[1]-positive. In blast crisis, some blasts had intracytoplasmic

IgM, which is characteristic of pre-B cells. That B cells from patients in
the chronic phase were also Ph¹-positive was shown by Martin *et al.*
(1980), who established Epstein–Barr virus (EBV)-transformed B-lym-
phoblastoid cell lines from a patient with Ph¹-positive CML who was also
heterozygous for glucose-6-phosphate dehydrogenase (G6PD) isozymes.
Nine of 74 cell lines were Ph¹-positive and of G6PD type B, which was
the isozyme type of the myeloid leukemia clone. Moreover, each cell line
expressed a single immunoglobulin class, thus providing further evidence
for their monoclonal nature. Bernheim *et al.* (1981) also showed more
directly that some B cells have a Ph¹ chromosome. In sIgM-positive cells
that were stimulated with pokeweed mitogen or nocardia opaca antigen,
seven of eight patients had a Ph¹ chromosome. In unstimulated cultures,
all cells were Ph¹-positive and they lacked sIgM; they were considered
to be granulocytes or monocytes. The question as to when the translocation occurs in relation to the process of malignant transformation will
be discussed below (p.38).

ACUTE NONLYMPHOCYTIC LEUKEMIA (ANLL) *DE NOVO*

There have now been numerous reports on cytogenetic analyses with
banding techniques of relatively large series of unselected patients with
ANLL as well as of single cases of selected patients (Mitelman and Levan,
1978; First International Workshop on Chromosomes in Leukemia,1978;
Sandberg, 1980; Second International Workshop on Chromosomes in
Leukemia, 1980; Rowley and Testa, 1982; Larson *et al.*, 1983). Abnormal
karyotypes have been reported in approximately 50% of all patients with
ANLL *de novo* whose bone marrow cells were examined with banding
techniques. At the Fourth International Workshop on Chromosomes in
Leukemia (1984), 354 (54%) of 660 patients with *de novo* ANLL examined
had chromosome abnormalities. The incidence of cytogenetic abnormalities will be significantly greater when techniques for culturing leukemic
cells and for obtaining prophase and prometaphase chromosomes are used
by more laboratories. In fact, many laboratories are currently finding that
at least 80% of patients have an abnormal clone, and Yunis *et al.* (1981)
have suggested that virtually every patient may have an abnormal karyotype. The most frequent abnormalities are a gain of chromosome 8 and
a loss of 7; these are seen in most subtypes of ANLL, although there are

some interesting differences in the frequency of these changes in some of the subtypes (Rowley *et al.*, 1982; Fourth International Workshop on Chromosomes in Leukemia, 1984). This discussion will emphasize certain specific aberrations that not only occur frequently, but also appear to be of exceptional biological interest. These include two translocations that are each specifically associated with a particular type of leukemia, another translocation that is associated with proliferation of a particular cell type, and two related abnormalities that are especially common in other types of acute leukemia. The two translocations are t(8;21), seen with rare exceptions only in acute myeloblastic leukemia with maturation (AML-M2), and t(15;17), seen only in acute promyelocytic leukemia (APL-M3). Myeloblasts and promyelocytes are two sequential stages in normal granulocyte differentiation (Fig. 1). The third translocation, t(6;9), is associated with an increase in the number of marrow basophils in ANLL. The rearrangements of 11q are more variable and can be translocations, deletions, or duplications involving 11q23–q24 preferentially. They are most commonly seen in acute monocytic leukemia (AMoL-M5), but have been reported in acute myelomonocytic leukemia (AMMoL-M4) and in AML-M2. Recently an association between increased numbers of bone marrow eosinophils and a deleted chromosome 16, or morphological and cytochemical abnormalities of marrow eosinophils, acute myelomonocytic leukemia (AMMoL-M4), and an inverted chromosome 16 has been identified.

Chromosome Gain and Loss

Although the karyotypes of patients with ANLL may be variable, both the nonrandom gain and loss of chromosomes and involvement in structural rearrangements are evident. The number of individual chromosomes gained or lost in 354 patients with clonal abnormalities of 660 patients studied at the Fourth International Workshop on Chromosomes in Leukemia (1984) is shown in Fig. 3. With the exceptions of chromosome 16, which was never observed as a gain, and 1, which was never lost, each of the autosomes and sex chromosomes contributed to the numerical changes. Some chromosomes are clearly overrepresented as gains or losses, while others are underrepresented. Thus, a gain of chromosome 8, the most frequent abnormality seen in ANLL, was found in 47 patients (13.3%). Gain of chromosomes 1–3, 5, 10, 12, 14, 15, 17, 18, 20, X, and Y were infrequently seen. Loss of chromosome 7, another frequent nu-

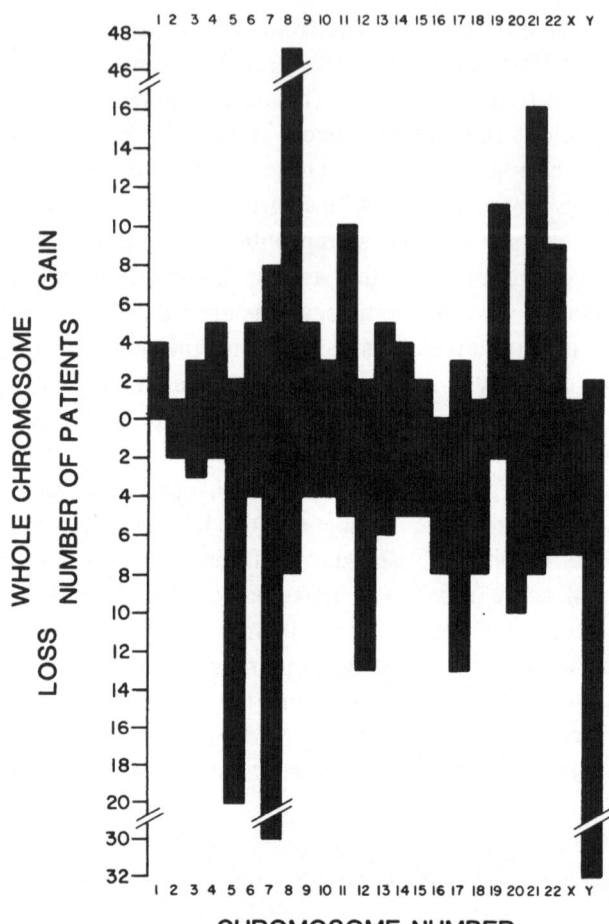

Fig. 3. Histogram illustrating the frequency of whole chromosome gain and loss in 660 patients with ANLL *de novo* studied at the Fourth International Workshop on Chromosomes in Leukemia (1984).

merical change, was observed in 30 (8.5%) patients, and loss of one chromosome 5 was noted in 20 cases (5.6%). A gain of either of these chromosomes is rarely observed. Those chromosomes that were seldom observed as losses include chromosomes 2–4, 6, 9, 10, and 19. It is interesting to note that gains or losses of the other autosomes seldom occurred as the sole abnormality. Thus, these abnormalities were likely to represent secondary events occurring in clonal evolution, rather than primary chromosomal changes.

Loss of the Y chromosome, the second most frequent numerical change in this summary, and X chromosome often occurred in association with an 8;21 translocation. Of the 32 males with a missing Y, 28 had a t(8;21). Loss of a Y as a sole abnormality has been described; however, the significance of this abnormality is somewhat uncertain, because a missing Y has also been reported in bone marrow cells of hematologically normal males, particularly those over the age of 60. Moreover, the t(8;21) in AML-M2 is associated with a younger median age. These observations have led Pierre and Hoaglund (1972) to suggest that the missing Y may represent a normal aging phenomenon of human bone marrow cells.

Structural Rearrangements

The distribution of chromosomes involved in structural rearrangements in the patients studied at the Fourth Workshop is illustrated in Fig. 4. Translocations and deletions accounted for most of the rearrangements observed. The most frequently rearranged chromosome was 17; abnormalities of this chromosome were noted in 53 patients, 43 of whom had the t(15;17). Likewise, the majority of cases with rearrangements of chromosomes 8, 15, or 21, the three next most frequently altered chromosomes, resulted from the two specific translocations t(8;21) and t(15;17). A deletion of 5q was identified in 25 patients, and rearrangements of 11q, primarily translocations, were also particularly frequent. Structural rearrangements involving chromosomes 2, 4, 19, 20, X, and Y were seen infrequently.

The 8;21 Translocation in Acute Myeloblastic Leukemia (AML-M2)

Kamada *et al.* (1968) suggested that a subgroup of ANLL patients may be characterized by an abnormality most likely representing a translocation between a C- and a G-group chromosome. The precise nature of this abnormality was resolved by Rowley (1973*b*), who determined that it was a balanced translocation between chromosomes 8 and 21 [t(8;21)(q22;q22), Fig. 5a]. The frequency with which this translocation occurs varies from one laboratory to another, but 25 of 249 (10%) abnormal cases reviewed by Rowley and Testa (1982) had this rearrangement. A similar incidence of the t(8;21) was reported in patients reviewed at both the First and Fourth International Workshops on Chromosomes in Leu-

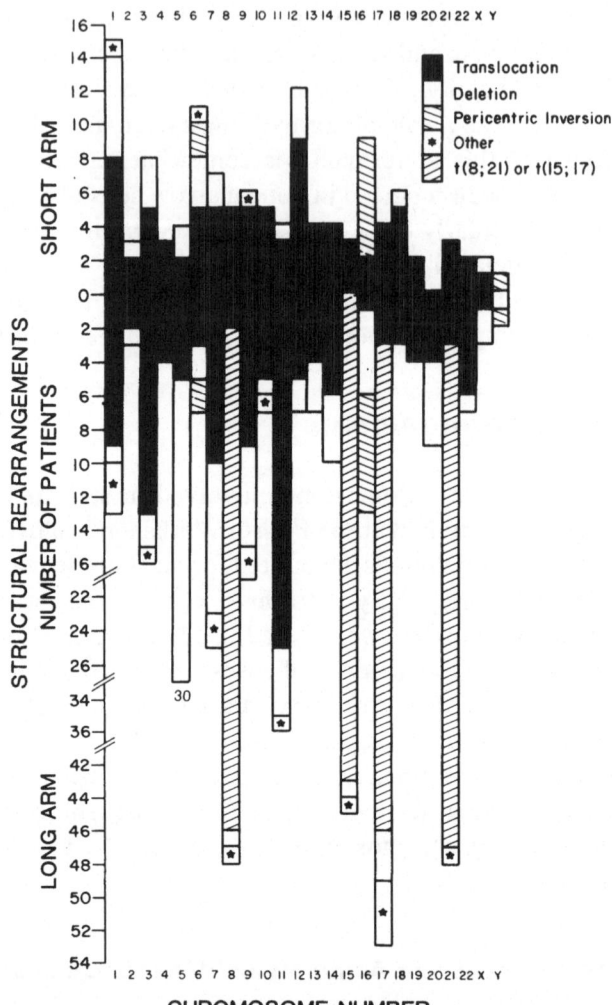

Fig. 4. Histogram illustrating the frequency of structural rearrangements in 660 patients with ANLL *de novo* (Fourth International Workshop on Chromosomes in Leukemia, 1984).

kemia (1978, 1984); 11 of 139 (7.9%) and 44 of 353 (12.5%), respectively, ANLL patients with abnormal karyotypes had a t(8;21). In the review by Rowley and Testa, the t(8;21) was found to be the most frequent abnormality in children with ANLL, being reported in 17% (10 of 60) of karyotypically abnormal cases. When only patients with AML-M2 are considered, 18% (41 of 226) of patients in the Fourth Workshop had a t(8;21).

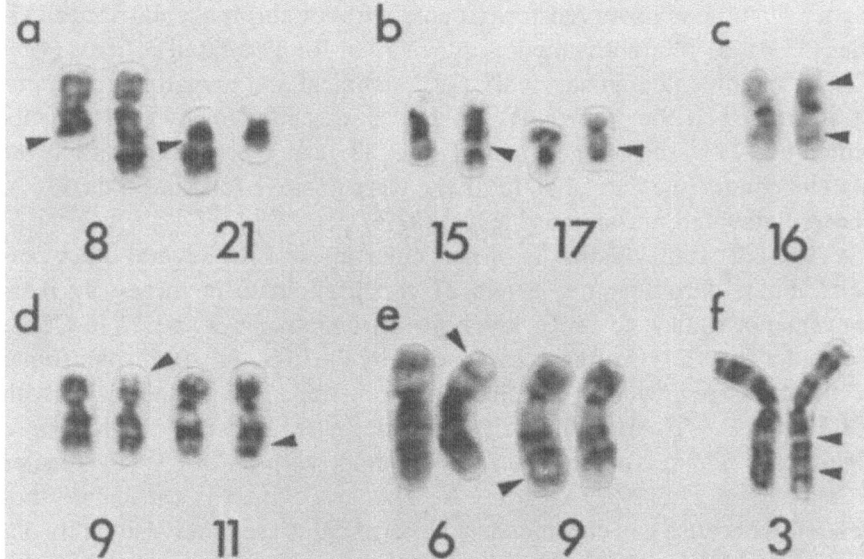

Fig. 5. Partial karyotypes from trypsin-Glemsa-banded metaphase cells depicting nonrandom chromosomal rearrangements observed in ANLL *de novo*. The chromosomal breakpoints are identified with arrowheads. (a) t(8;21)(q22;q22), AML-M2. The abnormal chromosomes 8 and 21 are on the left in each pair. (b) t(15;17)(q22;q11), APL. The rearranged chromosomes 15 and 17 are on the right in each pair. (c) inv(16)(p13q22), AMMoL. The inverted chromosome 16 is on the right. (d) t(9;11)(p22;q23). The abnormal chromosomes 9 and 11 are on the right in each pair. (e) t(6;9)(p23;q34). The abnormal chromosome 6 is on the right of pair 6. The rearranged chromosome 9 is on the left of pair 9. (f) inv(3)(q21q26). Inverted chromosome 3 is on the right.

    The abnormality initially appeared to be restricted to patients with a diagnosis of M2 leukemia (acute myeloblastic leukemia with maturation) according to the FAB classification. However, 7% (3 of 44) of patients analyzed at the Fourth Workshop whose cells had a t(8;21) and adequate bone marrow material available for cytological review had a diagnosis of M4 leukemia (acute myelomonocytic leukemia).

    Of clinical importance is the favorable prognosis associated with this cytogenetic abnormality. Data on the survival of 48 patients with the t(8;21) were reviewed at the Second Workshop; the median survival of the entire group was 11.5 months, which was much longer than that for patients with other chromosomal abnormalities. At the Fourth Workshop, the percentage of patients with a t(8;21) who entered a complete remission (CR) was 77% and the median survival was 13 months; these values are higher than those observed for patients without chromosomal abnormalities (55% CR, 10 months median survival) or for all treated patients (47% CR, 11 months median survival). Of the clinical and hematologic parameters studied at the Fourth Workshop, it was noteworthy that patients with a t(8;21) were younger (median age, 38 years), presented with lower platelet counts (median 28 $\times$ 10^9/liter), were positive for Auer rods (91%), showed elevated muramidase levels (82%).

The 8;21 translocation is of particular interest for several other reasons. First, chromosomes 8 and 21 can participate in three-way rearrangements similar to those involving chromosomes 9 and 22 in CML. Second, the t(8;21) is often accompanied by the loss of a sex chromosome; of the cases reviewed at the Second Workshop, 32% of the males with t(8;21) were $-Y$, and 36% of the females were missing one X. These figures are higher for the Fourth Workshop, with 28 of 33 (85%) males $-Y$ and 8 of 11 (73%) females $-X$. This association is particularly noteworthy because sex chromosome abnormalities are otherwise rarely observed in ANLL. Third, this translocation has never been reported as a constitutional abnormality or in other malignant diseases (J. D. Rowley, unpublished observations). Thus, it may be lethal in all cells except granulocytes.

The 15;17 Translocation in Acute Promyelocytic Leukemia (APL- M3)

A structural rearrangement involving the long arms of chromosomes 15 and 17 in APL (M3) was first recognized by Rowley et al. (1977). For many years, the precise breakpoints involved in this translocation were controversial; however, recently, with the use of elongated chromosomes, the rearrangement has been defined as t(15;17)(q22;q21) (Fig. 5b) (Kaneko and Sakurai, 1977; Fourth International Workshop on Chromosomes in Leukemia, 1984; Larson et al., 1984). Of the 80 patients with APL who were reviewed at the Second Workshop, 33 (41%) had a t(15;17) alone (23 cases) or with other abnormalities, seven had other types of chromosomal changes, and 40 had a normal karyotype. With improved techniques, including widespread use of bone marrow culture, only 15 of 61 (25%) patients analyzed at the Fourth Workshop had a normal karyotype. Forty-three patients (70%) had a t(15;17) and three had other abnormalities. This rearrangement was not found in patients with any other type of leukemia or a solid tumor. Two cases with complex translocations involving chromosomes 15 and 17 and either 2 or 3 were reported. Thus, the same pattern of variation of a specific translocation can involve the t(15;17) as well as the t(9;22) and the t(8;21). The usefulness of these variant translocations will be illustrated in a later section.

A number of clinical characteristics associated with APL have been noted. Specifically, patients with APL tend to be younger than other ANLL patients, to have bleeding problems, particularly disseminated intravascular coagulation (DIC), and to have a poor response to current therapy. Analysis of APL patients at the Fourth Workshop revealed a higher frequency of DIC (71% of patients) and a lower platelet count (median 21×10^9/liter), leukocyte count (median 6×10^9/liter), and percent blasts in the peripheral blood (median 8%), and a high frequency of Auer rods (85%).

By morphological criteria, acute promyelocytic leukemia is comprised of two subtypes, namely the common hypergranular and the microgranular variant. In the variant form of APL (M3V), typical hypergranular promyelocytes are seen in low numbers and a significant proportion of promyelocytes show a paucity of granules. The granules may be too small to be seen by light microscopy, although they are present when the cells are examined ultrastructurally (Testa et al., 1978). The t(15;17) is found in both types of APL, and in fact the variant category was identified largely on the basis of the clinical features and the presence of the translocation.

The second interesting feature of APL relates to the difficulty in demonstrating the t(15;17). There initially appeared to be an unusual geographic distribution of APL cases showing this translocation, in that the proportion of patients with the t(15;17) varied from laboratory to laboratory. In our experience, all 27 patients with APL whom we have studied had a t(15;17) (Larson et al., 1984). However, in three patients, no abnormal metaphase cells were observed when marrow cells were studied directly; 9–64% of marrow cells had a t(15;17) when the cells were cultured for 24 hr (Waghray et al., 1981). Similar observations have been reported by others (Knuutila et al., 1981; Yunis, 1982). The reason for this difficulty in obtaining mitoses in cells with the translocation is not known. However, Berger et al. have presented evidence that the translocation is present only in myeloblasts and promyelocytes, whereas the erythroid cells are normal. In their investigations, the mitotic cells observed in direct preparations were primarily erythroblasts; therefore, chromosomally abnormal promyelocytes may not be identified if only metaphase cells from direct preparations are analyzed (Berger *et al.*, 1980*a*).

Inv(16) and del(16q) in Acute Myelomonocytic Leukemia (AMMoL-M4)

Another clinical–cytogenetic association recently identified involves myelomonocytic (M4) leukemia with abnormal eosinophils. Arthur and Bloomfield (1983) described five cases (three with AML-M2 and two with AMMoL-M4 leukemia) in which the bone marrow contained an excess of eosinophils (8–54%); all five patients had a deleted chromosome 16 [del(16)(q22)]. Le Beau *et al.* (1983) reported on a related entity in 18 patients, all of whom had M4 leukemia with eosinophils that showed alterations of morphology, cytochemical reactions, and ultrastructure, including the presence of large and irregular basophilic granules, and a positive reaction with periodic-acid-Schiff and chloroacetate esterase. Many of these patients did not have an increased percentage of marrow eosinophils; one-third had fewer than 5% eosinophils. All patients had an inversion of chromosome 16, inv(16)(p13q22) (Figs. 5c and 6). The breakpoint in the long arm for the del(16) and for the inv(16) is the same. Among our M4 patients, 23% have an inv(16). Similar morphological features were observed in three patients studied by Tantravahi *et al.* (1984). This subgroup of M4 patients had a good response to intensive therapy; 13 of 17 (76%) treated patients entered a CR. Although the median survival has not yet been reached (median followup 65 weeks), this value is well over the 29-week survival realized by treated AMMoL patients who do not have this chromosomal rearrangement (CR, 34%) (Larson *et al.*, 1983).

The strong correlation between abnormal eosinophils and structural rearrangements of chromosome 16 was confirmed at the Fourth Workshop. Of 25 patients with M4 and more than 5% marrow eosinophils, ten had either a del(16)(q22) or an inv(16); 11 appeared to have a normal karyotype, and four had other abnormalities. Of ten patients with M4 and structurally abnormal eosinophils, seven had an abnormality of chromosome 16 and the others appeared to have a normal karyotype. The chromosomes in these three cases were quite contracted, and thus a subtle rearrangement of chromosome 16 could easily have been overlooked. In fact, an abnormality of chromosome 16 was noted in four Workshop patients with M4 and increased or abnormal eosinophils when the karyotypes were reviewed further. It is clear, therefore, that this relatively

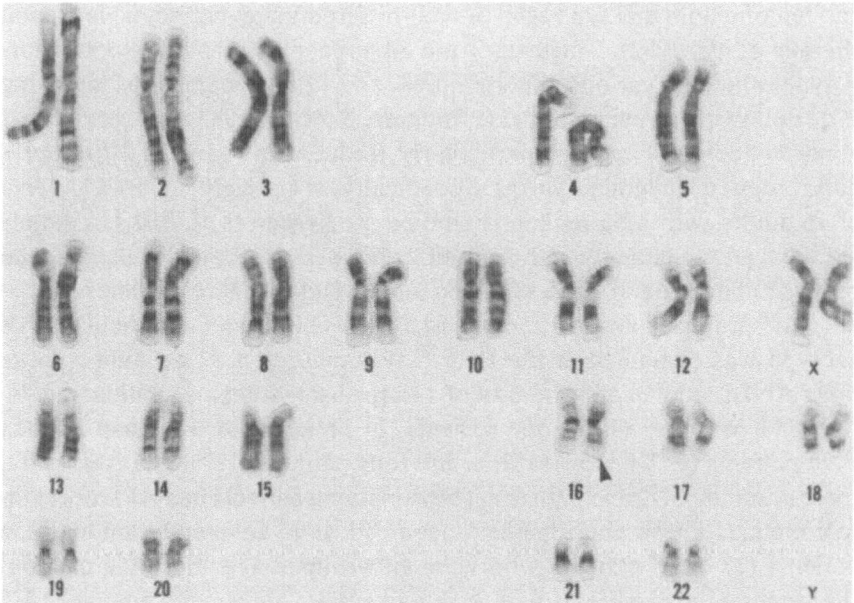

Fig. 6. Karyotype of a trypsin-Giemsa-banded metaphase cell illustrating the inv(16)(p13q22). This rearrangement is associated with AMMoL characterized by morphological and cytochemical abnormalities of bone marrow eosinophils.

common, but subtle chromosomal aberration was undetected in the past, because of poor morphology. Moreover, the inv(16), along with the t(8;21) in AML-M2, is associated with morphological alterations that are so characteristic that both these specific chromosomal abnormalities, which define a subset of AMMoL and AML-M2, respectively,can be predicted on the basis of morphological features alone.

Structural Alterations of 11q in Acute Monocytic Leukemia (AMoL-M5)

In addition to the consistent translocations described earlier, a new chromosome–morphology relationship has recently been described. Berger *et al.* (1980*b*) presented ten cases of acute monocytic leukemia (AMoL-M5) that had an unexpectedly high incidence of rearrangements of the long arm of chromosome 11. They recently reported on 34 patients, 24 of whom had type M5a or poorly-differentiated monocytic leukemia and ten of whom had type M5b or well-differentiated monocytic leukemia (Berger *et al.*, 1982). Thirteen of the 34 appeared to have a normal karyotype, nine had various abnormalities, and 12 had aberrations involving 11q. Following a review of these findings, Rowley (1983*a*) suggested that abnormalities of 11q were particularly frequent in children with poorly differentiated leukemia (type a). Specifically, six of eight children and five of 16 adults with M5a leukemia studied by Berger *et al.* had 11q abnormalities. Of ten patients with well-differentiated monocytic leukemia, one of three children and none of seven adults had 11q abnormalities.

The proposed association of 11q abnormalities and a particular FAB subtype was examined at the Fourth Workshop. Of 33 patients with *de novo* ANLL and an abnormality of 11q [translocations, 21 patients; deletions, 11 patients; i(11q), one patient], 21 patients, or 64%, had AMoL. Five patients (15%) had AMMoL and four patients (12%) had AML (M2, three patients; M1, one patient). The remaining patients had APL or erythroleukemia. These abnormalities occurred more frequently among M5a patients (15 of 18 patients who were subgrouped as either M5a or M5b) than among those patients with M5b leukemia. Conversely, among 32 M5 patients without abnormalities of chromosome 11, there were no significant differences in the frequency of M5a (18 patients) vs. M5b (14 patients) patients. Correlation of the morphological classification and breakpoint of 11q revealed that in 86% of M5 cases with an abnormal 11q, the breakpoint was in q23 or q24. Overall, 78% of the rearrangements involving 11q23 occurred in M5 patients. Thus, the incidence of 11q abnormalities was significantly higher in M5 patients than in other types of ANLL. Moreover, a structural abnormality of any type involving 11q23 was found to be significantly associated with the M5 subtype of ANLL, and particularly with M5a.

Aberrations of 11q differ from the t(8;21) and t(15;17) in three ways. First, the breakpoint in 11q usually involves band 11q23–q24, but can also occur in 11q13–q14; in Berger's series, 11q23–q24 was affected in nine patients and 11q13–q14 in three others. In the Fourth Workshop, 24 of the 33 breaks in chromosome 11 occurred in 11q23–q24; the others usually involved 11q13–q14. Second, the other chromosome involved in the translocation is variable, although 9p and 19 appear to be affected more often than others. A specific translocation between chromosomes 9 and 11 was described by Yunis *et al.* (1981) in a patient with AML and by Kaneko *et al.* (1982*b*) in a child with AMoL [t(9;11)(p22;q23), Fig. 5d]. Hagemeijer *et al.* (1982) noted this translocation in three patients with poorly-differentiated AMoL and proposed a specific association between this translocation and acute leukemia of the M5 subtype. Finally, 11q aberrations have been reported in patients with acute leukemia other than AMoL-M5. In a series of children reported by Kaneko *et al.* (1982*b*) a translocation involving 11q was seen in a patient with AML-M2, although the cytochemical reaction of the leukemic cells was of the monocytic type. It may be that the chromosome analyses have revealed a spectrum of morphological features in AMoL not heretofore suspected. Such morphological variability may be analogous to that noted in APL, in which the M3 variant or microgranular type was identified in large measure because of the consistent t(15;17) seen in the leukemic cells (Testa *et al.*, 1978).

The 6;9 Translocation in ANLL with an Increased Number of Basophils

A translocation involving chromosomes 6 and 9 [t(6;9)(p23;q34), Fig. 5e] was first described by Rowley and Potter (1976) in two patients, but no common features were detected. We have subsequently studied three additional patients and examined bone marrow slides from these five patients and from four others with this translocation (Pearson *et al.*, 1985). Eight of these nine patients had an increase in the number of basophils in the bone marrow ranging from 1.5 to 12%; the normal value is 0.2%. Because the marrow in all biopsy specimens was hypercellular, this represented a marked increase in the total basophil count. The basophils appeared to be morphologically normal. Only five of 163 ANLL patients whom we have studied had increased numbers of marrow basophils (>1%) in the absence of t(6;9). Of the nine t(6;9) patients, five were classified as AML-M2, three as AMMoL-M4, and one as AML-M1. The median age was 38 years, which is lower than that of other ANLL patients. As a group, patients with a t(6;9) have responded poorly to intensive remission induction therapy. Of all reported cases, only two of 11 (27%) treated patients had a complete remission. This finding contrasts with that noted at the Fourth Workshop, in which 57% of intensively treated patients had a CR. It is of interest that the breakpoint in chromosome 9 is in the same band as the t(9;22) in CML, and that a marked increase in basophils is a regular feature of Ph[1]-positive CML. It is possible that the break in both translocations is in the same region of the DNA, and thus that a gene related to the regulation of basophil proliferation may be located in this segment of 9q34.

Other Consistent Abnormalities in ANLL

Several other nonrandom chromosomal abnormalities have been recognized in ANLL. In general, these abnormalities are less appreciated than the other nonrandom abnormalities described above, in that they either occur less frequently or they are not limited to a particular FAB subtype. Rowley and Potter, (1976) described a patient with AMMoL and thrombocythemia in whom a translocation involving chromosome 3 homologues had occurred, and a second such case was subsequently described (Sweet *et al.*, 1979). It was therefore postulated that the long arm of chromosome 3 contains genes that function in regulating thrombopoiesis. A number of patients have since been described with ANLL and associated megakaryoctye and platelet abnormalities who have either a translocation (3;3) [t(3;3)(q21;q26)] or an inversion [inv(3)(q21q26), Fig. 5f]

Currently, variant translocations have been reported in Burkitt lym- (Bernstein *et al.*, 1982).

A deletion of chromosome 20 [del(20)(q11)] has been described in patients with ANLL as well as in patients with myeloproliferative disorder, polycythemia vera, and the myelodysplastic syndromes (Rowley and Testa, 1982). This particular rearrangement is not limited to any subtype of ANLL. Rearrangements of chromosome 1 leading to trisomy or partial trisomy for 1q, specifically for 1q25–1q32, is not an infrequent finding in ANLL (Rowley, 1977). Similar chromosome changes are a consistent finding in other hematologic diseases and even in solid tumors of various types.

Prognostic Significance of Chromosomal Abnormalities in ANLL

As early as 1973, Sakurai and Sandberg (1973), using conventional staining methods, demonstrated that the karyotypic pattern of bone marrow cells is correlated with survival in patients with ANLL. That is, patients with only normal metaphase cells (NN) had a longer survival (11.5 months) than did patients who had a mixture of normal and abnormal metaphase cells (AN; 10.3 months) or those who had only abnormal metaphase cells (AA; 3.2 momths). More recent studies, based on series of patients studied with banding techniques, have shown similar findings; however, these differences in median survival appeared to be limited to particular FAB subtypes of ANLL. Of the AML (M1 and M2) patients reviewed at the First Workshop, a substantially longer median survival (8 months) was found for NN patients as compared to those who were AA (3.5 months); patients who were AN had an intermediate survival (5 months). No such differences, however, were found in patients with AMMoL or AMoL.

These earlier observations of the ability of initial karyotype classification to predict outcome have recently been questioned by Larson et al. (1983). In their consecutive series of 148 patients with ANLL de novo, these investigators found a statistically significant difference in median survival based upon karyotype subgroup (NN, AN, AA) only for AML patients (NN, 24 patients, 12 months; AN, 26 patients, 9.5 months; AA, 5 patients, 1.8 months; $p = 0.01$). However, when the median survival for 25 AML patients who had received modern intensive remission induction therapy were compared according to the initial cytogenetic subgroup, no significant differences were observed ($p = 0.89$).

The response to intensive remission induction therapy for patients with ANLL was also investigated at the Fourth Workshop; the results are somewhat different than those obtained when all patients are considered. When 305 optimally treated patients were classified according to the presence of normal and abnormal metaphases, a significant difference in median survival was noted (NN, 15 months; AN, 10 months; AA, 10 months; $p = 0.02$). Significant differences in CR rate and survival were also noted when patients were classified according to the specific abnormality. Interestingly, patients in whom no abnormality was identified did not respond unusually well to treatment nor have the longest survivals. Patients with t(8;21), +21, hypodiploidy, or t(15;17) had the highest remission rate. The longest median survivals were seen in patients with −7 or del(7q), t(15;17), and hypodiploidy. Patients with abnormalities of chromosome 5 [−5 or del(5q)] did particuarly poorly. It is noteworthy that patients with −7 or t(15;17), who in other series have not responded well to therapy, showed a favorable prognosis. Whether or not this reflects the small sample size [−7, seven patients; t(15;17), 16 patients] or an improved response using modern therapy is uncertain.

In summary, many aspects of the medical management of patients with ANLL have changed during the last decade. As the use of more effective remission induction chemotherapy and supportive care in-

Table IV. Correlation of Karyotype and Survival of 660 Patients with ANLL *de Novo*[a]

Karyotype	Number of patients	Complete remission: Percent of patients (median duration of remission, months)	Median survival,[b] months
Normal	307	45 (13)	10
−5 or del(5q)	29	28 (4)	4
−7 or del(7q)	28	21 (25+)	3
Abnormal 5 and 7	21	20 (—)	3
t(15;17)	43	40 (10)	3
t(8;21)	44	77 (10)	13
11q abnormality	29	21 (6)	8
+8	36	22 (8)	6
+21	12	67 (19+)	10
46, abnormal	67	31 (13)	5
>46 chromosomes	31	16 (12)	4
<46 chromosomes	13	46 (6)	5

[a] Data from Fourth International Workshop on Chromosomes in Leukemia (1984).
[b] Difference in survival is significant ($p = 0.0002$).

creases, the ability of initial karyotype grouping into NN, AN, and AA to predict outcome may decrease further. On the other hand, actual prognostic significance may lie with the specificity of chromosomal abnormalities in that some abnormalities are associated with a particularly good or poor prognosis (Table IV).

ACUTE NONLYMPHOCYTIC LEUKEMIA INDUCED BY TREATMENT

The occurrence of acute nonlymphocytic leukemia (ANLL) in patients who have previously received cytotoxic therapy, either radiation and/or chemotherapy, for a prior disease is being recognized with increasing frequency (Rowley et al., 1981). It would appear reasonable to consider most, if not all, of these leukemias as being induced by the therapy. Radiation is well recognized for its leukemogenesis potential, and many of the drugs used to treat patients are alkylating agents that are also known for their mutagenic activity. Several investigations of the clinical and cytogenetic features of patients with secondary ANLL have been reported (Rowley et al., 1981; Grünwald and Rosner, 1982; Pederson-Bjergaard and Larsen, 1982; Sandberg *et al.*, 1982; Greene *et al.*, 1983; Rowley, 1983*b*; Fourth International Workshop on Chromosomes in Leukemia, 1984). In the following section we will summarize the findings in our own series of 63 patients with therapy-related ANLL or dysmyelopoietic syndrome (DMPS).

Of the 63 previously treated patients, 23 had Hodgkin disease (HD), 10 had non-Hodgkin lymphoma (NHL), 5 had multiple myeloma (MM), 1 had hairy cell leukemia, 21 had various solid tumors, and 3 had had a renal transplant. Thirty-one of the patients had received both radiotherapy and chemotherapy (RT, CT) prior to the development of their second malignancy, 21 patients had only chemotherapy, and 11 patients had only radiotherapy; the median time between the original diagnosis and the diagnosis of bone marrow dysfunction (BMD) was 61.5, 50.3, and 33.0 months, respectively. The time to BMD was not associated with the nature of the primary disease or the type of primary therapy. Nineteen patients presented with DMPS, 15 patients with ANLL, and 29 patients with DMPS that later evolved into ANLL. As a group, patients with therapy-related ANLL respond poorly to remission induction therapy. Of the 29 patients who received a standard Ara-C-based induction regimen, only six patients entered a complete remission.

In contrast to our series of patients with *de novo* ANLL, in which 54% of patients had clonal chromosomal abnormalities, 61 of 63 (97%) patients with therapy-related malignancies were chromosomally abnormal (Larson *et al.*, 1983). More importantly, one or both of two consistent changes were noted in 55 of 61 patients with abnormalities (Table V). Fourteen patients had loss of one chromosome 5 (six patients) or an interstitial deletion of the q arm (eight patients) and 24 patients had loss of one chromosome 7 (22 patients) or a del(7q) (two patients). An additional 17 patients had abnormalities of both chromosomes 5 and 7. A comparison of the frequency of abnormalities for each chromosome in *de novo* and secondary ANLL revealed that chromosomes 1, 4, 5, 7, 12, 14, and 18 were significantly involved more frequently in the latter group of patients (Fig. 7). Of the six patients with abnormalities involving chromosomes other than 5 and/or 7, it is noteworthy that two patients had a gain of chromosome 8 as their sole abnormality and both patients with secondary APL had the t(15;17)(q22;q21).

A comparison of the results of cytogenetic analysis with clinical findings revealed that chromosome abnormalities were unrelated to age, sex, or mode of primary therapy; however, abnormalities of chromosome 5

Michelle M. Le Beau and Janet D. Rowley

TABLE V. Relationship of Initial Disease and Karyotype of Leukemic Cells

Disease	Number of patients	Number with given chromosome abnormality				
		−5 or del(5q)	−7 or del(7q)	−5 or del(5q) and −7 or del(7q)	Other	Normal chromosomes
Malignant lymphoma	33	4	11 (1)	14	3	1
Other lymphoproliferative	6	2 (1)[a]	3	1	0	0
Solid tumors	21	8 (7)	8	2	3	0
Renal transplants	3	0	2 (1)	0	0	1
Total	63	14	24	17	6	2

[a] Parenthesis indicate number of patients with a deletion.

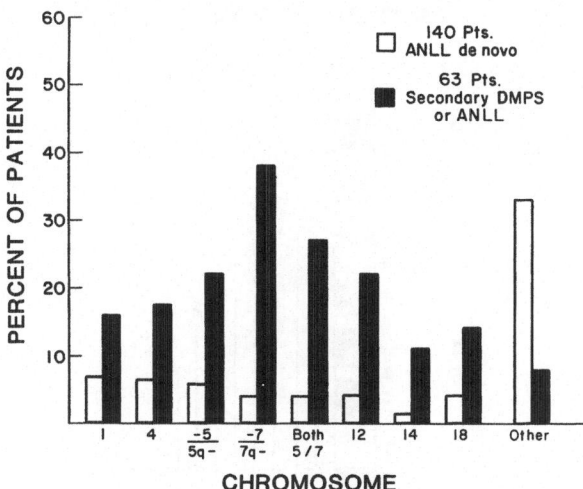

Fig. 7.   Comparison of the frequency of specific chromosomal abnormalities in secondary and *de novo* ANLL.

were correlated with the presence of DMPS ($p = 0.02$). Moreover, deletions of 5q were more frequent in patients whose initial disease was carcinoma, whereas loss of 5 was observed more frequently in patients with HD, NHL, or the other lymphoproliferative disordes ($p = 0.02$).

Those patients with secondary ANLL who have deletions of 5q or 7q are particularly important because by analysis of the breakpoints we can determine whether certain segments are consistently lost, and, if so, whether a particular segment or critical region is lost in all patients. By studying the breakpoints in 17 patients with an interstitial deletion of 5q, we have identified the critical region as 5q23–q32 (Fig. 8). The identification of the critical regions is relevant because the genes related to the malignant transformation are likely to be located in these regions.

The identification of specific chromosomal abnormalities in secondary ANLL has significant implications for our understanding of the etiology of ANLL *de novo*. Specifically, one can ask whether patients who are thought to have ANLL *de novo* who have loss of chromosome 5 or 7 might actually represent patients whose leukemia was induced by exposure to some mutagenic agent. Although this question cannot be completely answered as yet, two lines of evidence suggest that the answer may be positive. The first of these comes from a retrospective study of the correlation between karyotype and occupational exposure in ANLL,

CRITICAL REGION

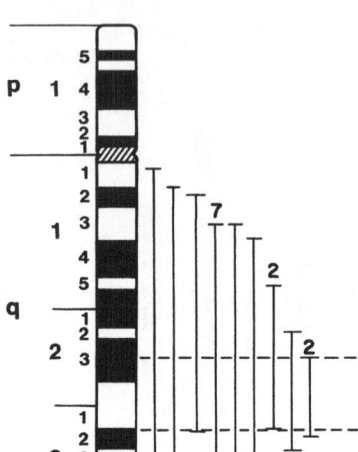

5
5q23-q32

Fig. 8. Diagrammatic representation of the banding pattern of chromosome 5, illustrating
the chromosomal breakpoints of interstitial long-arm deletions observed in 17 patients with
secondary ANLL. The smallest segment that is consistently deleted, or the critical region,
is 5q23–q32.

and the second from studies of childhood ANLL. The following discussion
will focus only on the former.

   Mitelman *et al.* (1978, 1981) reported on a retrospective study of 162
patients with ANLL *de novo*; 52 had a history suggesting occupational
exposure to chemical solvents, insecticides, or petroleum products,
whereas 110 had no such known exposure. Only 32% of the nonexposed
group had clonal chromosomal abnormalities, as compared to 75% in the
exposed group. There was a distinctly nonrandom pattern of changes in
the exposed group, with 79% of chromosomally abnormal (60% of all
patients) cases having at least one of four specific abnormalities: −5 [or
del(5q)], −7 [or del(7q)], +8, or +21. Only 54% of patients with abnormalities in the nonexposed group (17% of all patients) had any of these
changes. Golomb *et al.* (1982) confirmed these findings and in their series

of 74 patients with ANLL, 25 of 58 nonexposed patients (43%) had clonal abnormalities, as compared to 12 of 16 (75%) exposed patients. A−5 or del(5q) was observed in 4 of the 12 (33%) exposed patients and in 4 of the 25 (16%) nonexposed patients. A loss of chromosome 7 or del(7q) was detected in 7 of the 12 (58.3%) abnormal exposed patients and in 5 of the 25 (20%) abnormal nonexposed patients. Both of these differences are significant ($p < 0.05$). At least one of these two changes was present in 8 of the 12 (66.7%) exposed patients, but only in 7 of the 25 (28%) nonexposed patients. When the abnormal nonexposed patients were subdivided into groups "without hobbies" and "with hobbies," 3 of 18 patients (16.7%) in the first group vs. 3 of 7 patients (43%) in the second group displayed one or both of these aberrations. When the type of exposure was considered, it was noted that five of the six abnormal patients exposed to petroleum products (83.3%) had monosomy for chromosome 7, and three of the five abnormal patients exposed to chemicals (60%) had monosomy of chromosome 5. A gain of chromosome 8 or 21 was seen only in nonexposed patients who had no hobby-related exposure. The specific translocations were also detected primarily in the nonexposed group. Of the four patients who had a t(8;21) and the five who had a t(15;17), three and four, respectively, were nonexposed.

ACUTE LYMPHOCYTIC LEUKEMIA (ALL)

It has been reported that the most useful prognostic indicators in ALL, the most frequent leukemia in children, are age, WBC count, and immunologic markers. Patients who are between 3 and 7 years of age, with a WBC count of less than 10,000/mm^3, and whose leukemic cells have non-T, non-B surface membrane markers have the best prognosis. Metaphase chromosomes from ALL patients are often of poor morphology with indistinct bands, making an accurate analysis difficult. For this reason, there have been fewer reports of chromosome patterns in ALL than in ANLL. Remarkable improvements, however, have been made in recent years, and it is now possible to correlate the karyotype with other recognized prognostic factors, and to show that cytogenetic studies can increase the precision of other prognostic features (Third International Workshop on Chromosomes in Leukemia, 1981; Secker-Walker, 1984). Moreover, it was rigorously demonstrated for the first time at the Third Workshop that the karyotype is an important independent prognostic factor in ALL. Of utmost importance, however, is the ability to define subsets of patients with ALL on the basis of certain genetic (chromosome) changes and then to relate these changes to various functional and immunologic studies. In this way, we will gain a much more sophisticated and accurate understanding of the interrelationship of the various subsets of lymphoid cells.

This review includes data on the chromosome patterns of 33 ALL patients studied at the University of Chicago, on patients described in recent reports, and on 330 patients evaluated at the Third Workshop. Early studies suggested that cytogenetic abnormalities occurred in about one-half of the patients with ALL and that among aneuploid patients, hyperdiploidy was predominant. The study of 330 ALL patients (173 adults, 157 children) at the Third Workshop revealed that a higher proportion, 65%, of the patients had clonal abnormalities. Also, of the 213 aneuploid patients, 35% were pseudodiploid, 25% were hyperdiploid, and only 7% were hypodiploid. Similarly, analysis of 33 patients studied by Kaneko and Rowley (1981) also showed a high incidence of aneuploidy (70%), and pseudodiploidy was predominant (13/23 aneuploid patients). Although a number of karyotypic changes, many of which are complex, have been observed in patients with ALL, certain abnormalities recur. Those abnormalities observed most frequently are described in the following sections.

The 8;14 Translocation

A reciprocal translocation involving the long arms of chromosomes 8 and 14 has been detected in a high proportion of Burkitt tumors of both African and non-African origin, independent of whether they are Epstein–Barr virus (EBV)-positive or -negative (Zech et al., 1976; Kaiser-McCaw et al., 1977). An apparently identical translocation [t(8;14)(q24;q32), Fig. 9a] has been observed in ALL patients whose leukemic cells have B-cell markers and in patients with L3-type leukemic cells, indicating that Burkitt lymphoma and most B-cell ALL of the L3 type are probably different manifestations of the same disease. Sixteen patients with this rearrangement were studied at the Third Workshop (7.4% of all cases with abnormalities). In this group, there was an excess of males over females, and of adults over children. Most notable was the finding that, with one exception, all tested cases had B-cell markers, and all but one case in which markers were not studied were FAB-type L3. In the exceptional patient,

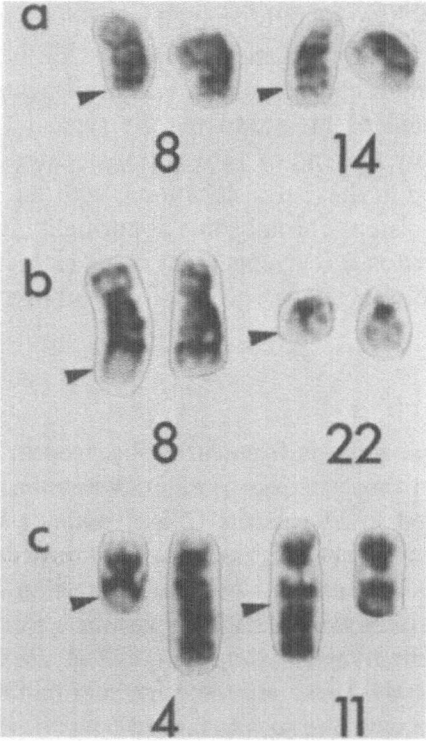

Fig. 9. Partial karyotypes of trypsin-Giemsa-banded metaphase cells from three patients with lymphoid malignancies. The chromosomal breakpoints are identified with arrowheads. The rearranged chromosomes are on the left of each pair. (a) t(8;14)(q24;q32) in Burkitt lymphoma and B-cell ALL. (b) Variant translocation, t(8;22)(q24;q11), in Burkitt lymphoma and B-cell ALL. (c) t(4;11)(q21;q23) observed in ALL.

the leukemic cells had a pre-B-cell phenotype and the morphology of the leukemic cells was of the L1 type; however, the morphology changed to L3 at relapse. This group of patients had a high incidence of central nervous system involvement at diagnosis and a poorer prognosis (CR rate, children 83%, adults 44%; median survival, 5 months) than did any other group of patients classified according to chromosome patterns.

Currently, variant translocations have been reported in Burkitt's lymphoma [t(2;8)(p12 or p13;q24); t(8;22)(q24;q11), Fig. 9b] [see Rowley and Testa (1982) for references]. Both variant translocations as well as t(X;8)(p23;q24) have been found in ALL patients with the L3 subtype. Moreover, complex three-way translocations have also been observed affecting the t(8;14). We recently studied a patient with B-cell ALL who had a complex translocation (Kaneko *et al.*, 1982*c*). In the leukemic cells, most of the long arm of chromosome 5 was translocated to 8 and the end of 8 was translocated to 14, producing the typical 14q+ marker chromosome; presumably the end of 14 was translocated to 5. Chromosome 8 is always involved in these translocations, with the breakpoint in band 8q24. Thus the consistent chromosome abnormality in some B-ALL and in Burkitt lymphoma is a rearrangement of 8q rather than 14q. The significance of these observations will be discussed in a later section.

14q+

A 14q+ chromosome is frequently observed in malignant lymphomas, particularly in those of B-cell origin (Mitelman, 1981). This abnormality was observed in 15 patients (7% of patients with abnormalities) studied at the Third Workshop; the 14q+ did not result from a translocation of the terminal segment of chromosome 8 in any of these cases. As observed in patients with t(8;14), there was an excess of males over females and of adults over children. One-half of the patients had non-T, non-B immunologic markers, and the other half had B-cell markers. The 14q+ chromosome was due to a balanced translocation in six cases, in four of which the donor chromosome was identified as number 11. This particular translocation is one of the common abnormalities seen in malignant lymphoma of the follicular small cell type, suggesting that there is a relationship between it and ALL with the 14q+ chromosome (Fukuhara *et al.*, 1978). The median survival for patients with a 14q+ was 9 months.

The 4;11 Translocation

A translocation involving the long arms of chromosomes 4 and 11 [t(4;11)(q21;q23), Fig. 9c] has been observed in a small percentage of patients with ALL (Van den Berghe *et al.*, 1979; Prigogina *et al.*, 1979; Parkin *et al.*, 1982). Of 216 ALL patients with chromosomal abnormalities studied at the Third Workshop, 18 ((8.3%) had this rearrangement. These patients had very high leukocyte counts (median WBC, 183,000/mm³), which is considered to be a poor prognostic factor. The leukemic cells were L1 type in seven patients, L2 type in seven, and L3 type in one patient. Of eight patients in whom immunologic markers were tested, seven had non-T, non-B ALL, and one had T-cell ALL. These patients had a very poor prognosis; the complete remission rate was 67%, and the median survival was 7 months. One-half of the patients were adults and the other half were children, most of whom were less than 1 year old. The association of the 4;11 translocation with neonatal or early-childhood ALL is particularly interesting in view of the low incidence of ALL in this age group (acute leukemias in this age group are usually of the myeloid type). There has been considerable confusion regarding the nature of the leukemic cells with a t(4;11). Parkin *et al.* (1982) characterized the morphological and ultrastructural features of this leukemia as consisting of mixed monocytic and lymphoid cell populations with lymphoid-appearing blasts that ultrastructurally and cytochemically may manifest myeloid markers. These findings led these authors to suggest that the t(4;11)-associated acute leukemia represents a proliferation of an early myeloid progenitor cell.

Near-Haploid ALL

The occurrence in ALL of leukemic cells with a near-haploid number of chromosomes is rare; seven such cases have been reported (Rowley and Testa, 1982). Of these seven cases, four were males and three were females. Five patients were children or adolescents and two were adults. These seven patients had a remarkably consistent chromosome pattern. The chromosome number of the near-haploid clone ranged from 26 to 36 (median, 28). In addition to a haploid set, +21 was seen in all patients, +10 or +18 in six, +X or +Y in five, +6 in four, and +1, +19, or +22 in three. Four patients had a variable percentage of cells that contained double the number of chromosomes of the near-haploid line. Of the two patients for whom immunologic markers were tested, both had non-T, non-B ALL; one was identified as having common ALL. The median survival for these seven patients was 9 months. Thus, ALL with near haploidy may be a unique subgroup of ALL with a prognosis that is poor compared with that for other types of non-T, non-B ALL.

Hyperdiploidy with 50–60 Chromosomes

The leukemic cells of some patients with ALL are characterized by a gain of many chromosomes and few structural abnormalities. Chromosome numbers usually range from 50 to 60, and a few patients may have up to 65 chromosomes. Although identical karyotypes are unusual, certain additional chromosomes are commonly seen. Among 30 hyperdiploid patients (14% of patients with abnormalities), including 22 children and eight adults evaluated at the Third Workshop, +21 was seen in 22, +6 in 15, +18 in 14, +14 in 11, and +4 or +10 each in ten patients. It is interesting that some of these chromosomes, particularly 10, 18, and 21, are also seen as additional chromosomes in patients with near-haploidy.

The median age of the 22 children with this abnormality was 3 years, and that of all 30 patients was 5 years, which was less than that of patients with other abnormalities. The WBC count in patients with hyperdiploidy was low, with a median of $6000/mm^3$. The L1 and L2 types of leukemic cells were seen in about equal numbers, and all patients had non-T, non-B ALL. The complete remission rate and the median survival for these 30 patients were 86% and 34 months, respectively. Thus, in patients who have hyperdiploidy with more than 49 chromosomes, all of the previously recognized factors, including age between 3 and 7 years, low WBC count, and non-T, non-B markers, that indicate a good prognosis are present. It should also be emphasized that the median survival of the hyperdiploid patients, including both children and adults, is longer than that of patients with a normal karyotype.

The Ph[1] Chromosome in ALL

The Ph[1] chromosome, resulting from a reciprocal translocation between chromosomes 22 and 9, is seen in patients with ALL, as well as in patients with CML. Thirty-nine Ph[1]-positive patients (18% of patients with abnormalities) were evaluated at the Third Workshop; 30 were adults and nine were children. The incidence of Ph[1]-positive patients with ALL was 5.7% for children and 17.3% for adults. Thus, the Ph[1] chromosome is the most frequent rearrangement in adult ALL. Thirty-six patients had the typical t(9;22), and the remaining three had variant translocations. The incidence of the variant form was 8%, which is similar to that observed in CML patients. About one-half of the patients showed abnormalities in addition to the Ph[1] chromosome. These additional changes were quite variable, and the usual changes seen in the acute blastic phase of CML were absent except for +8 in one case. The Ph[1]-positive patients had a high leukocyte count (median WBC count, $34,000/mm^3$), and all had non-T, non-B ALL. The complete remission rate was 55%. The median survival was 9 months, indicating a poor prognosis for these patients. By identifying this chromosomal abnormality, one can detect individuals in the non-T, non-B category who have a poor prognosis.

MALIGNANT LYMPHOMA (ML)

Surprisingly, there are far fewer cytogenetic studies of lymphomas using banding techniques than are available for leukemia; nonetheless, these investigations have shown that nearly all non-Hodgkin lymphoma (NHL) patients have clonal abnormalities, and more importantly, that the observed nonrandom abnormalities are associated with specific histological types (Fukuhara et al., 1978; Sandberg, 1981; Kaneko et al., 1982a; Yunis et al., 1982; Bloomfield et al., 1983). Malignant cells from patients with NHL, both small cell and large cell lymphomas, generally have modal numbers in the diploid range, whereas about 70% of patients with Hodgkin disease have a modal number in the triploid, tetraploid, or higher range. The incidence of karyotypic abnormalities is high in lymphoma patients. For example, only one of 27 patients with ML of various histological types studied by Fukuhara et al. (1978) had a normal karyotype, whereas Kaneko et al. (1982a) observed aneuploidy in each of 22 patients with NHL. It is noteworthy that Bloomfield et al. (1983) identified abnormalities in all 84 patients with B-cell NHL studied but only in seven of ten patients with T-cell NHL. Patients with NHL often have complex karyotypes.

Burkitt Lymphoma

Manolov and Manolova (1972) identified a consistent abnormality in the cells of five of six fresh Burkitt lymphomas and in seven of nine cultured cell lines. These investigators noted an additional band at the end of the long arm of one chromosome 14 (14q +). Zech et al (1976) first observed that, in all metaphase cells of adequate quality, the end of one chromosome 8 was consistently absent, and they suggested that the missing part of chromosome 8 was translocated to chromosome 14 [t(8;14)(q24;q32), Fig. 9a]. The t(8;14) has also been observed in nonendemic Burkitt tumors from America, Europe, and Japan. Thus, there is no doubt that the t(8;14) is a highly characteristic chromosome anomaly in Burkitt tumors. This translocation was identified in Burkitt tumors that lack any markers positive for EBV, as well as in EBV-positive tumors. It should be noted that the t(8;14) has been observed also in other lymphomas, particularly those of the small noncleaved cell (non-Burkitt) and large cell immunoblastic type (Yunis *et al.*, 1982; Bloomfield *et al.*, 1983).

As additional Burkitt tumors were examined, it became apparent that at least two other, related translocations could occur. All three translocations involved chromosome 8 with a break in the same band, 8q24. One variant translocation involved chromosome 2 with a break in the short arm [(2;8)(p13;q24)], and the other involved chromosome 22 with a break in the long arm in the band that is affected in CML [t(8;22)(q24;q11), Fig. 9b]. As discussed earlier, these same translocations have been seen in some patients with B-cell ALL.

Other Non-Hodgkin Lymphomas

A second translocation that occurs in the majority of patients with a particular type of lymphoid malignant disease is a t(14;18)(q32;q21). This was first identified by Fukuhara *et al.* (1978) in six of ten patients with poorly differentiated lymphocytic lymphoma, now called "malignant lymphoma, follicular, predominantly small cleaved cell" (FSC) in the International Classification System (Non-Hodgkin's Lymphoma Pathologic Classification Project, 1982). Fukuhara's finding was recently confirmed by Yunis *et al.* (1982), who noted a t(14;18) in each of 11 patients with FSC, as well as in five of eight other patients with follicular lymphoma of different cell types. Bloomfield *et al.* (1983) also found a t(14;18) in 22 of 91 lymphoma patients with aneuploidy; the great majority had follicular lymphoma. In addition to the t(8;14) and t(14;18), a third translocation in NHL involving chromosome 14 [t(11;14)(q13;q32)] has been described (Fukuhara *et al.*, 1978). A specific chromosome gain (+12) has been noted in four of 11 patients with small cell lymphocytic lymphoma (Yunis *et al.*, 1982), and a deletion of 6q was particularly frequent in patients with large cell lymphomas (Bloomfield *et al.*, 1983).

THE BIOLOGICAL SIGNIFICANCE OF CONSISTENT CHROMOSOMAL ABNORMALITIES

When Do Chromosomal Rearrangements Occur?

This question was considered in great detail by Rowley (1980) and here we reiterate only some of the pertinent conclusions. We do not know how consistent structural rearrangements occur, but there are at least two possibilites. The rearrangements may be random, but selection may act to eliminate the vast majority that do not provide the cell with a proliferative advantage. Alternatively, certain changes may occur preferentially, and thus may be the ones that we see. These two phenomena are not entirely mutually exclusive, since regardless of whether rearrangements occur randomly or whether certain rearrangements occur preferentially, a selective advantage over normal cells almost invariably must occur. Although there is some evidence that proximity between chromosomes within the interphase cell may be a contributing factor, we favor the first alternative. Also, in our view, the fact that the immunoglobulin gene undergoes extensive DNA rearrangements as B cells mature is unrelated to the t(8;14) in Burkitt lymphoma. Based on our present knowledge (or lack thereof), the genes involved in the translocations in myeloid leukemias do not undergo similar DNA rearrangements.

An equally important question is, when in the process of malignant transformation of a particular cell do translocations or other chromosomal aberrations occur? All available evidence from the study of carcinogenesis suggests that this is a multistage process. As is best illustrated by the blast crisis of CML, some chromosome changes occur as part of the further evolution of the malignant phenotype; they are, therefore, relatively late events. But what about the occurence of the t(9;22) in CML, for example? In an individual patient, does the Ph[1] occur in a single normal cell which becomes the progenitor of the leukemic clone (translocation as a primary or sole event in pathogenesis of CML), is there expansion of the clone, possibly a leukemic one, in which a translocation occurs in one of these already abnormal cells (translocation is one of several events), or is the translocation a secondary or unrelated event, occurring in an already malignant cell (unlikely mechanism)? This question is not easily resolved, because of the lack of independent markers for the leukemic cell. Fialkow et al. (1981) recently presented additional evidence supporting the middle concept. They used data from the report by Martin et al. (1980) on EBV-induced B-cell lines. Of the 72 B-cell lines established from this patient, 63 were Ph[1]-negative. Of these 63 lines, 18 were G6PD type A and 45 were type B. The expected ratio was 1 : 1, and this difference in frequency was significant ($p < 0.001$). Moreover, karyotypic analysis of the Ph[1]-negative cell lines revealed chromosome abnormalities, some of which were clonal, in eight of 33 evaluable lines with B-type enzyme, compared to zero of 14 lines with the A-type G6PD ($p < 0.05$). They concluded that this patient had an abnormal population of B-lymphoid cells that were Ph[1]-negative and had the same G6PD phenotype as the leukemic clone, and that these genetically unstable B cells arose from the same clone of stem cells that gave rise to the Ph[1]-positive leukemia. This notion is supported by observation of rare patients with CML whose marrow cells appeared to be Ph[1]-negative at diagnosis, but later became Ph[1]-positive. On the other hand, the observation of Kamada and Uchino (1982)that atomic bomb survivors who were followed regularly had virtually 100% Ph[1]-positive cells prior to the development of clinically evident CML indicates that the Ph[1] aberration can be a very early event in the disease process. Fialkow and Singer (1984) described two other patients who were G6PD heterozygotes, one with myelodysplasia and one with ANLL who was thought to be in complete remission. In each patient, the malignant clone had an abnormal karyotype; in the patient with myelodysplasia, 21 of 24 EBV-transformed B-cell lines had the same G6PD phenotype as the malignant clone; however, none was chromosomally abnormal. In the second patient, the chromosomally normal myeloid cells during remission had the same G6PD phenotype as did the leukemic cells prior to therapy.

The data from these three patients imply that the initial event is expansion of a chromosomally normal clone, and that the chromosome abnormality occurs in a cell belonging to this clone. What is required for resolution of this issue is a reliable marker for leukemic cells, or for preleukemic "initiated" cells, that is independent of the karyotype. One could then correlate the karyotype with this marker to determine how many cells with a normal karyotype were positive for the marker.

Defining the Critical Recombinant Chromosome

It is now apparent that the sites of consistent translocations pinpoint chromosome segments that contain genes critically involved in malignant transformation. Isolation and analysis of these segments of DNA have a high research priority. The evidence in Burkitt lymphoma is exciting and clearly points the way for future research in this area. The loci for the immunoglobulin genes are on the three chromosomes, other than chromosome 8, that are involved in translocations in Burkitt lymphoma. Thus, the locus for the heavy chain complex is on chromosome 14, that for the κ light chain is on chromosome 2, and that for the λ chain is on chromosome 22. Moreover, with the use of chromosome hybridization *in situ*, the κ light chain genes have been mapped to the short arm of chromosome

2 (band 2p12–13), the heavy chain gene has been mapped to 14q32, and the λ light chain gene has been mapped to 22q11 [reviewed in Rowley (1982), ar-Rushdi *et al.* (1983), Klein (1983), and Leder *et al.* (1983)].

An even more direct association between translocation types and gene function has been reported by Lenoir *et al.* (1982). They analyzed the type of immunoglobulin produced either in Burkitt tumor cell lines or in fresh tumor cells, and they correlated this information with the karyotype of the tumors. All three lines with a t(2;8) expressed κ light chains, and all five cell lines with a t(8;22) expressed λ light chains. Of 17 cell lines with t(8;14), nine were κ- and eight were λ-producers. An exception to this correlation, namely, a Burkitt tumor with a t(8;22) whose cells produced IgMκ, raises the question of whether the translocation event is intimately associated with the usual DNA rearrangement that is required to produce a functional immunoglobulin gene, or whether the two are independent. These data must be considered in the context of the observation by a number of investigators that the functional immunoglobulin gene locus is not the one involved in the translocation. However, the immunoglobulin gene on the 14q+ is transcribed, and thus mRNA from this gene can be detected.

There are two recombinant chromosomes in each translocation, and it would appear useful to determine which is the critical recombinant, that is, which of the two chromosomes contains the essential gene rearrangement (Rowley, 1982). As has been indicated earlier, each of the three common translocations in myeloid leukemia, t(9;22), t(8;21), and t(15;17), also occurs in a variant form in a limited number of patients, and one can use these variants to determine whether one recombinant chromosome is constant in these variant forms. In Fig. 10, the constant recombinant is enclosed in a box. Based on the data shown, the critical event leading to malignant transformation in these types of myeloid leukemia is related to the movement of 9q next to 22q in CML, that of 21q to 8q in AML, and that of the end of 17q to 15q in APL. The findings, in a patient with AMMoL and eosinophilia, with an inv(16) as well as a translocation of chromosome 1 to the same 16 [t(1;16;16)(q32;p13;q22)] suggests that the movement of 16p13 to band 16q22 (rather than the complementary recombinant) is the critical gene rearrangement (de la Chapelle and Lahtinen, 1983). A similar analysis of a variant translocation involving three chromosomes in B-cell ALL indicates that the important change is the movement of 8q to 14q (Rowley, 1982; Kaneko *et al.*, 1982c).

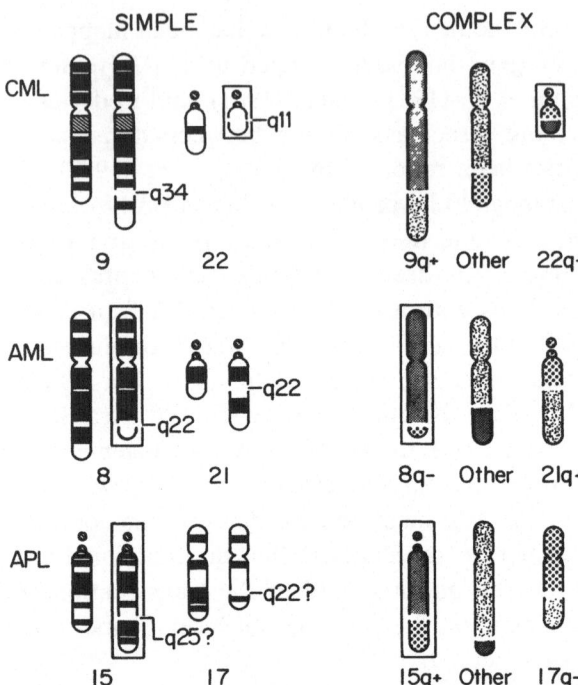

Fig. 10. Left: Diagrammatic representation of the breakpoints and the chromosome exchange in the simple consistent translocations in CML, AML, and APL. Right: Schematic drawing of the breakpoints and the typical pattern of chromosome exchange observed in the complex variants affecting each of these translocations. The other chromosome involved in these complex rearrangements is variable. For each type of leukemia, the rearranged chromosome that is consistently involved in both the simple and complex translocations is enclosed in a box. [Reprinted with permission from Rowley (1982).]

Chromosomal Localization of Cellular Oncogenes

One of the most exciting revelations in the past year has involved the cellular oncogenes and their chromosomal location. Much of the excitement derives from the observation that many oncogenes are located in the bands that are involved in consistent translocations (Rowley, 1983c; Human Gene Mapping 7, 1984) (Fig. 11). Of particular interest are c-*myc*, c-*mos*, and c-*abl*; these oncogenes have been localized to the breakpoints of chromosomes 8 and 9 that are involved in the t(8;14), t(8;21), and t(9;22), respectively. These three rearrangements are discussed in more detail later in this section.

The specific rearrangements of the c-*myc* gene and the immunoglob-

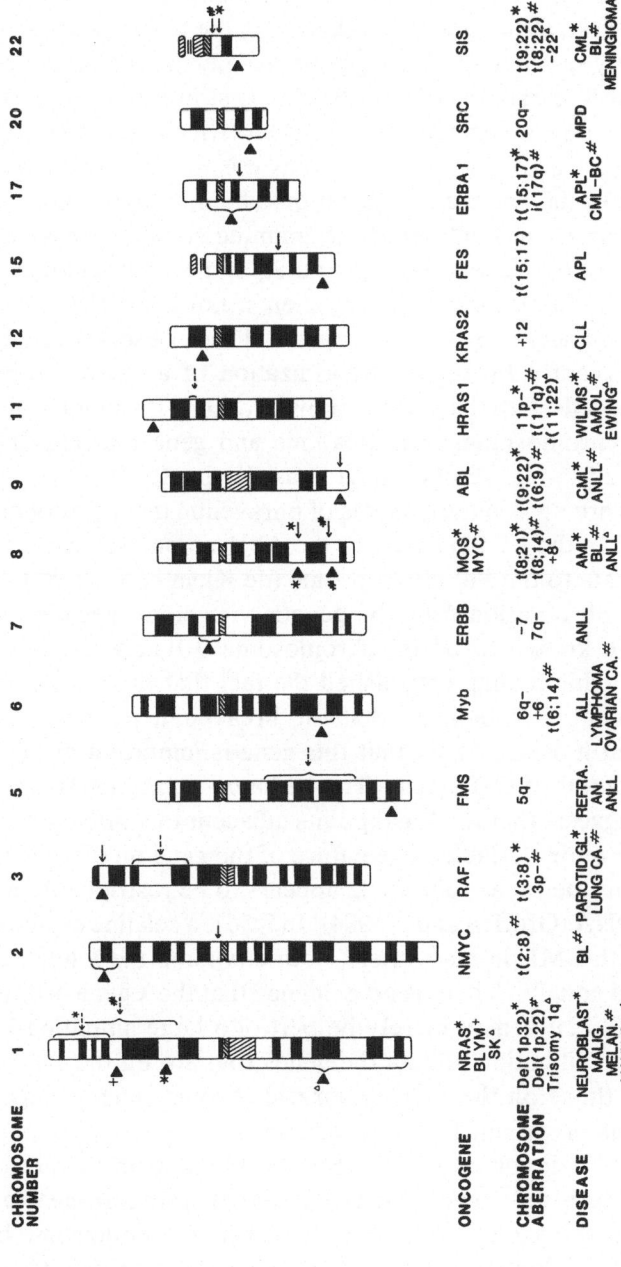

Fig. 11. Diagram of chromosomes containing known cellular oncogenes; the number is above each chromosome, and the oncogenes, karyotypic aberrations, and neoplastic diseases associated with these aberrations are indicated below the chromosomes. The arrow head (▶) to the left of each chromosome indicates the band carrying the cellular oncogene; the arrows to the right of a chromosome identify specific bands involved in consistent translocations (←) or deletions (←) observed in patients having the disorders listed. Abbreviations: REFRA. AN., refractory anemia; CLL, chronic lymphocytic leukemia; MPD, myeloproliferative disorders.

ulin (Ig) loci have been considered in detail by Leder *et al.* (1983) and ar-Rushdi *et al.* (1983), and only a few of their pertinent conclusions will be considered here. First, although the breakpoint in the Ig heavy chain gene is within a relatively restricted DNA segment, usually the constant region, the break adjacent to c-*myc* may be within the first intron of the gene in some cases, but may be at some distance in others. Second, in the t(8;14), the break is in the 5' region of c-*myc*, whereas it is in the 3' region in the t(2;8) and t(8;22). In the variant translocations, then, c-*myc* is not translocated to a chromosome containing the immunoglobulin genes (chromosome 2 or 22); rather, c-*myc* remains on 8q and the immunoglobulin genes are relocated. In all three rearrangements, however, the 5' region of the Ig gene is adjacent to the c-*myc* gene. These observations have been confirmed recently by *in situ* hybridization of a c-*myc* probe to Burkitt lymphoma cells with the various translocations. It should be noted that comparable chromosomal translocations and gene rearrangements have been observed in mouse plasmacytomas (Klein, 1983).

Investigators are now in the process of unraveling the mystery of the Ph[1] translocation. In the t(9;22) in CML, the Abelson oncogene has been shown to translocate to the Ph[1] chromosome (de Klein *et al.*, 1982). This was an important observation from the genetic viewpoint, because c-*abl* was the first gene known to be on chromosome 9 that was shown to translocate to 22. This finding established the fact that the translocation is reciprocal. Recent data indicate that the breakpoint in 9q34 is very close to c-*abl*, and it seems likely that this gene is important in the malignant transformation of CML cells (Heisterkamp *et al.*, 1983). Preliminary evidence suggests that the breakpoints adjacent to c-*abl* in different CML patients are quite variable. The nature of the gene on chromosome 22 is unknown, but the breakpoint in 22 appears to be restricted to a 5.8-kb region of the DNA (Groffen *et al.*, 1984). In K562, a cell line established from a patient with CML in blast crisis, both c-*abl* and the λ light chain gene are amplified equally. There is no evidence that the λ gene is directly involved in the t(9;22); it may merely be part of a large amplified DNA sequence. This amplification affects the genes that are on the Ph[1] chromosome and not those on the 9q + reciprocal chromosome as was predicted on the basis of variant Ph[1] translocations.

Whether c-*abl* is involved in the t(6;9) in ANLL with an increased number of basophils is unknown. The breakpoint in chromosome 9 in this translocation is in the same band, 9q34; however, a chromosome band contains about 10^7 nucleotide pairs, and therefore the breakpoints in the two translocations could be quite far apart. The c-*mos* gene is located on band 8q22; its relationship to the t(8;21) in AML is currently unknown. It was assumed for some time that c-*fes*, known to be on chromosome 15, was involved in the t(15;17) in APL, but such is not the case. First, we know that c-*fes* is not on the 15q+ chromosome (Sheer *et al.*, 1983). Moreover, c-*fes* has been localized to the end of chromosome 15 and thus is at some distance from the breakpoint (Harper *et al.*, 1983). Cells from patients with APL have also been examined for involvement of the Erb A1 oncogene, which has been located on chromosome 17 (Sakaguchi *et al.*, 1983). No rearrangement of the DNA of this oncogene has been detected (C. M. Croce, personal communication), and in somatic cell hybrids prepared from cells with the t(15;17), Erb A1 has been shown to be present on the der(17), localizing this oncogene to 17p11–17q21 (Sheer *et al.*, 1984). Thus, in a number of leukemias and lymphomas, chromosomal regions previously defined by cytogeneticists as sites of consistent rearrangements are found to be at or near the sites of oncogenes.

Specificity of Chromosomal Rearrangements

The evidence presented in this review clearly demonstrates the remarkable specificity of certain chromosome rearrangements for particular subtypes of leukemia or lymphoma. The mechanism or mechanisms by which this specificity is achieved are unknown. In an earlier consideration of this problem, Rowley noted that the specificity implied that a particular rearrangement provided a proliferative advantage only to a particular cell lineage, and only at a particular stage in differentiation within that lineage (Rowley, 1977). In addition to this specificity of chromosomal rearrangements for particular cell types, there appears to be a limited number of chromosomal regions involved in these rearrangements. Mitelman (1984) has identified 61 chromosomal regions that were the breakpoints in abnormalities observed in human tumors. Only structural rearrangements that were noted as the sole abnormality in at least two patients with the same disease were considered. It is particularly noteworthy that these 61 regions were infrequently observed as the breakpoints in the structural aberrations identified in isolated somatic cells from healthy individuals with normal chromosomal complements.

Recent experiments by a number of investigators may shed light on some of the factors that contribute to the specificity of translocations. Croce and his associates have studied the expression of the c-*myc* and immunoglobulin genes in somatic cell hybrids between Burkitt lymphoma cells containing a t(8;14) and a variety of cell types, including a mouse myeloma, a lymphoblastoid line, and fibroblasts (ar-Rushdi *et al.*, 1983; Nishikura *et al.*, 1983). In each hybrid cell system, subclones were available that contained either the normal or the translocated member of each chromosome pair, namely chromosome 8, the 8q−, 14, and the 14q+ chromosome. In the hybrid with the myeloma, both the human c-*myc* on the 14q+ chromosome and the normal immunoglobulin on 14 were expressed at levels 5–20 times higher than those in controls. In the hybrid with the lymphoblastoid cell line, the translocated c-*myc* was expressed at intermediate levels; this was also true for the functional immunoglobulin gene in these cells. Finally, in hybrids with fibroblasts, neither the translocated c-*myc* nor the immunoglobulin genes were transcribed. The uninvolved c-*myc* on the normal chromosome 8 was not expressed either in the Burkitt lymphoma parent or in any of the hybrids.

Two conclusions can be drawn from this series of observations. First, the cell type in which the particular gene is located has a profound influence on the level of expression of that gene. Second, the level of expression of the two genes involved in the Burkitt translocation is regulated in a coordinate fashion. That is, the expression of each is high, intermediate, or low depending on the cell type, and the level of expression is the same for both genes in any particular cell type.

Recent data of Kelly *et al.* (1984), however, indicate that c-*myc* can be expressed in fibroblasts under certain circumstances. In Balb/C-3T3 fibroblasts stimulated to proliferate by addition of platelet-derived growth factor, the level of c-*myc* increased approximately 40-fold within 3 hr. Similar rapid increases in c-*myc* mRNA were observed in resting B and T lymphocytes stimulated with the appropriate mitogens. This increase in c-*myc* mRNA synthesis occurred in the stimulated cells and, in fact, was enhanced if cycloheximide as well as the mitogen was added. In these experiments, the level of c-*myc* mRNA was lower in stationary-phase fibroblasts than in unstimulated lymphocytes.

If the results of such an analysis of the t(8;14) are generally applicable to other translocations, then some of the hypotheses proposed earlier regarding the specificity of chromosome aberrations can be refined further (Fig. 12) (Rowley, 1977). Moreover, one can make certain predictions regarding gene expression that would explain the specificity of the chromosomal rearrangements discussed in this review. Translocations or inversions bring together two genes that are normally far apart and are under

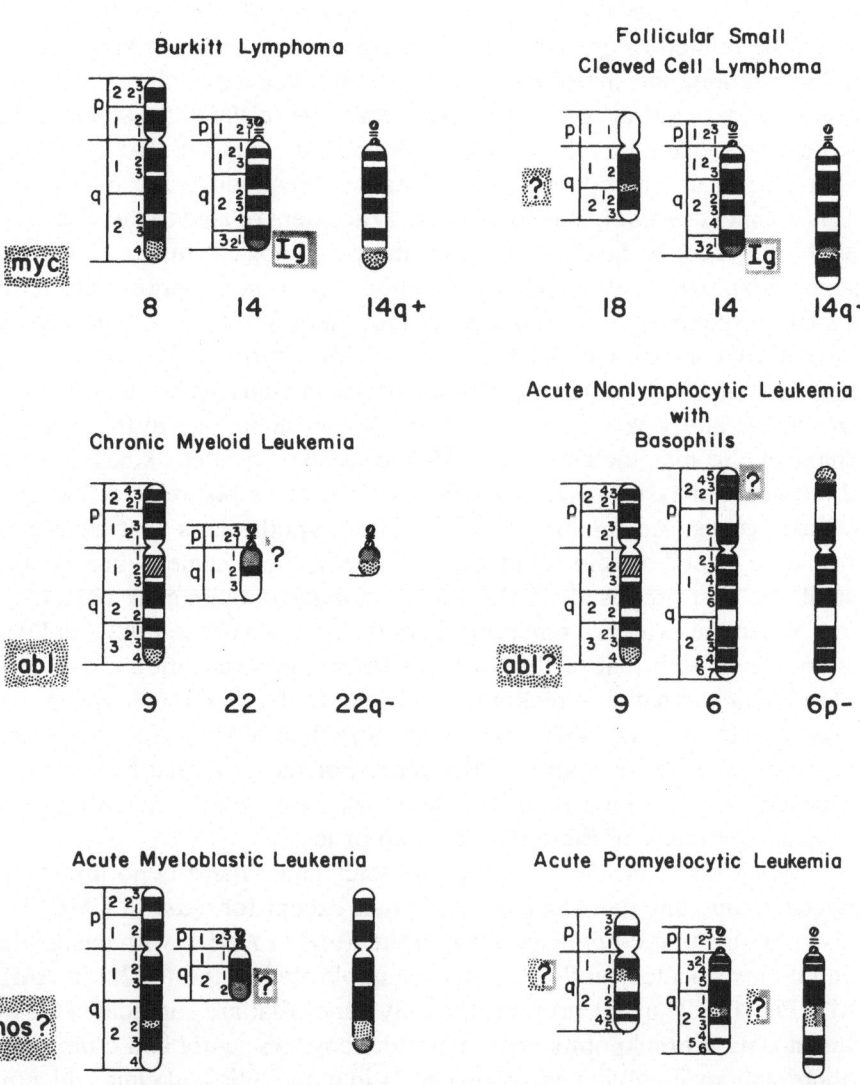

Fig. 12. Diagram illustrating various specific translocations in lymphomas and myeloid leukemias. The potential growth factors or oncogenes are indicated in regions stippled with large dots and the cell-specific genes by regions with small dots. Uncertainty about the nature of the relevant genes is indicated by a question mark.

different regulatory control. This may also be true for deletions that may be interstitial rather than terminal. As a general rule, one of these genes would be related to growth control in a particular cell type and stage of differentiation, and the other gene would produce a protein whose function played a central role in the same cell type in the same stage of differentiation. Thus far, the only growth-controlling genes that have been identified in association with translocation breakpoints are oncogenes. This is almost certainly due to a historical accident related to the discovery of these genes; in the future, when the physiological function of these genes is known, they should be identified by a more appropriate term. As Heisterkamp *et al.* (1983) have noted, there is extensive homology in the nucleic acid and amino acid sequence of the tyrosine phosphorylation region of c-*abl* and of corresponding regions of some other oncogenes (v-*src*, v-*yes*, and v-*fes*), as well as more distant homology to the catalytic chain of the mammalian cyclic AMP-dependent protein kinase. All of these genes may represent members of a diverse but related family of cellular genes. An important facet of the hypothesis is that each gene would be turned on and off in a coordinate fashion, namely, in a manner similar to that proposed for the c-*myc*–immunoglobulin gene complex.

When the evidence emerging from the analysis of the t(9;22) in CML is combined with that of the t(8;14), a further generalization can be proposed, namely that the breakpoints adjacent to the gene regulating growth may be extremely variable (varying by more than 50 kb) and may be either in the 5′ or in the 3′ region of the gene. For the gene that has a critical cell- and stage-specific function, the breakpoints will be much more restricted, generally of the order of 10 kb or less.

When one considers the myeloid leukemias, there is no direct evidence linking any gene to any breakpoint except for c-*abl* in CML. It is also possible that c-*abl* is involved in the t(6;9) in ANLL with basophilia, and c-*mos*, located on 8q22, could be implicated in the t(8;21) in AML-M2 (Fig. 12). Thus, at present, the only genes that are candidates for the translocation breakpoints are the protooncogenes, c-*abl* and c-*mos*. The abnormalities involving chromosome 11 in monocytic leukemia add a further dimension of complexity. In the framework of the growth-controlling gene–cell function-specific gene hypothesis, Rowley (1983*a*) has proposed that band 11q23 (or less often 11q13) is the locus for a growth-regulating factor (or oncogene) and that 9p21 (or bands on other chromosomes involved in the translocation) is the locus for the cell type-specific or cell stage-specific gene. This suggests, then, that there are a number of genes that function in the same genetic pathway as that on 9p21, any one of which could act as the cell-specific switch for the growth-regulating gene on 11q23. It should be noted that translocations involving 11q23 or 11q13 also occur with some frequency in various lymphoid malignancies; in lymphoid disorders, however, different chromosomes are involved in the translocations, of which chromosomes 4 and 14 are the most common. Whether the same growth-regulating gene on 11q is involved in these translocations will only be established when these genes have been precisely identified. Thus far, we have no information regarding the identity of any genes related to specialized functions in myeloid cells, analogous to the immunoglobulin genes in B cells. Moreoever, there is no evidence indicating whether all of these genes belong to the same general class, or whether they differ in different stages of cell development. However, because the chromosomal rearrangements precisely define the chromosomal location of these genes, this information might allow us to clone the genes, to determine their sequence, and possibly to identify them through DNA data banks, independent of other experimental approaches. This scenario might appear to be somewhat fanciful; however, now that the breakpoint of the t(9;22) has been cloned and the sequences of chromosome 22 that are adjacent to the breakpoint are available for analysis, the future is upon us.

REFERENCES

Alimena, G., Dallapiccola, H., Gastaldi, R., Mandelli, F., Brandt, L., Mitelman, F., and Nilsson, P. G., 1982, Chromosomal, morphological and clinical correlations in blastic crisis of chronic myeloid leukemia, a study of 69 cases, *Scand. J. Haematol.* **28**:103–117.

ar-Rushdi, A., Nishikura, K., Erikson, J., Watt, R., Rovera, G., and Croce, C. M., 1983, Differential expression of the translocated and the untranslocated c-*myc* oncogene in Burkitt lymphoma, *Science* **222**:390–393.

Arthur, D. C., and Bloomfield, C. D., 1983, Partial deletion of the long arm of chromosome 16 and bone marrow, eosinophilia in acute nonlymphocytic leukemia: A new association, *Blood* **61**:994–998.

Bennett, J. M., Catovsky, D., Daniel, M. T., Flandrin, G., Galton, D. A. G., Gralnick, H., and Sultan, C., 1976, Proposals for the classification of the acute leukemias, French–American–British (FAB) Co-operative Group, *Br. J. Haematol.* **33**:451–458.

Berger, R., Bernheim, A., and Flandrin, G., 1980a, Absence of chromosome abnormalities and acute leukemia: Relationships with normal bone marrow cells, *C. R. Acad. Sci. Paris* **290D**:1557–1559.

Berger, R., Berhneim, A., Weh, H. J., Daniel, M.-T., and Flandrin, G., 1980b, Cytogenetic studies on acute monocytic leukemia, *Leuk. Res.* **4**:119–127.

Berger, R., Bernheim, A., Sigaux, F., Daniel, M.-T., Valensi, F., and Flandrin, G., 1982, Acute monocytic leukemia chromosome studies, *Leuk. Res.* **6**:17–26.

Bernheim, A., Berger, R., Preud'homme, J. L., Labaume, S., Bussel, A., and Barot-Ciorbaru, R., 1981, Philadelphia chromosome positive blood B lymphocytes in chronic myelocytic leukemia, *Leuk. Res.* **5**:331–339.

Bernstein, R., Pinto, M. R., Behr, A., and Mendelow, B., 1982, Chromosome 3 abnormalities in acute nonlymphocytic leukemia (ANLL) with abnormal thrombopoiesis: Report of three patients with a "new" inversion anomaly and a further case of homologous translocation, *Blood* **60**:613–617.

Bloomfield, C. D., Arthur, D. C., Frizzera, G., Levine, E. G., Peterson, B. A., and Gajl-Peczalska, K. J., 1983, Nonrandom chromosome abnormalities in lymphoma, *Cancer Res.* **43**:2975–2984.

Boveri, R., 1914, *Zur Frage der Entstehung Maligner Tumoren*, Fischer, Jena.

Cannelos, G. P., Whang-Peng, J., and De Vita, V. T., 1976, Chronic granulocytic leukemia without the Philadelphia chromosome, *Am. J. Clin. Pathol.* **65**:467–470.

Caspersson, T., Gahrton, G., Lindsten, J., and Zech, L., 1970, Identification of the Philadelphia chromosome as a number 22 by quinacrine mustard fluorescence analysis, *Exp. Cell Res.* **63**:238–244.

de Klein, A., Geurts van Kessel, A. H. M., Grosveld, G., Bartram, C. R., Hagemeijer, A., Boatsma, D., Spurr, N. K., Heisterkamp, N., Groffen, J., and Stephenson, J. R., 1982, A cellular oncogene is translocated to the Philadelphia chromosome in chronic myelocytic leukemia, *Nature* **300**:765–767.

de la Chapelle, A., and Lahtinen, R., 1983, Chromosome 16 and bone-marrow eosinophilia, *N. Engl. J. Med.* **309**:1394.

Fialkow, P. J., 1974, The origin and development of human tumors studied with cell markers, *N. Engl. J. Med.* **291**:26–35.

Fialkow, P. J., and Singer, J. W., 1984, Tracing development and cell lineages in human hemopoietic neoplasia. in: *Leukemia* (Dahlem Konferenzen) (I. L. Weissman, ed.), pp. 203–222, Springer, Verlag, Berlin.

Fialkow, P. J., Martin, P. J., Najfeld, V., Penfold, G. K., Jacobson, R. J., and Hansen, J. A., 1981, Evidence for a multistep pathogenesis of chronic myelogenous leukemia, *Blood* **58**:158–163.

First International Workshop on Chromosomes in Leukemia, 1978, Chromosomes in acute nonlymphocytic leukaemia, *Br. J. Haematol.* **39**:311–316.

Fourth International Workshop on Chromosomes in Leukemia, 1984, A prospective study of acute nonlymphocytic leukemia, *Cancer Genet. Cytogenet.* **11**:249–360.

Fukuhara, S., Rowley, J. D., Variakojis, D., and Sweet, D. L., 1978, Banding studies on chromosomes in diffuse histiocytic lymphomas: Correlation of 14q+ marker chromosome with cytology, *Blood* **52**:989–1002.

Gahrton, G., Lindsten, J., and Zech, L., 1974, Involvement of chromosomes 8, 9, 19, and 22 in Ph[1] negative chronic myelocytic leukemia in the chronic or blastic stage, *Acta Med. Scand.* **196**:355–360.

Golomb, H.M., Alimena, G., Rowley, J. D., Vardiman, J. W., Testa, J. R., and Sovik, C., 1982, Correlation of occupation and karyotype in adults with acute nonlymphocytic leukemia, *Blood* **60**:404–411.

Greene, M. H., Young, R. C., Merrill, J. M., and De Vita, V. T., 1983, Evidence of a treatment dose response in acute nonlymphocytic leukemias which occur after therapy of non-Hodgkin's lymphoma, *Cancer Res.* **43**:1891–1898.

Groffen, J., Stephenson, J. R., Heisterkamp, N., de Klein, A., Bartram, C. R., and Grosveld, G., 1984, Philadelphia chromosomal breakpoints are clustered within a limited region, bcr, on chromosome 22, *Cell* **36**:93–99.

Grünwald, H. W., and Rosner, F., 1982, Acute myeloid leukemia following treatment of Hodgkin's disease, *Cancer* 50:676–683.

Hagemeijer, A., Hählen, K., Sizoo, W., and Abels, J., 1982, Translocation (9;11)(p21;q23) in three cases of acute monoblastic leukemia, *Cancer Genet. Cytogenet.* 5:95–105.

Hagemeijer, A., Bartram, C. R., Smith, E. M. E., van Agthoven, A. J., and Bootsma, D., 1984, Is the chromosomal region 9q34 always involved in variants of the Ph[1] translocation? *Cancer Genet. Cytogenet.* 13:1–16.

Harper, M. E., Franchini, G., Love, J., Simon, M. I., Gallo, R. C., and Wong-Staal, F., 1983, Chromosomal sublocalization of human c-*myb* and c-*fes* cellular onc genes, *Nature* 304:169–171.

Heisterkamp, N., Stephenson, J. R., Groffen, J., Hansen, P. F., de Klein, A., Bartram, C. R., and Grosveld, G., 1983, Localization of the c-*abl* oncogene adjacent to a translocation breakpoint in chronic myelocytic leukaemia, *Nature* 306:239–242.

Human Gene Mapping 7, 1984, *Cytogenet. Cell Genet.* 37:1–666.

ISCN, 1978, An international system for human cytogenetic nomenclature, *Cytogenet. Cell Genet.* 21:309–404.

Kaiser-McCaw, B., Epstein, A., Kaplan, H. S., and Hecht, F., 1977, Chromosome 14 translocations in African and North American Burkitt's lymphoma, *Int. J. Cancer* 19:482–486.

Kamada, N., and Uchino, H., 1982, Chronologic sequence in appearance of clinical and laboratory findings characteristic of chronic myelocytic leukemia, *Blood* 51:843–850.

Kamada, N., Okada, K., Ito, T., Nakatsui, T., and Uchino, H., 1968, Chromosome 21–22 and neutrophil alkaline phosphatase in leukaemia, *Lancet* 1:364.

Kaneko, Y., and Rowley, J. D., 1981, Correlation of karyotype with prognosis in acute lymphocytic leukemia (ALL), *Proc. Am. Soc. Clin. Oncol.* 22:338.

Kaneko, Y., and Sakurai, M., 1977, 15/17 translocation in acute promyelocytic leukemia, *Lancet* 1:961.

Kaneko, Y., Abe, R., Sampi, K., and Sakurai, M., 1982a, An analysis of chromosome findings in non-Hodgkin's lymphomas, *Cancer Genet. Cytogenet.* 5:107–121.

Kaneko, Y., Rowley, J. D., Maurer, H. S., Variakojis, D., and Moohr, J., 1982b, Chromosome pattern in childhood acute nonlymphocytic leukemia (ANLL), *Blood* 60:389–399.

Kaneko, Y., Rowley, J. D., Variakojis, D., Chilcote, R. R., Check, I., and Sakurai, M., 1982c, Correlation of karyotype with clinical features in acute lymphoblastic leukemia (ALL), *Cancer Res.* 42:2918–2929.

Kelly, K., Cochran, B. H., Stiles, C. D., and Leder, P., 1984, Cell-specific regulation of the c-*myc* gene by lymphocyte mitogens and platelet derived growth factor, *Cell* 35:603–610.

Klein, G., 1983, Specific chromosomal translocations and the genesis of B-cell derived tumors in mice and men, *Cell* 32:311–315.

Knuutila, S., Vuopio, P., Elonen, E., Siimes, M., Kovanen, R., Borgstrom, G. H., and de la Chapelle, A., 1981, Culture of bone marrow reveals more cells with chromosomal abnormalities than the direct method in patients with hematologic disorders, *Blood* 58:369–375.

Larson, R. A., Le Beau, M. M., Vardiman, J. W., Testa, J. R., Golomb, H. M., and Rowley, J. D., 1983, The predictive value of initial cytogenetic studies in 148 adults with acute nonlymphocytic leukemia: A 12 year study (1970–1982), *Cancer Genet. Cytogenet.* 10:219–236.

Larson, R. A., Kondo, K., Vardiman, J. W., Butler, A. E., Golomb, H. M., and Rowley, J. D., 1984, Every patient with acute promyelocytic leukemia may have a 15;17 translocation, *Am. J. Med.* 76:827–841.

Le Beau, M. M., Larson, R. A., Bitter, M. A., Vardiman, J. W., Golomb, H. M., and Rowley, J. D., 1983, Association of inv(16)(p13q22) with abnormal marrow eosinophils in acute myelomonocytic leukemia: A unique cytogenetic–clinicopathologic association, *N. Engl. J. Med.* **309**:630–636.

Leder, P., Battey, J., Lenoir, G., Moulding, C., Murphy, W., Potter, H., Stewart, T., and Taub, R., 1983, Translocations among antibody genes in human cancer, *Science* **222**:765–771.

Lenoir, G. M., Preud'homme, J. L., Bernheim, A., and Berger, R., 1982, Correlation between immunoglobulin light chain expression and variant translocation in Burkitt's lymphoma, *Nature* **298**:474–476.

Manolov, G., and Manolova, Y., 1972, Marker band in one chromosome 14 from Burkitt lymphomas, *Nature* **237**:33–34.

Martin, P. J., Najfeld, V., Hansen, J. A., Penfold, G. K., Jacobson, R. J., and Fialkow, P. J., 1980, Involvement of the B-lymphoid system in chronic myelogenous leukaemia, *Nature* **287**:49–50.

Mayall, B. H., Carrano, A. V., Moore, D. H., II, and Rowley, J. D., 1977, Qualification by DNA-based cytophotometry of the 9q+/22q− chromosomal translocation associated with chronic myelogenous leukemia, *Cancer Res.* **37**:3590–3593.

Mitelman, F., 1981, Marker chromosome 14q+ in human cancer and leukemia, *Adv. Cancer Res.* **34**:141–170.

Mitelman, F., 1984, Restricted number of chromosomal regions implicated in aetiology of human cancer and leukemia, *Nature* **310**:325–327.

Mitelman, F., and Levan G., 1978, Clustering of aberrations to specific chromosomes in human neoplasms. III. Incidence and geographic distribution of chromosome aberrations in 856 cases, *Hereditas* **89**:207–232.

Mitelman, F., Brandt, L., and Nilsson, P. G., 1978, Relation among occupational exposure to potential mutagenic/carcinogenic agents, clinical findings and bone marrow chromosomes in acute nonlymphocytic leukemia, *Blood* **52**:1229–1237.

Mitelman, F., Nilsson, P. G., Brandt, L., Alimena, G., Gestaldi, R., and Dallapiccola, B., 1981, Chromosome pattern, occupation, and clinical features in patients with acute nonlymphocytic leukemia, *Cancer Genet. Cytogenet.* **4**:197–214.

Nishikura, K., ar-Rushdi, A., Erikson, J., Watt, R., Rovera, G., and Croce, C. M., 1983, Differential expression of the normal and of the translocated human c-*myc* oncogenes in B cells, *Proc. Natl. Acad. Sci. USA* **80**:4822–4826.

Non-Hodgkin's Lymphoma Pathologic Classification Project, 1982, National Cancer Institute-sponsored study of classifications of non-Hodgkin's lymphoma: Summary and description of a working formulation for clinical usage, *Cancer* **49**:2112–2135.

Nowell, P., and Hungerford, D. A., 1960, A minute chromosome in human chronic granulocytic leukemia, *Science* **132**:1197.

O'Riordan, M. L., Robinson, J. A., Buckton, K. E., and Evans, H. J., 1971, Distinguishing between the chromosomes involved in Down's syndrome (trisomy 21) and chronic myeloid leukemia (Ph[1]) by fluorescence, *Nature* **230**:167–168.

Parkin, J. L., Arthur, D. C., Abramson, C. S., McKenna, R. W., Kersey, J. H., Heideman, R. L., and Brunning, R. D., 1982, Acute leukemia associated with the t(4;11) chromosome rearrangement: Ultrastructural and immunologic characteristics, *Blood* **60**:1321–1331.

Pearson, M. G., Vardiman, J. W., Le Beau, M. M., Rowley, J. D., Schwartz, S., Kerman, S. L., Cohen, M. M., Fleishmann, E. W., and Prigogina, E. L., 1985, Increased numbers of marrow basophils may be associated with a t(6;9) in ANLL *Am. J. Hemat.* **18**:393–403.

Pederson-Bjergaard, J., and Larsen, S. O., 1982, Incidence of acute nonlymphocytic leukemia, preleukemia, and acute myeloproliferative syndrome up to 10 years after treatment of Hodgkin's disease, N. Engl. J. Med. 307:965–971.

Pierre, R. V., and Hoaglund, H. C., 1972, Age-associated aneuploidy: Loss of Y chromosome from human bone marrow cells with aging, Cancer 30:889–894.

Prigogina, E. L., Fleischman, E. W., Volkova, M. A., and Frenkel, M. A., 1978, Chromosome abnormalities and clinical and morphologic manifestations of chronic myeloid leukemia, Hum. Genet. 41:143–156.

Prigogina, E. L., Fleischman, E. W., Puchkova, G. P., Kulagina, O. E., Najakova, S. A., Balakirev, S. A., Frenkel, M. A., Khvatova, N. V., and Peterson, I. S., 1979, Chromosomes in acute leukemia, Human. Genet. 53:5–16.

Pugh, W. C. Pearson, M. G., Rowley, J. D., and Vardiman, J. W., 1983, Philadelphia-negative chronic myelogenous leukemia: A morphologic reassessment, Br. J. Haematol. 60:457–467.

Rowley, J. D., 1973a, A new consistent chromosomal abnormality in chronic myelogenous leukemia identified by quinacrine fluorescence and Giemsa staining, Nature 243:290–292.

Rowley, J. D., 1973b, Identification of a translocation with quinacrine fluorescence in a patient with acute leukemia, Ann. Genet. 16:109–112.

Rowley, J. D., 1977, Mapping of human chromosomal regions related to neoplasia: Evidence from chromosomes 1 and 17, Proc. Natl. Acad. Sci. USA 74:5729–5733.

Rowley, J. D., 1980a, Chromosome abnormalities in cancer, Cancer Genet. Cytogenet. 2:175–198.

Rowley, J. D., 1980b, Chromosome changes in acute leukemia, Br. J. Haematol. 44:339–346.

Rowley, J. D., 1980c, Ph[1]-positive leukemia, including chronic myelogenous leukemia, Clin. Haematol. 9:5586.

Rowley, J. D., 1982, Identification of the constant chromosome regions involved in human hematologic malignant disease, Science 216:749–751.

Rowley, J. D., 1983a, Consistent chromosome abnormalities in human leukemia and lymphoma, Cancer Invest. 1:267–280.

Rowley, J. D., 1983b, Chromosome changes in leukemic cells as indicators of mutagenic exposure, in: Chromosomes and Cancer: From Molecules to Man (J. D. Rowley and J. E. Ultmann, eds.), pp. 140–159, Academic Press, New York.

Rowley, J. D., 1983c, Human oncogene locations and chromosome aberrations, Nature 301:290–291.

Rowley, J. D., and Potter, D., 1976, Chromosomal banding patterns in acute leukemia, Blood 47:705–722.

Rowley, J. D., and Testa, J. R., 1982, Chromosome abnormalities in malignant hematologic diseases, Adv. Cancer Res. 36:103–148.

Rowley, J. D., Golomb, H. M., and Dougherty, C., 1977, 15/17 translocation, a consistent chromosomal change in acute promyelocytic leukemia, Lancet 1:549–550.

Rowley, J. D., Golomb, H. M., and Vardiman, J. W., 1981, Nonrandom chromosome abnormalities in acute leukemia and dysmyelopoietic syndrome in patients with previously treated malignant disease, Blood 58:759–767.

Rowley, J. D., Alimena, G., Garson, O. M., Hagemeijer, A., Mitelman, F., and Prigogina, E. L., 1982, A collaborative study of the relationship of the morphologic type of acute nonlymphocytic leukemia with patient age and karyotype, Blood 59:1013–1022.

Sakaguchi, A. Y., Zabel, B. U., Grzeschik, K.-H., Law, M. L., and Naylor, S. L., 1984, Human proto-oncogene assignments. Human Gene Mapping 7, Cytogenet. Cell Genet. 37:572.

Sakurai, M., and Sandberg, A. A., 1973, Prognosis in acute myeloblastic leukemia: Chromosomal correlation, *Blood* **41**:93–104.

Sandberg, A. A., 1980, *The Chromosomes in Human Cancer and Leukemia*, Elsevier/North-Holland, New York.

Sandberg, A. A., 1981, Chromosome changes in the lymphomas, *Hum. Pathol.* **12**:531–540.

Sandberg, A. A., Abe, S., Kowalczyk, J. R., Zedgenidze, A., Takeuchi, J., and Kakati, S., 1982, Chromosomes and causation of human cancer and leukemia. L. Cytogenetics of leukemias complicating other disease, *Cancer Genet. Cytogenet.* **7**:95–136.

Secker-Walker, L. M., 1984, The prognostic implications of chromosomal findings in acute lymphoblastic leukemia, *Cancer Cytogenet. Cell Genet.* **11**:233–248.

Second International Workshop on Chromosomes in Leukemia, 1980, *Cancer Genet. Cytogenet.* **2**:89–113.

Sheer, D., Hiorns, L. R., Stanley, K. F., Goodfellow, P. N., Swallow, D. M., Povey, S., Heisterkamp, N., Groffen, J., Stephenson, J. R., and Solomon, E., 1983, Genetic analysis of the 15;17 chromosome translocation associated with acute promyelocytic leukemia, *Proc. Natl. Acad. Sci. USA* **80**:5007–5011.

Sheer, D., Hiorns, L. R., Spurr, N., and Solomon, E., 1984, Is c-*erb* A1 rearranged in the 15q+;17q− chromosome translocation associated with acute promyelocytic leukemia, *J. Cell. Biochem. Suppl* **8A**:74 (abstract 0184).

Sonta, S., and Sandberg, A. A., 1978, Chromosomes and causation of human cancer and leukemia. XXIV. Further studies on karyotypic progression in CML, *Cancer* **41**:153–163.

Sweet, D. L., Golomb, H. M., Rowley, J. D., and Vardiman, J. W., 1979, Acute myelogenous leukemia and thrombocythemia associated with an abnormality of chromosome No. 3, *Cancer Genet. Cytogenet.* **1**:33–37.

Tantravahi, R., Schwenn, M., Henkle, C., Nell, M., Leavitt, P. R., Griffin, J. D., and Weinstein, H. J., 1984, A pericentric inversion of chromosome 16 is associated with dysplastic marrow eosinophils in acute myelomonocytic leukemia, *Blood* **63**:800–802.

Testa, J. R., Golomb, H. M., Rowley, J. D., Vardiman, J. W., and Sweet, D. L., 1978, Hypergranular promyelocytic leukemia (APL): Cytogenetic and ultrastructural specificty, *Blood* **52**:272–280.

Third International Workshop on Chromosomes in Leukemia, 1981, *Cancer Genet. Cytogenet.* **4**:95–142.

Van den Berghe, H., David, G., Broeckaert-Van Orshoven, A., Louwagie, A., Verwilghen, R., Casteels-Van Daele, M., Eggermont, E., and Eeckels, R., 1979, A new chromosome anomaly in acute lymphoblastic leukemia (ALL), *Hum. Genet.* **46**:173–180.

Waghray, M., Egues, C., Rowley, J. D., Martin, P., and Testa, J. R., 1981, Methods of processing marrow samples may affect the frequency of detectable aneuploid cells, *Am. J. Hematol.* **11**:409–415.

Whang-Peng, J., Canellos, G. P., Carbona, P. P., and Tjio, J. H., 1968, Clinical implications of cytogenetic variants in chronic myelocytic leukemia (CML), *Blood* **32**:755–766.

Yunis, J. J., 1982, Comparative analysis of high-resolution chromosome techniques for leukemic bone marrows, *Cancer Genet. Cytogenet.* **7**:43–50.

Yunis, J. J., 1983, The chromosomal basis of human neoplasia, *Science* **221**:227–236.

Yunis, J. J., Bloomfield, C. D., and Ensrud, K., 1981, All patients with acute nonlymphocytic leukemia may have a chromosomal defect, *N. Engl. J. Med.* **305**:135–139.

Yunis, J. J., Oken, M. M., Kaplan, M. E., Ensrud, K. M., Howe, R. R., and Theologides, A., 1982, Distinctive chromosomal abnormalities in histologic subtypes of non-Hodgkin's lymphoma, *N. Engl. J. Med.* **307**:1231–1236.

Zech, L., Haglund, V., Nilsson, K., and Klein, G., 1976, Characteristic chromosomal abnormalities in biopsies and lymphoid cell lines from patients with Burkitt and non-Burkitt lymphomas, *Int. J. Cancer* **17**:47–56.

Chapter 2

An Algorithm for Comparing Two-Dimensional Electrophoretic Gels, with Particular Reference to the Study of Mutation

Michael M. Skolnick* and James V. Neel

Department of Human Genetics
University of Michigan Medical School
Ann Arbor, Michigan 48109

INTRODUCTION

Concerns over the possible mutagenic effects of exposure to chemicals and radiation resulting from human activities, which surfaced so strongly in the 1950s, continue essentially unabated. Regulations and legislation in which genetic considerations play a significant role are being promulgated, and litigation concerning possible genetic damage from exposures resulting from human activities is in the courts. While animal models, particularly those employing the house mouse, have been essential in preliminary evaluations of the potential magnitude of the human risks, their potential for error in any precise evaluation of the magnitude of the issues is now apparent (Denniston, 1982; Kohn, 1983; Neel, 1983; Lyon, 1983). There is an urgent need for data on these risks derived from studies of human populations.

On the scale on which the experimental geneticist works, most human exposures would appear to be low. With respect to radiation, the two

---

* *Present address* for M. M. S: Department of Computer Science, Rensselaer Polytechnic Institute, Troy, New York 12181.

best-documented examples of "population" exposures thus far appear to be the aftermaths of the atomic bombings of Hiroshima and Nagasaki and of the Bravo thermonuclear test explosion at Bikini in 1954. In the former instance, the average conjoint gonadal dose to individuals who survived and later reproduced and who were within the zone of significant radiation has been estimated to be approximately 60 rem (Schull *et al.*, 1981), but this estimate is now in the process of a revision downward (Radiation Effects Research Foundation, 1983, 1984). With regard to the Bravo test, a relatively small group received a total γ surface dose from fallout deposited on the ground which has been estimated to range from 14 R (157 persons on Utrik) to 175 R (64 persons on Rongelap), with smaller groups on Ailingnae and Rongerik receiving intermediate doses. Additional γ exposures presumably resulted from fallout adhering to the skin, but the γ exposure from this is unknown. (There were in addition β emission exposures, but these emissions presumably did not penetrate beyond the skin.) The gonad dose, either as a direct consequence of fallout or from the ingestion of contaminating radionuclides following the incident, has never been estimated. Whether the recent Juarez episode will result in exposures of the magnitude experienced following the Bikini tests remains to be seen (Marshall, 1984).

The more notable examples of occupational or accidental exposures to potentially mutagenic chemicals are commonly thought to stem from the experiences of a subset of workers in the petrochemical industry or agriculture, the exposures in the latter resulting primarily from the use of herbicides or pesticides. The exposures incident to the use of Agent Orange during the Vietnam episode constitute a special case currently receiving intensive scrutiny. Perhaps the most ubiquitous exposure to a chemical mutagen, however, involves cigarette smoke, as judged by the results of an Ames test on the urine of heavy smokers (Yamasaki and Ames, 1977). In none of these examples of exposure to chemical mutagens is the gonad dose known, but, for that matter, gonad doses are not usually known in experimental studies of chemical mutagens. In citing these examples of a possible mutagenic exposure, we do not mean to imply a belief that a significant genetic risk exists; we mean only to identify those groups most commonly mentioned in discussions of exposures to mutagenic chemicals.

The radiation exposures currently causing the most concern appear to be much smaller than these just enumerated. For instance, in the U.S. two of the outstanding examples of public concern result from the exposure of service personnel and civilians to radioactive fallout resulting from the testing of atomic weapons in New Mexico. The exposures received by civilians remain highly debatable, but because the exposures of servicemen were monitored by film badges, data that should be reasonably accurate are available. These data indicate an average exposure to the approximately 250,000 servicemen who participated in the various test shots of about 0.5 rem. Congress has recently responded to the public concerns over the possible effects of these veterans' exposures by enacting legislation mandating a study of both the somatic and genetic effects of these exposures if such a study is found to be feasible (Public Law 98-160). We would put in the same category—of probably very low-level exposures—the exposures sustained in consequence of current methods for the management of toxic chemicals. But while these chemical exposures currently appear to be small, they are not as easily terminated as most of those mentioned earlier.

The costs of meeting the concerns created by these various exposures are potentially far more major than commonly realized. These stem from indemnification of individuals who received exposures now thought to be harmful, and from the implementation of standards set for the disposal of toxic waste, either radioactive or chemical. For instance, a driving consideration in the plan of the Environmental Protection Agency for the management of high-level radioactive waste [40 CFR part 191 (Proposed)] is the perceived health effects of this waste after storage. These estimates require extrapolation more than three orders of magnitude beyond experimental data, which data present very considerable uncertainties. Since the cost of each of the projected waste repositories is estimated at 6–7 billion dollars, and approximately a dozen are contemplated, the financial consequences of an overestimate of the risks involved in the storage procedures are not small.

While in this and other circumstances the protection of the public must be a driving concern, it is impractical to maintain an industrial society without some risks, which may simply be replacing other risks long present in the environment (Ames, 1983). For some years we have been suggesting that in view of the gravity of the societal issues involved, both psychological and financial, a carefully coordinated effort, preferably international, to study the various cohorts of children presumably at high risk of mutation might be indicated (Neel, 1981). The argument is that such a ''worst case'' approach should produce the perspective from which to deal with the implications of lesser exposures.

Two basic problems in the implementation of such proposed studies have been that not only, as noted above, are the exposures even in most of the "worst cases" very low by the standards of the experimental geneticist, but the various possible study cohorts are small and most studies would perforce be retrospective, with all the problems that arise in any attempt to recreate precise reproductive histories and outcomes. The first consideration leads to the problem of numbers, the second leads to the problem of bias.

With respect to the problem of numbers, the over-riding consideration is the rarity of mutation. Let us agree that the genetically "cleanest" study involves specific locus mutation rates. In humans the mutation rate per locus encoding for a protein product is of the order of 1×10^{-5}/locus per generation (Neel, 1983), but no one current technique will detect the complete spectrum of mutation at a given locus. What would currently be considered enormous numbers of observations are necessary to detect the increase in mutation rates it is reasonable to expect. For instance, we have calculated that in a situation where the observed spontaneous mutation rate was 4×10^{-6}/locus per generation (an estimate of what the electrophoretic approach might yield), it would require control and "exposed" samples of 18,000,000 observations each (observations, not people) to demonstrate an increase of 50% in the mutation rate in the exposed sample, with the type I (α) error set at 0.05 and the type II (β) error at 0.20 (Neel, 1971, 1986; Neel et al., 1984). A less ambitious approach, which we advocate for the immediate future, is a study that pools the results of examining the offspring of the most potentially mutagenized groups of parents to be identified anywhere, and uses the findings to set upper limits on the damage which might have been sustained. Now the numerical requirements are open-ended, depending on the certainty one wishes to achieve.

With respect to the problem of bias, the issue is especially acute when an attempt is made to employ congenital defect and physical disability as a measure of induced genetic damage in children. Both end points are highly complex from the genetic standpoint. If a prospective study can be established, as has been the case in the followup studies in Japan on atomic bomb effects (Neel and Schull, 1956), then the outcome of each pregnancy to a predetermined cohort of women can be determined by specially trained observers, and the products of these pregnancies define a second cohort which can be followed in time and space. Usually, however, the study will be in whole or part retrospective. Such a study is highly dependent upon the recall of the parties involved, and the comparison or control sample will seldom have the same motivations as a sample that believes itself to be at an increased risk. To some extent this bias can be obviated by recourse to hospital records and birth and death registrations, but the shortcomings of routine hospital records are well documented, and death as an indicator of genetic damage is a rather coarse sieve. What is needed in any retrospective (and prospective) study that meets current scientific standards is a battery of indicators that, while essentially nonprejudicial to survival, can readily be related to more serious effects.

An additional consideration in the design of any such studies is the desirability of indicator traits that can also be employed in animal models, and *vice versa*. One of the difficulties in the extrapolation from mice to humans has been how to reach inferences applicable to the human situation from the morphological impact of mutation at a relatively few selected loci in specially developed strains, or from the frequency of radiation-induced, inherited cataracts or skeletal malformation in strains specially selected as suitable for such studies. Fortunately, the explosion in the techniques of biochemical genetics of the past 30 years has now created the clear possibility of using as indicator traits specific changes in proteins for which homologues exist in man and mouse. In principle, as the DNA technologies continue to advance, similar considerations apply to the use of homologous DNA probes in the two species.

With all these considerations in mind, some 5 years ago we were attracted to the the the potential of the new two-dimensional polyacrylamide gel electrophoresis (two-dimensional) for the study of mutation. In this presentation we will review the progress made to date in bringing a system based on two-dimensional gels on line. Because of the need for very large numbers of observations mentioned earlier, and the enormous labor and potential error involved in scoring these gels by eye, from the outset a major effort has been directed toward the adaptation and/or development of computer algorithms which would facilitate the reading of these gels. We have recently described the total approach under development in some detail (Neel *et al.*, 1984). In this review we will devote little space to gel technology, but instead extend substantially the account of the algorithm under development and its validation, comparing our approach with the approaches of others attempting to automate the reading of such gels. We consider this a progress report only, on a very complex undertaking.

THE THEORY AND PRACTICE OF TWO-DIMENSIONAL GELS, WITH PARTICULAR REFERENCE TO THE STUDY OF MUTATION

In two-dimensional gels, the proteins of a cell type, tissue, or body fluid are solubilized in such a way as to dissociate multimeric proteins into their constituent polypeptides, and these are then separated in two dimensions, the first on the basis of charge by isoelectric focusing, the second on the basis of molecular weight by electrophoresis in the presence of sodium dodecyl sulfate. The basic technique, as developed by O'Farrell (1975), Klose (1975), and Scheele (1975), seems to undergo slight modifications in each laboratory that uses it; the specifics of our procedure are given in Neel et al. (1984). At the outset, the positions of the polypeptides on the gels were visualized either by autoradiography or staining with Coomassie brilliant blue. The highly sensitive silver-staining techniques developed several years ago by Merril et al. (1981), Sammons et al. (1981), and Wray et al. (1981) have now replaced in our laboratory the other two methods of visualizing the polypeptides, except for certain special purposes. Recently the Eastman Kodak Co. (1983) has announced a system of nickel staining for two-dimensional gels, the utility of which in our setting has not yet been validated. Comprehensive reviews of the current state of the two-dimensional art will be found in Special Issue (1982), Dunn and Burghes (1983), and Celis and Bravo (1984).

Two-dimensional gels are fragile. A problem common to most laboratories is localized stretching or actual physical breaks in the first-dimension "noodle" as it is being handled, and tears in the second-dimension slab gels. Even after "repair" this may result in distortions in the image which a human observer compensates for more readily than a computer algorithm, as will be discussed later. Furthermore, the pH gradient in the first dimension may vary slightly (and locally) from gel to gel. In principle, one should only use "perfect" gels, since, as we shall see, even these are not in complete register from individual to individual, but, for now, as we explore the robustness of the algorithms we are developing, we have tolerated occasional small imperfections of this type.

The most readily available and most informative material for studies of human mutation rates employing two-dimensional gels will be blood. As should be apparent from the Introduction, we feel a major challenge is to develop the ability to extract the maximum amount of reliable genetic information from every individual who enters into a study. To this end, our program, fully implemented, requires visualizing, on separate gels, the polypeptides of plasma, erythrocytes, platelets, lymphocytes, and polymorphonuclear leukocytes. The number of apparently different polypeptides *clearly* visualized on each of these gels varies from approximately 100 in a serum preparation to 500 in a lymphocyte preparation. (This is not necessarily the number of polypeptides to be scored; see section on Introduction of *a Priori* Knowledge.) The degree of overlap in the polypeptides visualized in the various preparations is unknown, but presumably considerable. (Henceforth the term "polypeptide" will be interchangeable with the term "spot.")

At the outset, a considerable effort has been directed toward exploring the extent and appearance of the genetic variation revealed on these gels. Illustrations of some of the forms in which genetic variants manifest themselves in our hands are to be found in Rosenblum *et al.* (1983, 1984). The index of heterozygosity for the polypeptides studied thus far in our laboratory [from preparations of erythrocyte lysate (without membrane), plasma, and platelets] is thus far 3.8 ± 0.3% (Rosenblum *et al.*, 1983, 1984; Hanash *et al.*, 1986). Others, working with other types of preparations, have on average detected less than half this amount of variation (McConkey *et al.*, 1979; Walton *et al.*, 1979; Smith *et al.*, 1981; Hamaguchi *et al.*, 1981, 1982a,b; Comings, 1982; Goldman and Merril, 1983). The reasons for the differences between studies are complex and not the primary concern of this presentation. The reasons for the lesser amount of variation recognized in these gels than in the more established one-dimensional electrophoretic studies of serum proteins and erythrocyte isozymes, for which the index of heterozygosity is at least 6%, are also complex and will not be pursued here. Suffice it to say at this point that on the basis of our experience with examining known genetic variants on two-dimensional gels (Wanner *et al.*, 1982; see also Anderson and Anderson, 1977), we suggest that at least 80% of the electrophoretic variants detected with 1DE systems especially developed for specific proteins are also detectable with two-dimensional gels. In addition, about 20% of the variants we have encountered thus far are in the molecular weight axis; it is not clear whether these would be detected with 1DE.

In several large-scale studies of mutation involving the application of 1DE technologies to humans (Neel *et al.*, 1980a,b, 1983), employing as many as 40 indicator proteins, familiarity with the types of variants to be expected is now at a level permitting the investigators to screen for rare (nonpolymorphic) variants, such as might be maintained by mutation pressure, with family material being collected only after the variant has been identified. These variants have a frequency of 1–2 per 1000 determinations. We suggest that, by contrast, in a program involving two-dimensional gels, for the time being it will be desirable for two reasons to collect the material in units of nuclear families. First, the nature of the genetic variation in these gels is still being defined; very often it will be helpful to have family material immediately available. Second, if "rare" variants are detected with the same frequency in the proteins visualized with two-dimensional gels as with 1DE (~1–2 per 1000), and if one is scoring *in toto* some 500 polypeptides per individual, then the probability that the investigator will *not* encounter a finding demanding an examination of the parents is approximately 0.998^{500}, or 0.37. Given this frequent a need for family studies, it seems more efficient to collect samples from the parents at the same time samples are collected from the propositi.

In this setting, a mutation will be defined as a "new" polypeptide in a child; i.e., a polypeptide not visualized in either parent. Any such finding must of course be confirmed with a repeat determination entailing an independent sample, to exclude all of the possible artifactual reasons for such a finding. However, even after confirmation such a polypeptide does of course permit alternative explanations. The first is a discrepancy between the stated and the true parentage; such discrepancy can now be detected with high accuracy [see discussion in Rothman *et al.* (1981)], and the gels themselves will contribute to this end. A second explanation, if one is working with newborn infants, as in a portion of our program, is the occurrence of fetal proteins; these can be identified with experience. A third possible explanation would be disease-related proteins, as may occur in some of the childhood leukemias (Hanash *et al.*, 1982). All these possibilities should be dealt with in the course of the kinds of detailed studies an apparent mutant would command.

We note in passing that few geneticists would be comfortable terminating their study of a putative mutation simply by excluding other alternative explanations for a new "blip" on a gel. One internal piece of evidence relevant to the occurrence of a mutation is the following: we may presume that in most instances of mutation, both parents will be homozygous for the normal allele, so that, in the absence of independently inherited regulatory mechanisms, the density on the gel (i.e., amount) of the polypeptide associated with this allele should be approximately half normal in the mutant individual. Conversely, the observation, in conjunction with an apparent mutation, of a nearby polypeptide half the staining intensity of the corresponding polypeptide in the parents should be a strong clue as to origin. In addition, current microbiochemical techniques permit the characterization of at least the more abundant of the proteins visualized on a two-dimensional gel, to the point where similarities can be sought between the "new" protein and the normal gene product of which it is presumed to be a variant. The ultimate test will be genetic, the transmission of this new trait. For the immediate future, this demonstration will have to be based on experimental material, such as the mouse; we would assign such a demonstration high priority.

With this background, we can now address the potential role of computer algorithms in the analysis of two-dimensional gels. To be sure, such gels can be scored by eye. However, given the large number of observations required in a study of mutation rates, indicated above, not only is scoring all these preparations an extremely onerous task, of a type conducive to a high turnover in laboratory personnel, but the fatigue and monotony factors could be a serious impediment to accurate results. This is a task for which computers are ideally designed if a suitable algorithm can be developed; the less operator intervention required in the execution of the algorithm, the better.

As we began to consider such an algorithm, it was obvious that genetic principles immediately provide certain guidelines for the algorithm. In the absence of the relatively uncommon and easily identified perturbations in the system discussed earlier, any polypeptide observed in a child must have a counterpart in one or the other (and most likely both) parents. On the other hand, a parent may well exhibit polypeptides not present in the child. In other words, the algorithm must be written to encompass genetic variation. However, to be effective in the search for mutation, it is not required that the algorithm be written to associate the various alleles of the genetic systems contributing to this variation.

There are also two "practical" constraints that become preconditions for the development of an algorithm. The first is the need to "threshold" the analysis of the gel at some "reasonable" level. The spots one sees on a stained gel range in amount from those barely visible after staining to those, such as albumin, that are smears that seriously interfere with the scoring of nearby spots. No spot visualized on a gel is suitable for scoring if it would not be clearly visible if halved in quantity. This necessitates first setting an appropriate threshold for a gel, then conducting the analysis at approximately half the intensity of the threshold value. The second constraint is that *ideally* each of the spots being scored with reference to mutation should be surrounded by a sufficient open area, relatively uncluttered by the occurrence of other spots, that there is a high probability of identifying a mutant derivative of that spot. Experience has shown that a one-charge change alters mobility by 3–6 mm in the IEF axis, the precise amount depending on the molecular weight (Wanner *et al.*, 1982; Asakawa *et al.*, 1985). The variants in the vertical axis thus far recognized exhibit smaller shifts in mobility. Thus the "ideal" polypeptide for such a study as this would be surrounded by a clear area 1 cm in diameter. This ideal is seldom fully realized. For instance, among the spots scored for genetic variants in two-dimensional gels of erythrocyte lysates, on the average, in a subset, 7% of the area in that circle was obscured by the presence of other polypeptides; the relative area within which a "new" spot would overlap with a preexisting spot to the degree that it was unrecognizable as such would be even greater (Rosenblum *et al.*, 1984). We will consider later strategies to meet these constraints.

It would be extremely desirable in any study of mutation to be able to detect mutations in consequence of which no protein product was formed. For the moment, our program is directed toward the detection of "qualitative" variants and mutations; we return to the detection of "quantitative" variation later.

THE GENERAL PROBLEM OF IMAGE COMPARISON

Designing an algorithm for the automated comparison of the types of images under consideration presents many challenges. Efficiency demands that somehow the enormous amount of information on a gel be reduced to certain essentials. There are no simple guidelines specifying exactly how much information is required to perform accurate comparisons on two or more gels. This problem is compounded further because of variability in the information being compared. All variations in the sensed environment must be classified either as real or not real (the latter is generally termed "noise"). Unfortunately, we often have a very limited understanding of the criteria by which noise can be distinguished from reality. Put another way, there is always some uncertainty in the criteria by which we (or a computer program or algorithm) judge some variations to be "real" rather than "noise." To the extent that the variability in an image is well understood or limited in scope, the problems in designing an image comparison algorithm are minimized. Further, to the extent that errors in distinguishing noise from reality are tolerable, the need for a sophisticated algorithm is lessened.

In the current state of the art, the variability of two-dimensional gels is neither well understood nor limited. Further, due to the rarity of the mutational events being sought, there is little tolerance for errors in distinguishing noise from reality. Thus, the proposed two-dimensional gel image comparison algorithm is designed to exhibit a high level of sophistication and "intelligence." For less demanding applications, simpler comparison algorithms would suffice.

Thresholding Spot Intensity

An image of a two-dimensional gel is initially produced by a digital image-sensing device (e.g., a video camera with A/D converter) and consists of a two-dimensional array of picture elements, or "pixels." The image digitized may be the gel itself or a derivative such as an autoradiogram or a photographic negative. Each pixel takes on a "gray-scale" value corresponding to the amount of light sensed at that location. A fundamental issue in digitization is that of resolution; i.e., the number of pixels comprising the length and width of the digitized image. If one samples with low resolution, then one has less information to process (increasing speed of execution), at the cost of certainty in the measurement procedures (a protein spot evaluated on a grid of 20×20 pixels can be measured more accurately than the same one measured at a resolution of 5 pixels). High resolution increases certainty at the cost of ever more information to process. In general, we lack information as to the optimal level of resolution. This is only the first of many sources of uncertainty. In addition, in terms of performing image comparisons, a major problem in representing image information as a sensed array of pixels is the large amount of space and time needed when processing pixels. If an image consists of n rows and n columns (where n is typically 1024), then n^2 pixels must be manipulated each time the image is processed. Thus, it is desirable to reduce the pixel-based information into a more economical form.

Pixel-based information is reduced by analyzing the image information into a set of "features." Measurements, specific to each type of feature, are made of an image and the results stored in the locations specific to each type of feature. Features of interest in two-dimensional gels may involve local maxima, measures of spot shape (involving such properties as concavity, convexity, and connectedness), and measures of spot "size" or "amount" (ranging from first approximations, such as the maximum intensity of a spot, to more precise estimates, such as the "normalized" volume of a spot). Each pixel on an image is measured to see if it is where a given feature is located. For a given feature, most locations on the image should return a value of zero; at a much smaller number of locations the feature measurement is nonzero. The image information can now be stored as a list of locations, which is more economical, since the number of nonzero locations is much less than n^2.

While feature measurements reduce the amount of information to be processed, problems exist related to the unreliability of low nonzero feature measurements. There are two reasons for this lack of reliability. First, an insignificant variation in an image's pixel pattern can match some true aspect of a feature, causing the feature measurement to be nonzero. Second, since different features can be similar in certain aspects, a feature which is similar to another feature can produce a (false) nonzero measurement. Either of these situations can result in the spurious detection of a feature. Generally, a threshold is applied to all feature measurements, in the hope that the unreliable nonzero values will fall below threshold. At the same time, sometimes a feature on one image, which should correspond to an above-threshold feature on another image, will produce a below-threshold measurement. This can happen when variations in the image pixel pattern (generally attributed to noise) degrade the fidelity with which the image pixel pattern reflects the feature being measured.

All these considerations point to a basic dilemma in setting a threshold for feature measurements in the analysis of a gel. If one sets the threshold at low values, then, among all the locations corresponding to a given feature, there will be locations corresponding to the detection of spurious features. If one sets the threshold at higher values, then above-threshold locations will more likely be corresponding locations of a feature, but correct locations of features degraded by noise will fall below threshold. There is generally no optimum threshold value that can guarantee that above-threshold locations will correspond to the valid features of the image and below-threshold locations will correspond to nonfeatures. No matter what threshold is chosen, there will usually be below-threshold locations that should have been detected and above-threshold features that should not have been detected.

This problem—of the variability of feature measurement with reference to a threshold—is a fundamental source of differences between images in the image comparison problem. It is not unusual to have corresponding features on two images result in feature measurements which on one image fall below threshold and on the other image fall above threshold. In other words, variations about a threshold result in apparent differences between processed images. In order to distinguish real versus threshold-related image differences, it is useful to have access to information on the feature measurements, as opposed to accessing only the above-threshold features. In order to discriminate real from noise-related variations about a feature measurement threshold, it is sometimes necessary to return to the original image pixel information or even to redigitize problematic regions at higher resolutions. The comparison algorithm to be described has mechanisms for distinguishing this fundamental source of discrepancies between images.

Adjusting for Positional Variations

In addition to gel-to-gel variability in the intensity of a given spot, a second fundamental source of image variability arises from the fact that even if, in a pair of gels, corresponding features fall above threshold (and are both "detected"), there may be variations in their precise locations. If their locations are not absolutely congruent, by what criterion will they be judged to correspond? We must again introduce some notion of noise. That is, some of the variation in spot position can be thought of as resulting from positional noise. Intuitively, positional noise should involve insignificant (or "small") variations in the positions of corresponding features. It is important, though, to reject one part of our common intuition of noise, namely that noise is insignificant in the sense of being easily ignored. This is true for human vision, since we are not conscious of the very complex ways in which we ignore noise, but it will become clear that compensating for noiselike variations is at the heart of the difficulties in automating image comparison. We must keep in mind that noise itself can be a complex phenomenon.

To define the role of positional noise in the comparison problem, consider what would be meant by having no positional noise. If there were no positional noise between the images being compared, then the locations of corresponding features would be identical. The images would be said to be in "registration." Positional noise can then be defined by the ways in which images can be out of registration; i.e., by the various factors which alter the locations of corresponding features so that they are no longer identical.

One of the simpler forms of positional noise arises when an image is out of registration with a counterpart due to a uniform translation affecting all the feature locations; i.e., due to the addition of a constant vector to all coordinates. Other simple noise models involve the multiplication of all coordinates by a scalar or the rotation of an image by some given angle. A distortion involving translation, rotation, and scaling can be modeled as a linear (trigonometric or affine) transformation. If, in addition to a linear model, it is assumed that there are no spurious or missing features in the images being compared, then linear programming algorithms exist (Baird and Steiglitz, 1982) capable of finding the parameters of the transformation that will put two images back into registration. In the general image comparison problem and, more particularly, in the problem of two-dimensional gel comparison, it is reasonable to assume the occurrence of spurious and/or missing spots. Algorithms for the calculation of a global translation, which are not adversely affected by spurious or missing features, have been developed (Kahl et al., 1980; Ranade and Rosenfeld, 1980). It is important to note that the output of the algorithm is a parametrized linear transformation which can be applied to one image (or more precisely, the list of derived feature coordinates) in order to bring it into registration with the other image being compared.

It is the general experience that two-dimensional gels do not yet exhibit the degree of uniformity necessary for a globally applied linear transformation to be useful in bringing gel images into correspondence. At the same time, within local regions of two-dimensional gel images the linearity assumption may be profitably applied. The problem then becomes one of identifying the regions of the images that can reasonably be put into correspondence with a linear transformation. The regions to be put into correspondence may be defined by human operators who indicate the locations of preselected pairs of corresponding "landmark" spots (Taylor et al., 1981; Miller et al., 1982). In this approach the landmark spots are selected to be approximately evenly spaced and serve to define both the regions in which the linear transformation will be applied and the parameters by which the local transformations will be estimated. Let us assume that the operator selects three pairs of corresponding spots which serve to define a triangular region on the two gels being compared. A linear transformation can be estimated by decomposing the differences in location between corresponding pairs of spots into the three components of translation, rotation, and scale. The locations of spots falling within the triangular regions are then subjected to the estimated transformation, resulting in pairs of spots in "near" registration—"near," since the linearity assumption is often a first approximation to the actual situation. A least squares fitting procedure is then used to determine the locations of corresponding spots within this triangular region.

The goal of the algorithms described above is to find a linear transformation that will put the two images into registration so as to minimize distortion. Since spurious or missing features can occur, an input parameter d is provided, which defines the maximum positional distortion allowable after the application of the transformation. This parameter d, which we will call a "noise radius," permits points to be considered in registration when, in actuality, they are out of registration by at most a distance d. Conversely, the least squares estimate of best acceptable matches rejects neighboring matches separated by a distance of d.

While some function to treat the noise radius is desirable, there is always uncertainty in its application. The algorithm must be designed so that the uncertainties introduced by such a positional noise function—by us termed Ω—are detected. In a certain sense, the positional noise function introduces problems analogous to those of the feature measurement threshold. It serves as an imperfect filter by which positional differences are judged to be real or not. As such, the positional noise function ensures that the results of the comparison algorithm are correct most of the time, but provision must be made to detect those cases in which the positional noise function has failed.

While it is useful to consider the issue of noise in terms of bringing the images into registration, it is not necessary to conceptualize all comparison algorithms as incorporating a parametrized function for putting the images (or subregions) into maximum registration. In general, as the positional noise model becomes more complex, the approach becomes one of explicitly finding the locations of corresponding features, without concern for finding a linear transformation that maps the corresponding features into registration (Barnard and Thompson, 1980; Barrow et al., 1977; Burr, 1981). In matching the spots of two-dimensional gels, some investigators (Lemkin and Lipkin, 1981b; Lemkin et al., 1982; Garrels, et al., 1984) have developed interactive algorithms which explicitly match pairs of spots based upon operator-defined matches of "landmark" spots. No attempt is made to find a linear transformation which explicitly brings spots (falling within the regions defined by the landmark spots) into correspondence. Lemkin and Lipkin (1981*b*) classify neighbors (of the operator-defined landmark matches) into matches having various degrees of certainty, based upon such criteria as the distance from the landmark matches and the amount of distortion encountered. Garrels *et al.* (1984) use a similar procedure of iteratively working out from the operator-provided landmark matches to their neighbors, on to the neighbor's neighbors, and so on. Common to both approaches is the initial determination of more certain matches, followed by resolution of less certain matches later (based upon the more certain match information). This is necessary due to the basic uncertainties underlying the processes producing positional distortions. This uncertainty is expressed, in all the above approaches, in a positional noise function. While, for the most part, these positional noise functions are adequate, there are situations where they can result in mismatches. The classification of matches according to their certainty is an attempt to develop mechanisms to detect mismatches; i.e., to maintain "match accuracy." The algorithms are designed to use contextual information to maintain accuracy in their match assignments, where contextual information is needed to resolve less certain matches. The problem of how to use context in maintaining accuracy is a fundamental problem, which will be the focus of much of the discussion in this chapter. We will argue for the need for (and sketch out) mechanisms for the maintenance of accuracy that represent more systematic approaches to these issues.

In the context of using two-dimensional gels for the estimation of the rate of human mutation, it is desirable to minimize the use of operator interaction (since requiring an operator to identify landmark matches over thousands of gel "families" would slow the procedure significantly). Accordingly, unlike the approaches just discussed, we have sought to develop a comparison algorithm that requires no operator intervention. (Most recently, Miller *et al.* (1984) has modified his algorithm to be free of operator intervention.) Instead, matching point pairs on images are identified by the similarity of their neighborhood patterns, much as one uses constellations to orient oneself around the night sky. As in the approaches of Garrels *et al.* (1984) and Lemkin and Lipkin (1981*b*), there is no attempt to produce a linear transformation to put the images or subregions into correspondence. At the same time, because of the accuracy requirements of the genetic application, the proposed algorithm employs mechanisms for using contextual information to maintain accuracy in a manner that sets it apart from the other approaches (Garrels *et al.*, 1984; Lemkin and Lipkin, 1981*b*; Miller *et al.*, 1984).

A SET OF ALGORITHMS FOR DETECTING POTENTIAL MUTATIONAL EVENTS

While the set of algorithms under development have very general applications, in this treatment we will describe only one use in detail: the comparison of "trios" of two-dimensional gel images for the purpose of estimating the rate of mutation. A "trio" (or in some contexts, what we shall call a "family") of two-dimensional gels will consist of gels derived from corresponding samples from a father, mother, and child. The output of these algorithms consists of a description of the extent of the qualitative correspondence of the spots on the three gel images. Of especial interest (for the purposes of estimating the rate of mutation) is the situation where a spot on a child's gel is determined not to match any spot on either the father's or mother's gel. The algorithms we have developed for this task can be described under the following five headings.

Estimating the Locations of Protein Spots

The input to the algorithms being developed is provided by feature measurement algorithms which list the x and y coordinates of each spot for each two-dimensional gel image. (Associated with each spot is a quantitative measure; currently, this consists of the pixel intensity at the associated spot coordinates.) Note that the x and y coordinates of corresponding spots on different gels may be different. There are two factors responsible for this: first, the lack of a completely reliable origin from which to initiate the measurements; and, second, positional distortions that put images out of registration (independently of whether a reliable origin point existed). Thus, the x and y coordinates of spots on one gel image are not related in any simple fashion to corresponding coordinates on other gel images. One can view the task of the comparison algorithm as that of "discovering" the relation between spot locations on different gels.

The algorithms we have used to perform feature measurements represent a different approach from those being used by others analyzing two-dimensional gels (Anderson *et al.*, 1981; Bossinger *et al.*, 1979; Garrels *et al.*, 1984; Lemkin and Lipkin, 1981*a*; Taylor *et al.*, 1980). These differences reside in the mathematical framework within which they are specified and in their dependence upon specialized image-processing hardware for efficient execution. The mathematical framework, known as mathematical morphology, is based upon a restricted class of cellular automata transformations as defined by Serra (1982, 1986) and Sternberg (1986). [Burks (1970) defined the mathematical framework of general cellular automata.] As applied to image processing, a cellular automata consists of an array of processing elements, each element corresponding to a digitized pixel on an image. Each processing element is set to a given state (initially corresponding to the gray-scale value of the amount of sensed light) and is programmed to change its state based upon the states of its immediately surrounding neighbors (eight neighbors in the rectangular array and six in the hexagonal array) and its own state. At each time step, all the states of the processing elements are altered in parallel so as to produce the next set of states over the array. Given the large number of processing elements (n^2, where n may equal 1024) it is necessary (for the sake of efficiency) to implement such algorithms in specialized hardware capable of performing the transitions from one state to the next in parallel. Our algorithms have been developed to run on such a computer (Sternberg, 1981, 1982); a more detailed description of these morphological algorithms than is appropriate here will be found in Skolnick *et al.*, 1986; Skolnick, 1986).

Common to both the morphological algorithms and the algorithms of other researchers is the existence of uncertainty in the reliability of the feature measurements. Basically, uncertainties arise both out of the trade-off between efficiency and accuracy and out of lack of knowledge of the criteria by which polypeptide moieties are distinguishable from artifacts. In addition, because of the unavailability in the past of fast feature-measurement algorithms (which depend upon specialized image-processing hardware), there has been a tendency to relegate feature measurements to a preprocessing step to image comparison. The pressure has been to design feature-measurement algorithms that process the images only once (at the beginning) and which thus must attempt to minimize the uncertainties in the feature-measurement process in the initial pass. Unfortunately, it is difficult to minimize these uncertainties. We suggest that these uncertainties are inherent to the feature-measurement process and that they can best be dealt with through an integration into the image comparison process.

Within the area of computer vision, feature-measurement algorithms are generally thought of as "low-level" procedures (Davis and Rosenfeld, 1981), which are then followed by "high-level" procedures that integrate the low-level information. Image comparison is generally thought of as a high-level problem. We will argue that the high-level process of image comparison can interact with, and help resolve, the inherent uncertainties in feature measurement. One of the primary objectives in the following consideration of the sequence of steps in the morphological algorithms for determining the location and size of protein spots is to transmit some sense of how uncertainties enter into the feature-measurement procedures. While we will not consider the feature-measurement algorithms of other investigators, they are also prone to the same sources of uncertainty.

The first step in the feature-measurement process involves the application of filters to the digitized image. The filters are designed to remove artifacts from the images (the "noise") in order to facilitate the detection and measurement of the protein spots (the "signal"). Recall that, as mentioned above, it is not easy to determine the precise boundaries between signal and noise. For example, consider the factors that determine the intensity of a pixel that is part of some spot: there is the general level of illumination at the time of digitization, the amount of staining occurring in a given region of a gel, the amount of stain associated with other spots (e.g., due to streaking), and the actual stain associated with a given spot. The intensity of the pixel is a single integer value. The problem of separating signal from noise involves the decomposition of this value into the appropriate components. Further, it is clear that one must consider neighboring pixel values to obtain enough context to perform the decomposition.

One filtering operation involves the removal of the background intensities of the image pixels, a process known as "background normalization." Generally, this information is considered to be "low-frequency" information, since the background illumination in an image tends to vary much more gradually than the changes in illumination associated with a spot. Uncertainty enters into background normalization in terms of the inability to specify criteria by which (or "the" frequency at which) background information can always be distinguished from the information of interest. Just as in the issue of resolution, we lack *a priori* information concerning the criteria guaranteed to distinguish spots from their background. Another filtering operation involves the removal of "high-frequency" noise from the sensed image. (The high-frequency variations in an image involve relatively abrupt or "random" changes in illumination relative to those associated with either spot or background intensities.) Again, the same issue arises: while we may know some useful criteria by which to distinguish signal from noise, there are always situations in which the distinction fails to work.

It is tempting at this point to suppose that, with the removal of the high- and low-frequency components in the pixel intensities, the resulting intensity values correspond to those of the actual spots. Unfortunately, there remain other forms of nonspot (or nonsignal) information. One example is that caused by streaking or tailing associated with the spots. Either *in vivo* or in the physical process of gel preparation, protein complexes of many types may be formed. These products may appear as streaks or trails on the gel images. The streaks must then be treated as noise in the sense that they (incorrectly) increase the intensity values of spots that happen to have coincided in position with the streaks. At the same time, there are reasons for treating streaks as useful information, as opposed to noise to be removed. For example, for accurate quantification the streak absorbance should be integrated into the absorbance of the protein from which it is derived. There is a potential conflict between the necessary removal of the streak information as noise and retaining the streak information for later use. The feature-measurement algorithms are meant to reduce the information to be dealt with. At the same time, information "thrown away" as noise can, in other contexts, be useful, a point to which we return later. Thus, these issues in streak removal support the general claim being made concerning the desirability of integrating the feature-measurement process into the comparison process (as opposed to relegating the feature measurement process to a preprocessing step). If the comparison algorithm is capable of efficiently reexamining the original image information in a more focused fashion (i.e., without having to reexamine the entire image), then it becomes possible to treat the same image information (e.g., streaks) as either noise or non-noise, depending upon the context.

After the filtering operations, the current morphological algorithm determines the locations of all local maxima in the filtered images. The locations of the local maxima determine the locations of the detected protein spots. At this point, two quite different types of errors may occur. On the one hand, two spots in close proximity may be discrete on one gel but confluent on another gel. In the latter case, the smaller spot will be perceived as a shoulder to the larger. The fact that there are confluent spots may not be detected in the current operation to detect local maxima either because there really is no second maximum within the confluence or because the process of removing high-frequency noise has eliminated an actual local maximum corresponding to the spot location. On the other hand, in the process of validating the operation of the algorithm (to be described later), we have become aware that very occasionally the result of filtering out a very intense streak through a spot is the creation of two local maxima on either side of the streak. Both types of errors are the result of inadequacies in our current feature-measurement algorithms. The first type results from differences between gels that are too subtle to detect using the current algorithm, whereas the second type is an artifact of the current algorithm itself. Other types of errors also can be introduced through the feature-measurement algorithms.

While feature-measurement errors result from inherent uncertainties in the criteria by which spots are distinguished from each other, information is available by which the number of these errors could be reduced. In the case of a "shoulder spot," even though the information on the local maxima may not be adequate for detection, there is shape information that can be used. That is, under some circumstances an isolated spot can be distinguished from a spot confluent with a second spot by such shape information as would be provided by taking an appropriate topographic slice (horizontally) through the image. A topographic slice of an isolated spot would be consistently convex, while that of a spot and a neighboring "shoulder" spot would often be concave in some regions, the concavity occurring at the intersection of two circular or elliptical slices.

The intent of these considerations is to indicate that additional feature measurements (beyond local maxima) would be useful in increasing our confidence in the ability of the feature-measurement algorithm to detect spots correctly. At the same time, the tradeoffs which operate within the issues of resolution and filtering are also important in this context. Thus, with each increase in complexity in the feature-measurement algorithms, we increase our confidence in these algorithms. However, at the same time, complete confidence in the algorithms is at best highly costly in terms of computation and, more likely, is unattainable. As we shall see, the comparison algorithm can provide information (relevant to the detection of errors arising in the feature-measurement procedures) that can be used in a selective manner to guide the algorithm to locations on images where it would be useful to look at more complex sets of feature measurements. The comparison algorithm can be used to determine the situations where more complex feature analysis is justified. The effects of feature-measurement errors on the accuracy of the comparison algorithm will be considered later.

Once the locations of spots are determined, an estimate of spot intensity must be made. This is a difficult problem, involving such issues as the appropriate model for spot intensity distributions (can a spot always be modeled as a Gaussian process?) and spot extents (when does one spot end and another begin?). Given our initial concern with qualitative differences between two-dimensional gels, until now we have chosen to avoid these issues. Currently, the quantitative measure provided to the comparison algorithm consists of the (background-normalized) intensity of the single location corresponding to the maximum density of each spot. This is a first, and imperfect, approximation to spot quantity. More sophisticated models of spot quantitation could be incorporated into the system. Other investigators (Bossinger, et al., 1979; Lutin et al., 1979; Taylor et al., 1980; Lemkin and Limkin, 1981a; Garrels et al., 1984) have considered the spot quantitation problem in greater detail.

We now consider the information currently being provided as input to the comparison algorithm. Figure 1 is a photograph of a two-dimensional gel prepared from the solubilized protein contents of a sample of human erythrocytes taken from a single individual (in this case, the father's gel in a family trio of gels). In all such gels the outlined section corresponds to the area analyzed. Figure 2 is the computer-generated image of this section. Figure 3, representing the spot locations produced by applying the feature-measurement algorithms to Fig. 2, is the input derived from the father's gel that is provided to the comparison algorithm (similar inputs are provided for the mother and child).

The father's, mother's, and child's input images (in the format illustrated in Fig. 3) are read by the comparison algorithm. Each input image is read across each line (from left to right) starting at the topmost line. In the order in which each spot is detected (defined by each nonzero pixel encountered as the input image is scanned), its location and maximum intensity are entered sequentially onto a list. Order on the list provides an identifying number for each spot. The x and y coordinates and the maximum intensity of the ith spot i_F from the list of spots from the father's gel are denoted, respectively, by $x(i_F)$, $y(i_F)$, and inten(i_F) (the prepara-

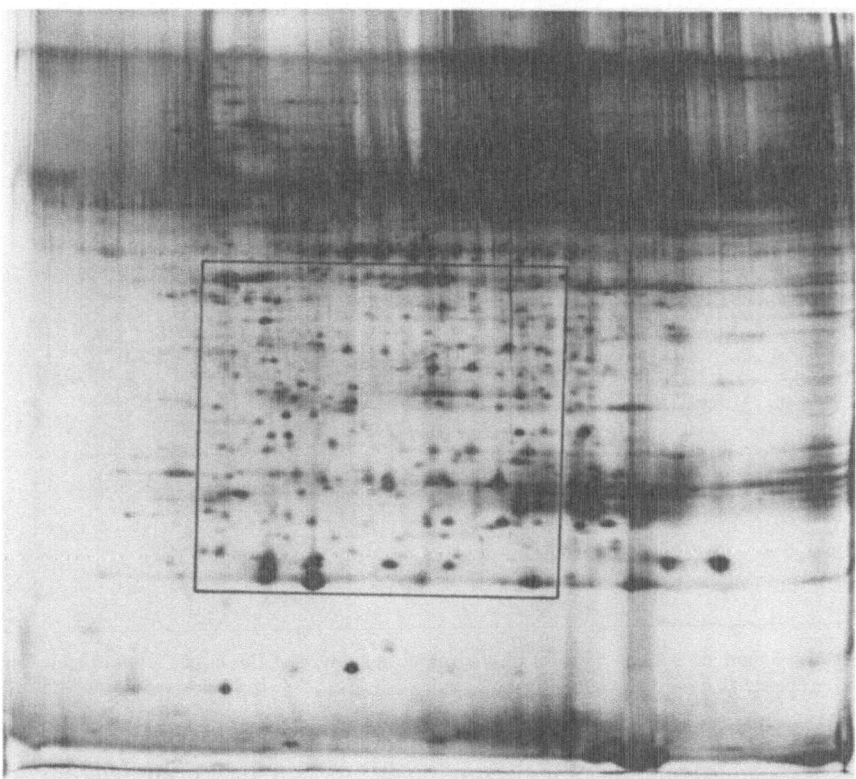

Fig. 1. Photograph of a two-dimensional gel prepared from the solubilized protein contents of a sample of human red blood cells.

tions of mother and child are denoted by the subscripts M and C, respectively). The subscript identifying the specific individual may be omitted, in which case the notation refers to any of the three family members. Note that the number i assigned to a spot is a function of the order in which it is read. Thus, corresponding spots on different gels will have different spot numbers. The task of the comparison alogrithm is to find the i_F, j_M, and k_C (where i, j, and k are generally different) that correspond to identical protein spots.

A threshold is applied to the estimated intensity of each spot. For the purpose of the gel application this threshold, SpotIntenThresh, is arrived at through an input parameter, InitNumSpots, which specifies the

Fig. 2.   Digitized section (from a photographic negative) of the father's two-dimensional gel prepared from red blood cell lysate.

(approximate) number of highest intensity spots to be considered for comparison. As the input images are scanned, a distribution is obtained based upon the number of spots of given intensities. Then, the intensity in this distribution at which the total count of spots of higher intensity is greater than or equal to InitNumSpots will be assigned to SpotIntenThresh. It is then determined, using the computed SpotIntenThresh, whether each spot is above or below threshold. Figure 4 shows the identifying numbers of all spots, both above and below threshold, superimposed on the father's gel image. Due to the limited gray-scale range that can be produced by the printer generating this image, some of the lowest level spots cannot be visualized, even though they are labeled. For example, spot numbers 74, 102, and 124 are labeled in Fig. 4 even though the corresponding gray-scale information is not apparent. It should be kept in mind, however, that is possible that such spots were spuriously detected and rightly fall below threshold. Figure 5 shows the above-threshold spots from the father. (Note that the relatively intense spot corresponding to spot number 96 on Fig. 4 did not fall above threshold. This is due to artifactual errors

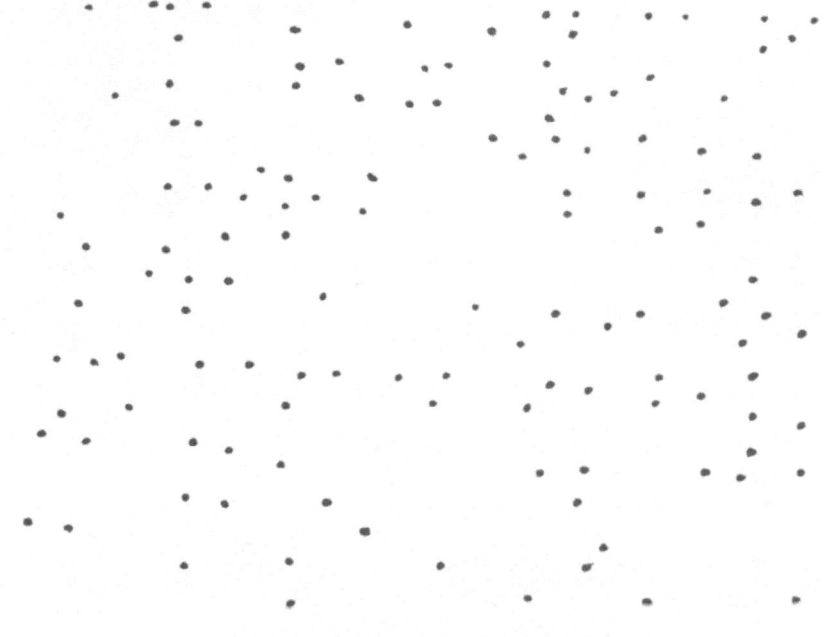

Fig. 3.   Input image from the father's gel.

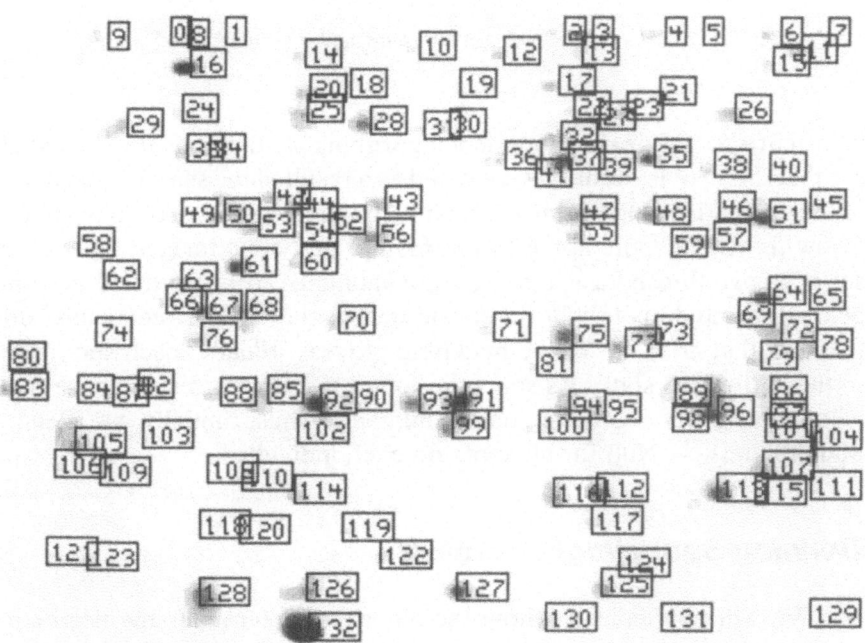

Fig. 4.   Illustration of system of assigning numbers to spots, from the father's gel.

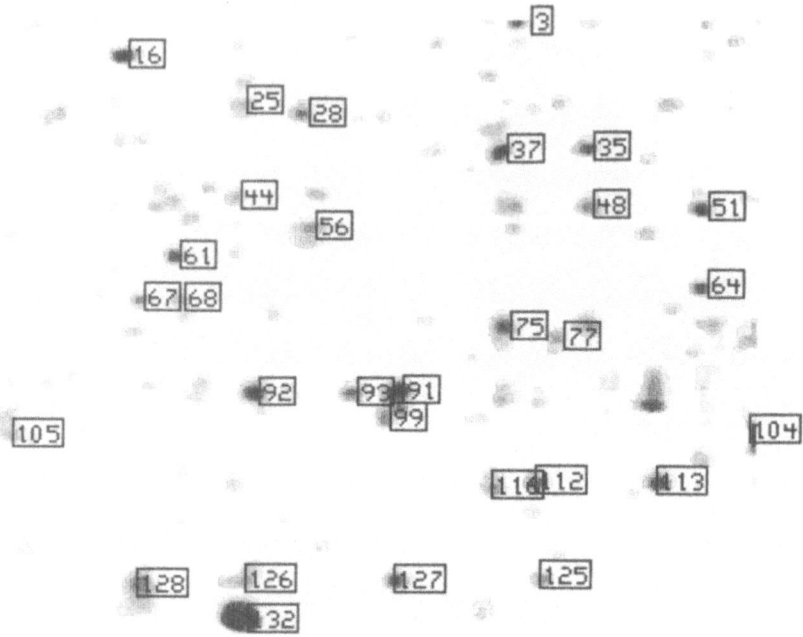

Fig. 5.   Thirty most intense spots forming nodes of initial father graph.

in the current feature-measurement algorithms. At the same time, we shall see that this spot is eventually detected as a result of the search procedures of the comparison algorithm.) Similar distinctions between the above- and below-threshold spots apply to the mother and child images. The initial set of above-threshold spots are the candidates to be matched and the below-threshold spots will be considered in the task of reconciling differences that arise out of the matching process. Finally, each spot is set to the null match state. As spots are found to be in correspondence they will be asigned a unique match number. Thus, initially we denote MatchState[i] = Null for all spots on each individual.

Defining Spot Neighborhoods

We will now consider how the algorithm determines the neighbors of each spot and how this information is used. The mathematical problems

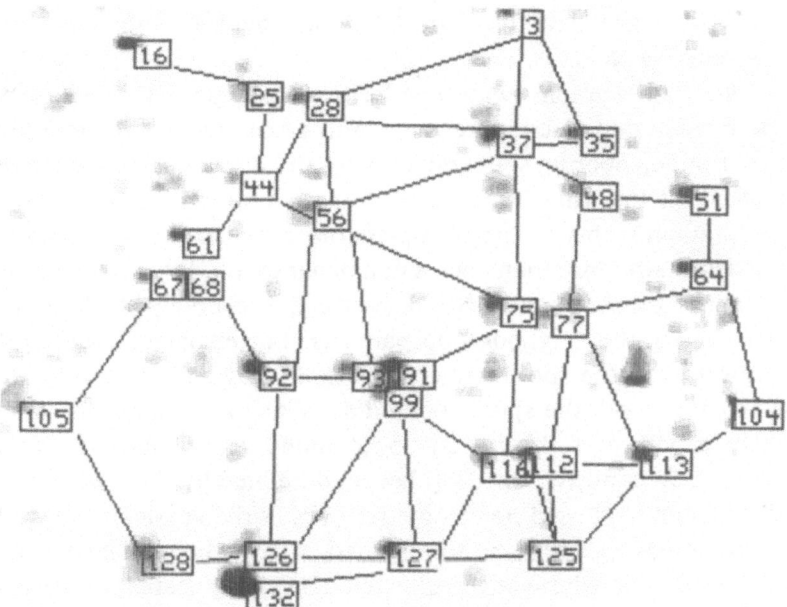

Fig. 6.   Gabriel graph of above-threshold spots superimposed on the father's gel section image.

in defining spot neighborhoods are addressed by the specialty of computational geometry, which *inter alia* concerns itself with algorithms for the construction of graphs connecting nodes on a plane [reviewed by Toussaint (1980)]. For our purposes, the graph nodes are the locations of all spots that exceed the SpotIntenThresh, as computed above. The graph edges coming out of each spot define, according to the graph construction criterion, the neighbors of each spot. After considerable experimentation, we have found a modified Gabriel-type graph (Gabriel and Sokal, 1969) to be particularly suitable in the generation of the neighbors of a point. The criterion for constructing a Gabriel graph is that two nodes are connected by an edge if and only if the circle defined by the diameter—which is also the potential edge—connecting the two nodes contains *no* other nodes of the graph. Figure 6 illustrates the superimposition of the Gabriel graph (derived from the above-threshold spots detected on the father's digitized image) on the image itself. (Note that some of the close nodes have no edges displayed between them. This is to avoid cluttering the display, and the reader can assume that edges in fact exist between close nodes. Also note that the node labels are placed to the right of their corresponding spots.)

The Gabriel graph always results in a planar graph (i.e., no two edges may cross), a rather severe restriction in a situation where increasing the number of neighboring spots might be useful in the determination of spot matches. At the same time, it is worth noting that an advantage of a Gabriel graph is that the graph's planarity provides a more visually comprehensible structure than does a nonplanar graph. Even more important, the Gabriel graph has the advantage of being relatively stable in the face of changes in the neighborhood patterns. For example, changes due to the lowering of the spot intensity threshold may add some new spots to the neighborhood; the spots counted as neighbors at the higher intensity threshold will (most likely) still be counted as neighbors at the lower threshold. In contrast, the neighborhood defined by the k nearest neighbors (a commonly used nongeometric neighborhood construct) is subject to undesirable variations in the defined neighborhood. These variations arise based upon where one begins to count (the k nearest neighbors) and whether new spots have appeared or dissappeared in the neighborhood (e.g., at a lower spot intensity threshold the additional spots in one quadrant of the neighborhood will affect the spots chosen as neighbors in the opposite quadrant). The geometric criterion of a Gabriel graph permits it to be relatively free from these types of variations.

Recall that the Gabriel graph criterion states that the number of nodes contained within the circle (defined by the potential edge *qua* diameter) must be zero. Obviously, the criterion can be generalized by letting the number of nodes contained within the circle be greater than zero. For example, a graph can be constructed that allows up to four neighbors to fall within the circle before the criterion of edge creation is violated (see Fig. 7). This generalization of the Gabriel graph generates more neighbors for each detected spot and thus provides more useful information for the comparison process. We have found that for our purposes a generalized Gabriel graph that permits up to ten neighbors to be contained within the circle defining the edge construction criterion is adequate. The comparison algorithm will be illustrated by displaying only the node labels. This is because the nonplanar edges (defining the neighborhoods of each spot) are visually uninformative and would clutter the representations to a confusing degree. In viewing the remaining figures, it should be kept in mind

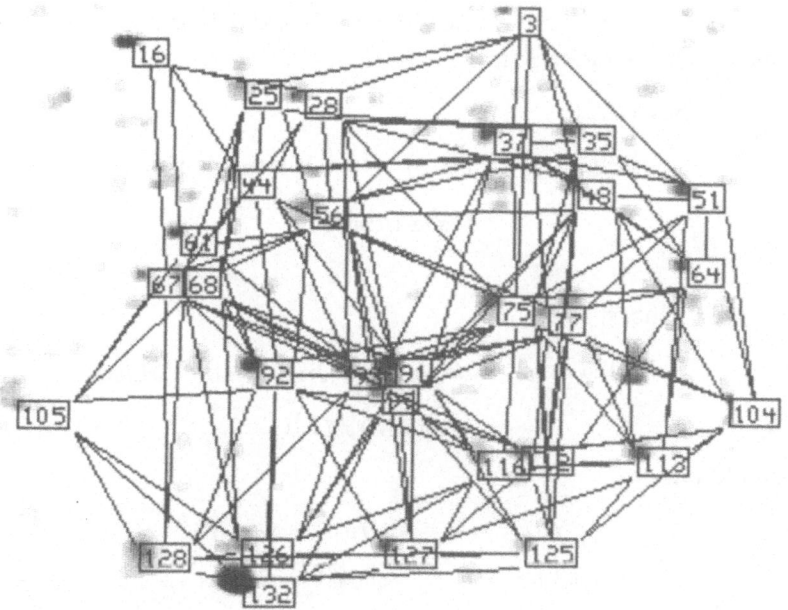

Fig. 7.   Generalized Gabriel graph of above-threshold spots superimposed on the father's gel section image.

that a neighborhood structure exists but is not illustrated. The neighbors of the ith node or spot are determined by the nodes of the graph edges coming out of the ith node and are denoted by Nhbrs[i].

Finding a Subset of Matching Spots

Spots on different gels are determined to match if the patterns of neighboring spot locations surrounding the matching spots are similar. This requires definition of a similarity function Sim, which measures the similarity of neighborhoods surrounding two spots from different images. Suppose we want to determine whether node i_F from a father's gel corresponds to node j_M from a mother's gel (i_F and j_M will be referred to as the "match candidates"). First, we define the "relative coordinates" as the coordinates of the neighbors of each match candidate, where the match candidates are considered to be origin points on orthogonal x, y

axes. Define the relative coordinates RelC as follows (note that "$\in$" stands for set membership):

let $r_F \in \text{Nhbrs}[i_F]$,

$$\text{RelC}_{i_F}[r_F] = (x(r_F) - x(i_F), y(r_F) - y(i_F))$$

$$= (x_0[r_F], y_0[r_F])$$

(1)

let $s_M \in \text{Nhbrs}[j_M]$,

$$\text{RelC}_{j_M}[s_M] = (x(s_M) - x(j_M), y(s_M) - y(j_M))$$

$$= (x_0[s_M], y_0[s_M])$$

In addition,

$$D(i_F, r_F) = (x_0[r_F]^2 + y_0[r_F]^2)^{1/2}$$
$$D(j_M, s_M) = (x_0[s_M]^2 + y_0[s_M]^2)^{1/2}$$

(2)

define, respectively, the distances of neighboring spots of the father and mother match candidates. These definitions can be represented graphically. The relative neighborhood (illustrated in Fig. 8 by a hypothetical example) is formed by considering each match candidate to be at the origin of a graph and determining the positions of the neighbors of each match candidate relative to the origin. In Fig. 8, relative neighbors of the spots of the father and mother that are match candidates are indicated respectively by an F or M placed at the appropriate locations. This relative neighborhood will be useful in understanding the definitions that follow.

A potential problem arises at this point. The absolute and relative image coordinates must be defined with respect to some specified image axes. In two-dimensional gels the borders of the image are subject to distortion and do not provide reliable axes. In practice, we provide for uniform axes across images by bringing the images being compared into correspondence visually (with respect to axes) on the graphics monitor which displays the digitized images. Both vertical and horizontal streaks and characteristic constellations of spots are used to align the digitized images along the same axes. In practice this has been found to result in an adequate correspondence of the axes of the images being compared. More generally, if such controls on the axes are not possible, it would be reasonable to consider the use of polar coordinates (as opposed to Carte-

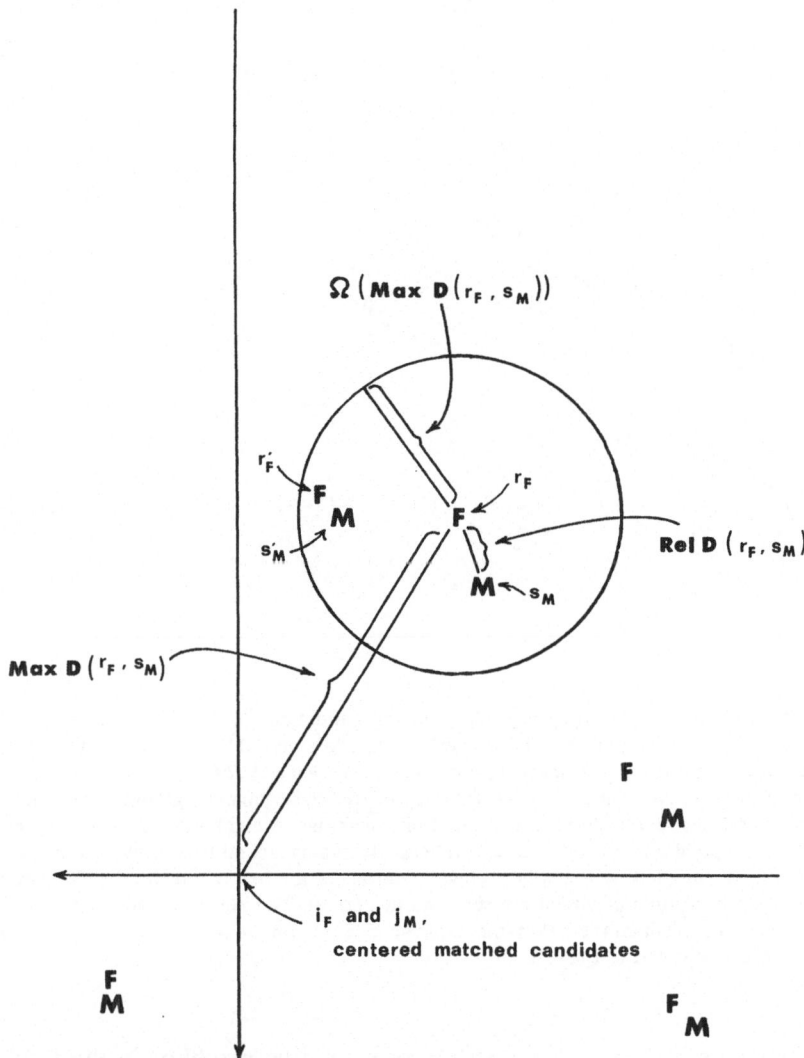

Fig. 8.   General form of relative neighborhood graph. Further explanation in the text.

sian coordinates); the present algorithm could be converted to the use of polar coordinates.

In addition to the hypothetical relative neighborhood shown in Fig. 8, we will consider in Fig. 9 the relative neighborhood of a particular set of match candidates selected from the images used to illustrate the al-

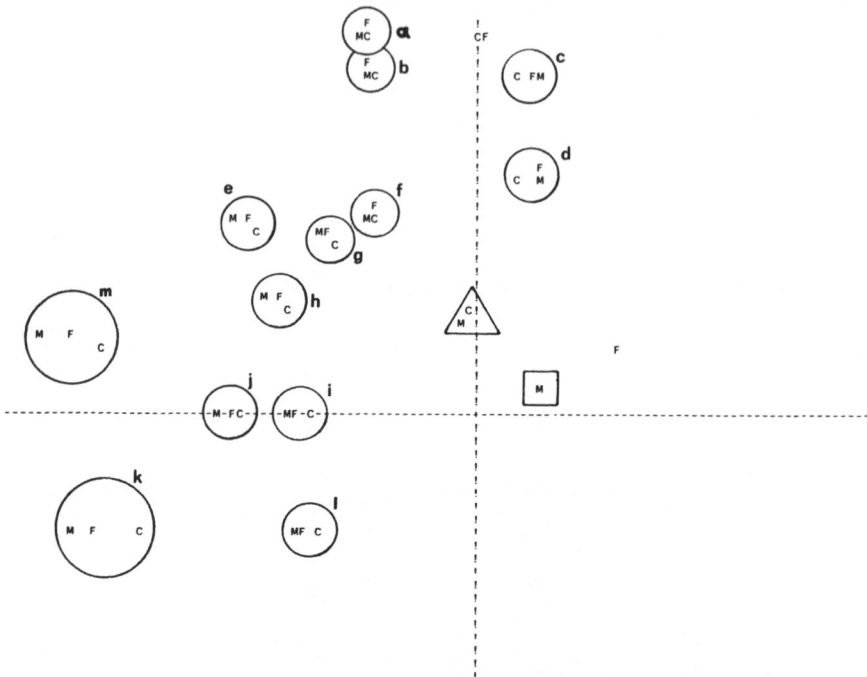

Fig. 9.   Relative neighborhood graph of match candidates: 113_F, from Fig. 5, and two apparently corresponding spots in mother's and child's gels, 114_M and 107_C. The location of neighbors from the father, mother, and child are labeled as F, M, or C respectively. Those eighbors of 113_F, 114_M, and 107_C that were considered to be "matching" under the similarity function and thus contributed to the count of "matching" neighbors (the match score) are labeled with solid circular outlines and letters which correspond to entries on Fig. 10. The neighbors surrounded by the solid triangle determined the below-threshold spot search on the father, the results of which are reported in Fig. 10. The neighbors surrounded by the solid square determined the below-threshold spot search on the father and child, the results of which are reported in Fig. 10.

gorithm. As in Fig. 8, the position of a relative neighbor in the father's or mother's gel is indicated by an F or M, respectively. (In addition, the position of a relative neighbor in the child's gel is indicated by a C.) To determine the node to which a given relative neighbor position corresponds, consider Fig. 10, which summarizes the calculations used to determine whether the match candidates—in this case 113_F, 114_M, and 107_C—meet these criteria. In the leftmost column of Fig. 10 are labels that correspond to the labeled circles around the relative neighbors in Fig. 9. To find the node numbers of the relative neighbors (and their relative

MATCH NUMBER 18

Fig. 9 label	Father		Mother		Child		F-M RelD	M-C RelD	F-C RelD
	Node#	Nhbr-Coords	Node#	Nhbr-Coords	Node#	Nhbr-Coords			
a	35	-28 129	33	-30 129	35	-28 126	2.00	3.61	3.00
b	48	-28 107	51	-29 106	52	-26 104	1.41	3.61	3.61
c	51	16 106	52	17 106	54	11 104	1.00	6.32	5.39
d	64	16 76	69	17 75	70	11 75	1.41	6.00	5.10
e	75	-59 60	77	-62 60	75	-56 59	3.00	6.08	3.16
f	73	-27 61	78	-29 60	76	-26 60	2.24	3.00	1.41
g	77	-39 56	81	-41 56	80	-37 54	2.00	4.47	2.83
h	134	-51 37	88	-54 37	87	-49 35	3.00	5.39	3.00
i	112	-46 0	113	-49 0	106	-43 0	3.00	6.00	3.00
j	116	-63 -2	119	-66 -1	109	-60 -3	3.16	6.32	3.16
k	127	-99 -38	133	-105 -36	116	-87 -38	6.32	18.11	12.00
l	125	-44 -37	134	-47 -36	115	-41 -37	3.16	6.08	3.00
m	99	-104 24	142	-112 25	123	-96 22	8.06	6.08	8.25

Average Num of Neighbor "matches" (the match score)   =   12.66

Below-Threshold spot search information from FNC Match Candidates 113 114 107

Search Father at relative coords. (-3, 32) and at absolute coords. (146,271) for radius of 10.06 :

Below threshold node number   96 added to Father graph

Search Father and Child at relative coords. (17, 10)
and at absolute coords. (168,291) and (165,298)(Father and Child respectively) with radius   5.70 :

Below threshold node number   107 added to Father graph
Virtual node number   124 added to Child graph

Fig. 10.   The match score computation and below-threshold spot search results for the eighteenth match. See. Fig. 9 for the graphical representation of this information.

coordinates) corresponding to the circled neighbors labeled on Fig. 9, consult the corresponding labeled row of Fig. 10. For example, the relative neighbors within circle h correspond to the node numbers 134_F, 88_M, and 87_C and their respective relative coordinates are $(-51,37)$, $(-54,37)$, and $(-49,35)$.

The next component in the similarity measure is the relative distance RelD between a neighbor from the father and a neighbor from the mother:

$$\text{RelD}(r_F, s_M) = \{(x_0[r_F] - x_0[s_M])^2 + (y_0[r_F] - y_0[s_M])^2\}^{1/2} \qquad (3)$$

The maximally distant neighbor is defined as

$$\text{MaxD}(r_F, s_M) = \max\{D(i_F, r_F), D(j_M, s_M)\} \qquad (4)$$

Finally, the similarity measure Sim is defined as

$$\text{Sim}(i_F, j_M) = \sum_{r_F} \sum_{s_M} \text{NMatch}(r_F, s_M) \qquad (5)$$

where

$$\begin{aligned}\text{NMatch}(r_F, s_M) &= 1 \qquad \text{if (6a) and (6b) are true} \\ &= 0 \qquad \text{if (6a) or (6b) is false}\end{aligned} \qquad (6)$$

and the conditions referred to in (6) are as follows:

$$\text{RelD}(r_F, s_M) < \Omega(\text{MaxD}(r_F, s_M)) \qquad (6a)$$

(where Ω is a noise function to be described below) and

$$\text{RelD}(r_F, s_M) < \text{RelD}(r_F', s_M)$$

$$\text{for all } r_F' \in \text{Nhbrs}[i_F] \text{ such that } r_F' \neq r_F$$

and $\qquad\qquad\qquad\qquad\qquad\qquad\qquad\qquad\qquad\qquad (6b)$

$$\text{RelD}(r_F, s_M) < \text{RelD}(r_F, s_M')$$

$$\text{for all } s_M' \in \text{Nhbrs}[j_M] \text{ such that } s_M' \neq s_M$$

{Note that s_M and r_F vary over $\text{Nhbrs}[i_F]$ and $\text{Nhbrs}[j_M]$, respectively, and that the NMatch function just defined is assumed to have access to the minimal RelD between all the neighbors under consideration, so that condition (6b) can be determined each time that NMatch is invoked to evaluate two relative neighbors}

The measure of similarity is essentially a cross-correlational measure of the locations of the neighboring spots relative to the match candidates.

That is, the match candidates (i_F and j_M) are centered at a common origin; the location of each neighbor (r_F and s_M) is plotted relative to the origin; and the measure essentially determines the degree of overlap between the neighboring spot locations relative to the match candidates. The cross-correlational measure currently used is a simple form (i.e., an indicator function) and could easily be made more complex. For example, it would be reasonable to consider a weighted measure based upon a criterion that favors relative neighbors that are closer to the match candidates than to those that are more distant. In general, while it may be useful to increase the complexity of the cross-correlational measure of neighborhood similarity, such effort can be misplaced. As we shall see (in the section on Improving the Accuracy of the Algorithm), cross-correlational measures have certain inherent uncertainties. While these uncertainties can be reduced, they cannot be eliminated.

The neighbor match function NMatch is an indicator function which returns a value of 1 if the neighboring nodes r_F and s_M are close enough to be considered "matching." It is important to be clear on our nomenclature at this point. The match candidates i_F and j_M are being judged by the similarity function Sim as to whether the neighboring nodes are in register to a degree that the match candidates can be considered as potential matches. Note that the neighboring nodes are considered as potential matches only for the purposes of judging the match candidates; the judgment as to whether the neighbors should in fact be considered to match is (currently, but not necessarily) an independent judgment, to be made later when they, too, are submitted to the similarity measure. Thus, quotes will be placed around "matching" when we are referring to potential matches of neighboring nodes used to compute NMatch.

Conditions (6a) and (6b) in the definition of NMatch provide the criteria for judging whether neighboring nodes are close enough to be considered "matching." Condition (6a) requires that the relative distance between the father and mother neighbors (r_F and s_M, respectively) be less than some specified noise radius. This noise radius $\Omega(\text{MaxD}(r_F, s_M))$ is a function of the farthest neighbor's relative distance from the centered father and mother match candidates, i_F and j_M, respectively. The positional noise characteristics of the images being compared are embodied in Ω. For example, Ω could map onto a constant value d, in which case neighboring nodes, no matter how distant from the origin provided by i_F and j_M, could not vary by more than d pixels in their relative distances from each other. On the other hand, it may be necessary to have Ω in-

crease as the distance from the "origin" increases. We have found this
latter case to be relevant to two-dimensional gel comparison. In the section concerning a more rigorous treatment of the positional noise function,
we will again discuss the determination of Ω. In the meantime, we note
that Fig. 27 (from that section) is the particular form of Ω used to process
the two-dimensional gels about which we will report. Finally, to return
to our discussion of NMatch, condition (6b) requires that the neighbors
being considered as close enough to be scored as "matching" (for the
purposes of computing Sim) also be the closest neighbors in the given
region.

Since NMatch is an indicator function, the similarity measure Sim
counts the number of neighbors of the match candidates that (according
to the noise function) can be considered as "matching." The similarity
measure is computed for i_F and all spots in the mother j'_M that are within
some maximum distance of the absolute image coordinates of i_F (the maximum distance is given by the input parameter MaxDistortion and will be
explained below). For each father and mother spot-pair a threshold, given
by the input parameter AccepNumMatches, is used to determine whether
there is a sufficient number of "matching" neighbors to consider the spot
pair as a potential match. (AccepNumMatches is set to 10 for all the gels
upon which we will report.)

Finally, the spot pair i_F and j_M that receives the greatest similarity
measure (greater than AccepNumMatches) is considered to form a pairwise match. Thus, the following conditions must be satisfied in order to
consider i_F and j_M to form a pairwise match:

$$\text{Sim}(i_F, j_M) > \text{AccepNumMatches} \tag{7a}$$

and

$$\text{Sim}(i_F, j_M) > \text{Sim}(i_F, j'_M) \tag{7b}$$

for all $j'_M \neq j_M$ satisfying

$$\{(x(i_F) - x(j'_M))^2 + (y(i_F) - y(j'_M))^2\}^{1/2} < \text{MaxDistortion} \tag{7c}$$

Pairwise matching nodes have a similarity measure that is greater than
AccepNumMatches [condition (7a)] and is greater than that produced by
any other pairing [condition (7b)]. Condition (7c) serves to limit, for the
sake of efficiency, the number of maternal spots considered as alternative
matches to the current maternal match candidate. If we are looking in
the mother's gel for match candidates for a given spot in the father's gel,

then it is only necessary to consider maternal spots that are within some maximum distance (with respect to the absolute image coordinates of the father's and mother's images) from the father's spot because, in general, an upper bound exists (corresponding to the input parameter, Max-Distortion, currently set equal to 60 pixels) on the nonregistration of matching spots on different images. For example, it serves no useful purpose to consider matches between spots in the upper right-hand corner of a paternal gel with spots in the lower left-hand corner of a maternal gel.

The matching node j_M from the mother is then used to search for further matches with nodes in the gel of the child, based upon the pairwise comparison procedure described above. If j_M is determined to match some node k_C from the child, then there is a *potential* match of i_F, j_M, and k_C. The reason the match is only potential is that up to this point all evidence for the match is based upon pairwise comparisons between the father and mother and between the mother and child. Since these pairwise comparisons are independent of each other, there is the need to verify that they are consistent with each other. First it must be verified that i_F corresponds to k_C. However, even though the correspondences are consistent, in the sense that i_F does not correspond to a different node in the child's gel than in the mother's, it is necessary to return to the original neighborhood patterns of the potential matches to verify their consistency. Thus, a new "match score" must be computed which reflects a consistent three-way application of the matching criteria used in the pairwise matchings of Sim.

Figures 9 and 10 illustrate the final match score of the particular match candidates being used to describe the algorithm: 113_F, 114_M, and 107_C. The relative neighbors considered to be "matching" under the similarity function and thus contributing to the count of "matching" neighbors (the match score) are labeled in Fig. 9 with solid circular outlines and letters (which in turn correspond to entries on Fig. 10). The neighbors surrounded by the square and triangle were involved in a search for below-threshold spots (see next section).

If the final match score is greater than AccepNumMatches, then the three nodes are given the same match state number and are added to the set of nodes corresponding to the intial subset of matching spots. The match state number is the number of matches determined at the current point of time in the running of the algorithm. Symbolically, MatchState[i_F], MatchState[j_M], and MatchState[k_C] are assigned a *current* match number; in this case MatchState[113_F], MatchState[114_M],

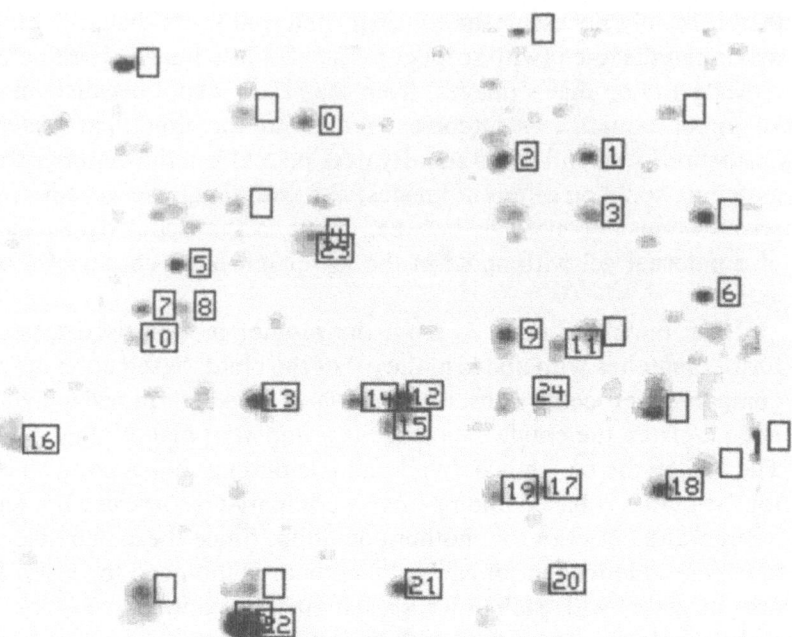

Fig. 11.   Father's match graph at the end of the first iteration.

and MatchState[107$_C$] are arbitrarily termed match set 18. See Figs. 11–13 for the initial set of match labels for the father, mother, and child respectively. Note that the empty boxes correspond to nodes not yet matched.

Iteration of Matching Step

The initial subset of matching spots forms the basis for an iterative process which progressively decreases the differences in the neighborhoods of the matched spots, so that the matching process can continue to find new matches. While the match score measures the neighborhood's similarities, information about the differences in the neighborhood patterns is also recorded. This information is used to search for below-threshold spots, which, if added to the graph structure, allow more matches to occur.

Consider the case where, at a certain relative displacement from the matched spots, there are "matching" spots in the preparations of the

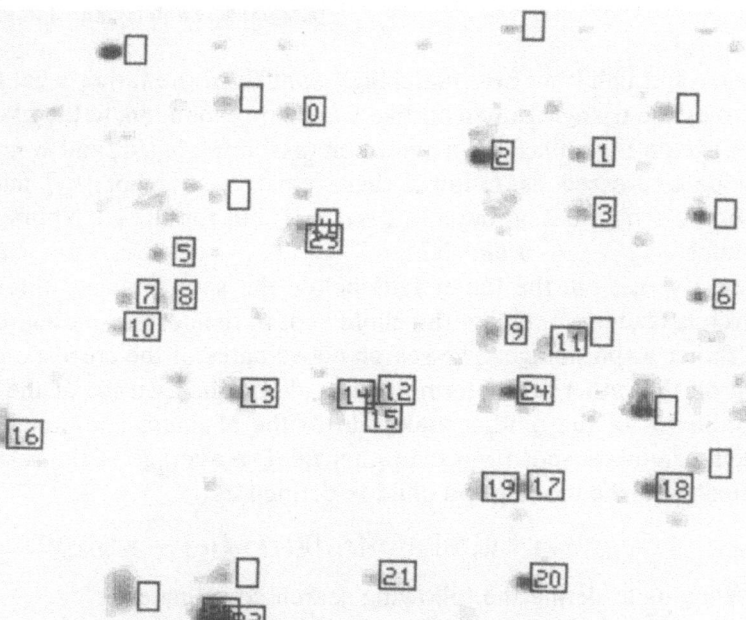

Fig. 12.   Mother's match graph at the end of the first iteration.

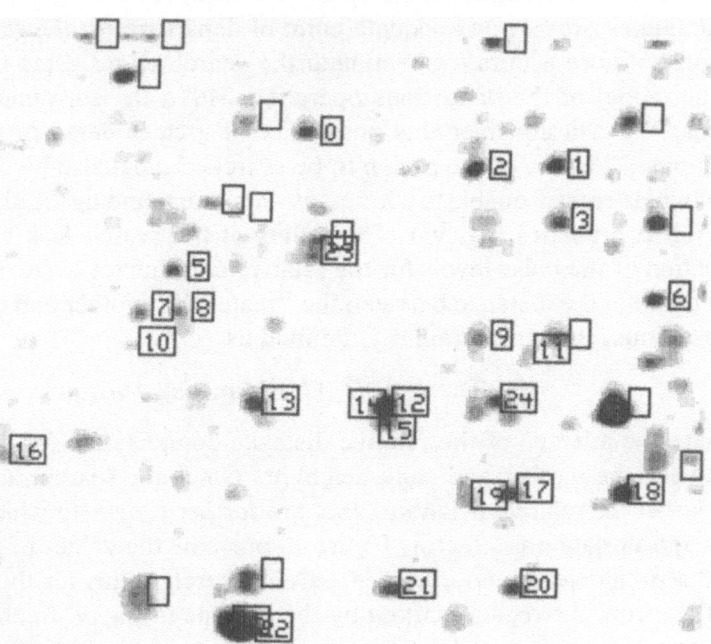

Fig. 13.   Child's match graph at the end of the first iteration.

mother and child but no "matching" spot from the father's gel (as indicated by the triangle drawn on Fig. 9 and corresponding to the first search message on Fig. 10). Such a condition (assuming i_F, j_M, and k_C matched) can be expressed as follows: there exist $t_C \in$ Nhbrs[k_C] and $s_M \in$ Nhbrs[j_M] such that NMatch (t_C, s_M) = 1, but for all $r_F \in$ Nhbrs[i_F] both NMatch (r_F, t_C) = 0 and NMatch (r_F, s_M) = 0. Since this can occur when a spot from the father falls below the spot intensity threshold, a search is made for a below-threshold spot in the corresponding region on the father's spot image. The search coordinates of the corresponding region on the father are determined by adding the average of the relative coordinates of the mother and child to the absolute coordinates of the match candidate spot from the father i_F. The average of the relative coordinates of the mother and child is defined as

$$(\bar{x}_F, \bar{y}_F) = ((x_0[t_C] + x_0[s_M])/2, (y_0[t_C] + y_0[s_M])/2)$$

allowing us to define the following search coordinates:

$$(x(i_F) + \bar{x}_F, y(i_F) + \bar{y}_F)$$

Generally, the search coordinates derived from the average of the relative coordinates provide an adequate point of departure. At the same time, it might be more accurate to estimate the search coordinates based upon some model of the distortions operative within the surrounding gel regions. We will consider this possibility in greater detail in subsequent sections. The area of the region to be searched must also be determined. It would seem reasonable to define it as a disk surrounding the displacement search coordinates $(\bar{x}_F, \bar{y}_F)$. The radius of the search disk should be a function of the noise levels for the relative coordinates of the mother and child and of the distance between the "matched" mother and child neighbors. Thus, the search radius is defined as

$$\text{RelD}(s_M, t_C)/2 + \Omega(\text{MaxD}(s_M, t_C))$$

where the average of the relative distance compensates for the distance between the mother and child neighbors (since the search radius should be larger for relative neighbors that are further apart), to which is added the appropriate noise factor. Figure 10 presents the values of the relative and absolute search coordinates and the search radius for the search resulting from the region marked by the triangle in Fig. 9. In an analogous manner, absolute coordinates and search region radii can be computed for the cases where there are "matching" neighbors from only a father and child or only a father and mother, in which case the search for below-threshold spots would occur on the mother and child, respectively.

The other class of searches occurs when there are spots in the neighborhood of one of the match candidates which "match" no other relative neighbors. Consider the case where at a certain relative displacement from the matching spots there is a neighboring spot from the mother but no "matching" neighbors from the father or child (as indicated by the square on Fig. 9 and the second search entry of Fig. 10). Such a condition can be expressed as follows: there exists $s_M \in$ Nhbrs[j_M] such that NMatch(s_M, r_F) = 0 for all $r_F \in$ Nhbrs[i_F], and NMatch(s_M, t_C) = 0 for all $t_C \in$ Nhbrs[k_C]. Since this can occur when corresponding spots in gels from the father and child fall just below the spot intensity threshold, a search is made for a below-threshold spot in the corresponding regions on the father's and child's spot images. The coordinates of the corresponding region on the father's and child's gels are determined by adding the relative coordinates of the neighboring spot in the mother's gel to the absolute coordinates of the match candidates from the father and child. The coordinates from which to search the gels of the father and child are, respectively,

$$(x(i_F) + x_0[s_M], y(i_F) + y_0[s_M])$$

$$(x(k_C) + x_0[s_M], y(k_C) + y_0[s_M])$$

and the radius of the disk defining the search regions is $\Omega(D(j_M, s_M))$. The values of the relative and absolute search coordinates and the search radius for the search resulting from the region marked by the square in Fig. 9 are given in the second entry of the search information of Fig. 10. In an analogous manner, absolute coordinates and search region radii can be computed for the cases where there are isolated neighbors from a mother or child, in which case the search for below-threshold spots would occur on the father/child and mother/father, respectively.

If a below-threshold spot is found within the region being searched, then it is added to the graph. If no such spot is found, then a "virtual node" is added to the graph; the virtual node can participate in future matching, but it is flagged so that it can be distinguished from observed data (consider Fig. 10 for the results of the searches from match 18). Note that the location of the virtual node is identical to the center coordinates of the search radius. This can result in distortions, since the location of the virtual node is based upon the average distance between relative neighbors. It may be the case that a more complex model of the relative neigh-borhood should guide the placement of the virtual nodes. For example, if all relative neighbors of the father tend to undergo some uniform shift with reference to the relative neighbors of the mother and child, then any virtual father nodes created should mirror that pattern. How such a more complex model is possible will be described latter, in the section on Improving the Accuracy of the Algorithm.

As matching nodes are found, the algorithm reconciles differences in the neighborhoods of the matched nodes, either by finding below-threshold spots or creating virtual spots. The matching process can then be repeated on all nodes that have not yet been matched. The newly entered below-threshold or virtual nodes can now participate in new matches and can contribute as new neighbors to the match score of other nodes. At each iteration of the algorithm new nodes are entered into the graph and then the matching procedure is reapplied. After a number of iterations each individual should have a graph which is essentially the union of the three graphs from which the trio started. (Theoretically the algorithm should compute the union. In practice, because of excessive gel-to-gel variations, the algorithm only approximates computing the union.) Figures 14–16 show the final match graphs for the father, mother, and child, respectively.

The search for below-threshold spots is made more complex by spots on image boundaries. Because images are not in registration, the search from an "unmatched" neighbor of a match on the image boundary of a given image can cause a search that extends beyond the boundaries of the other image. This condition is easily detected and the action currently taken is to remove such "unmatched" neighbors from the entire matching process. For example, some of the (as yet unmatched) spots at the top of Fig. 13 are removed for this reason; they are absent in Fig. 16.

Another, more fundamental complexity in searching for below-threshold spots concerns which neighbors of a match will be allowed to determine the search regions and, possibly, the location of virtual nodes. A spot whose "corresponding spots" are either below threshold or do not exist will be in the neighborhood of many different matches. If distortion increases with distance from any given match, then it is clearly undesirable to have searches governed by matches that are far away from the region(s) to be searched. This potential for error is tolerable when the search results in the detection of below-threshold spots, since the noise function Ω should be able to compensate for the effects of increased dis-

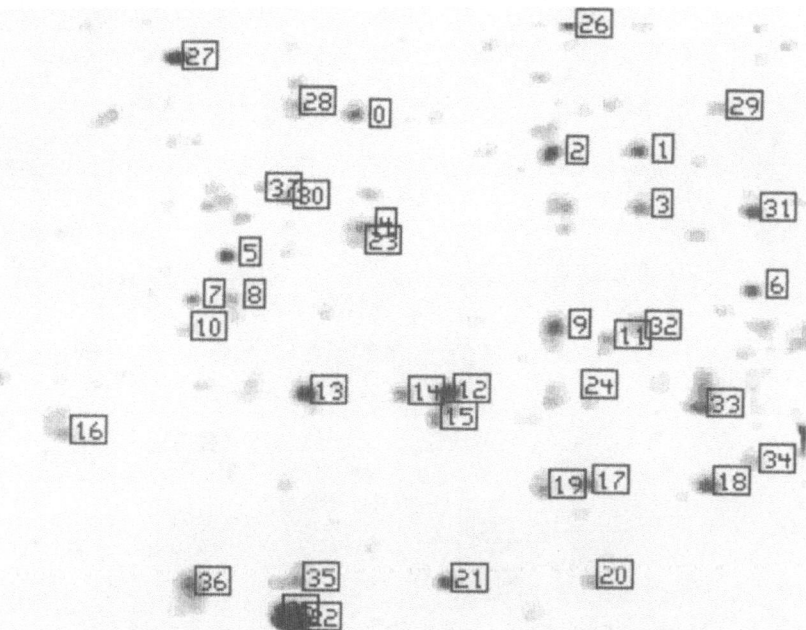

Fig. 14. Father's final match graph. Note that although this comparison began with the 30 most intense spots on each of the three gels, the creation of virtual nodes and recognition of below-threshold spots increased the final graph to 38 nodes. See Table II for the match categorizations corresponding to the match numbers of the graph.

tortion and should thus provide a search radius wide enough to find corresponding below-threshold spots. On the other hand, if no below-threshold spot is found, the coordinates of a virtual spot must be determined and it is important that these coordinates be minimally affected by noise. Thus, for these reasons, the comparison algorithm limits such searches to the nearest neighbors of a given match. This is a conservative strategy, some of whose implications will be examined in the section on Recovery from Mismatches.

All matches consist of some combination of above-threshold, below-threshold, and virtual nodes from the father, mother, and child. Clearly some kind of convenient shorthand for the various possible combinations is necessary. We have adopted the system given in Table I. Note that a spot is "observed" if it was one of the original above-threshold spots or if it was a below-threshold spot found in the search process. The final output of the comparison process as applied to the gel sections analyzed

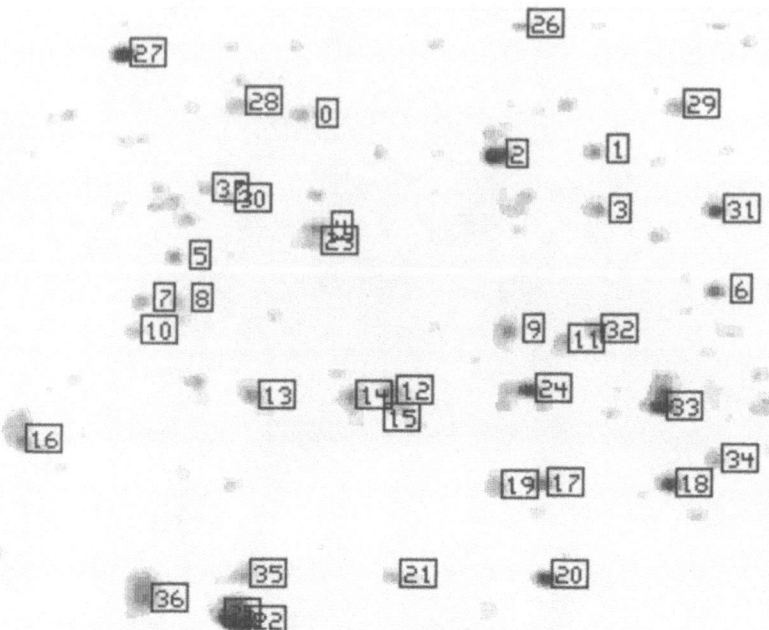

Fig. 15. Mother's final match graph. Explanation of match numbers as for Fig. 14.

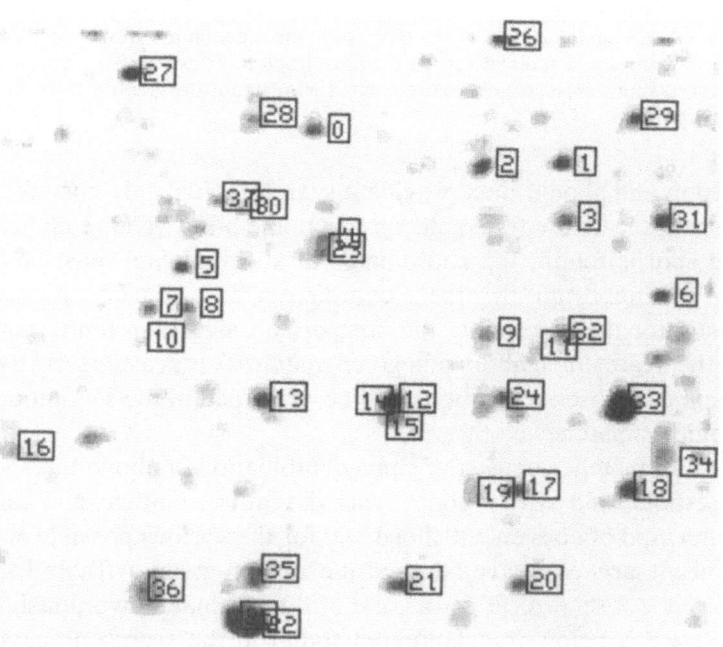

Fig. 16. Child's final match graph. Explanation of match numbers as for Fig. 14.

TABLE I. Match Category Names and Meanings

Category	Meaning
Family	Father, mother, and child observed
Childless	Father and mother observed, child was virtual spot
Fatherless	Mother and child were observed, father was virtual
Motherless	Father and child were observed, mother was virtual
Bachelor	Father was observed, mother and child were virtual
Spinster	Mother was observed, father and child were virtual
Orphan	Child was observed, father and mother were virtual

to this point is shown in Table II. Figures 14–16 can be compared with the categorizations of each match as indicated by Table II.

In addition to the qualitative categorizations, each output lists the maximum intensity of each spot. The spots with an intensity of zero correspond to the virtual spots. The spot intensities constitute an additional set of constraints that would be useful in increasing the certainty of gel comparisons. The current estimate of spot quantity is not a sufficiently reliable measure, but with further improvements in the feature-measurement algorithms we believe spot quantity not only could participate in the matching process, but could be made the basis for a search for a class of genetic variants characterized by half-normal spot quantity. In the section on Future Improvements to the Comparison Algorithm, we will consider how information on spot quantity could be integrated into the algorithm.

Recovery from Mismatches

The match score used to determine matches is basically a cross-correlation of the patterns of neighboring locations of spots. With any

TABLE II. Match Status Information for Gel Trio Illustrated in Figures 14–16
(30 Most Intense Spots)

Match number	Father		Mother		Child		Match type
	Node number	Inten	Node number	Inten	Node number	Inten	
0	28	107	26	100	27	128	Family
1	35	116	33	107	35	131	Family
2	37	120	38	139	37	127	Family
3	48	87	51	92	52	95	Family
4	56	92	55	107	61	96	Family
5	61	126	62	105	67	122	Family
6	64	107	69	107	70	118	Family
7	67	109	71	102	71	99	Family
8	68	93	72	91	72	103	Family
9	75	113	77	110	76	108	Family
10	76	77	79	93	79	56	Family
11	77	89	81	91	80	60	Family
12	91	129	93	105	92	142	Family
13	92	128	96	95	91	117	Family
14	93	95	97	92	122	0	Childless
15	99	87	142	0	123	0	Bachelor
16	105	92	104	98	101	78	Family
17	112	118	113	117	106	128	Family
18	113	129	114	135	107	129	Family
19	116	105	119	102	109	91	Family
20	125	99	134	137	115	131	Family
21	127	132	133	103	116	128	Family
22	132	145	140	154	121	120	Family
23	133	0	141	0	64	102	Orphan
24	134	0	88	105	87	94	Fatherless
25	135	0	143	0	120	111	Orphan
26	3	98	2	87	6	104	Family
27	16	125	11	156	14	142	Family
28	25	83	20	83	24	94	Family
29	26	73	23	90	19	113	Family
30	44	88	44	66	48	56	Family
31	51	112	52	131	54	114	Family
32	73	73	78	93	75	103	Family
33	96	64	99	98	89	129	Family
34	107	75	106	93	124	0	Childless
35	126	87	132	86	114	97	Family
36	128	87	136	96	117	72	Family
37	42	58	40	70	46	91	Family

cross-correlation function there is always the possibility that neighbor-hood patterns on two spots of the same gel will by chance be similar and result in high match scores, which in turn may result in false matches between gels. In this sense, cross-correlational measures tend to be "my-opic." Beyond this possibility, there is a fundamental tradeoff involving the setting of the match score threshold AcceptNumMatches. If AcceptNumMatches is high, then the algorithm will determine matches with a high degree of confidence. However, because the current match function is simply cumulative, too high a match score criterion could cause failure to determine matches that have less spots in their neighborhoods; e.g., a spot appearing on the image borders. On the other hand, if AccepNumMatches is low, then the algorithm will make more false matches. Thus, because of uncertainties due to the use of a cross-cor-relation measure and the application of a threshold on that measure to determine matches, it is desirable to verify matches. Furthermore, there

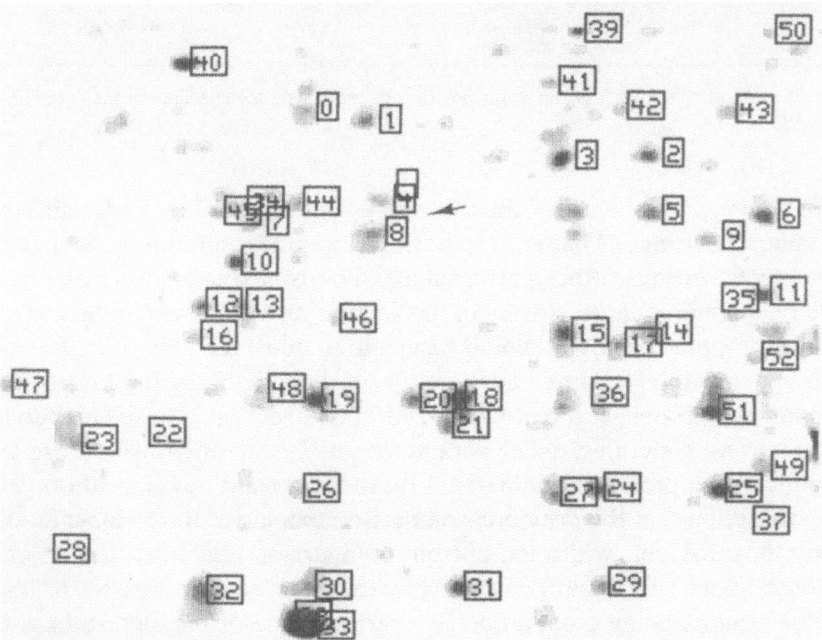

Fig. 17. Father's match graph resulting from a comparison that began with the 40 most intense spots. Note that the creation of virtual nodes and recognition of below-threshold spots increased the final graph to 55 nodes. The position of the inconsistent match discussed in the text is indicated by the arrow.

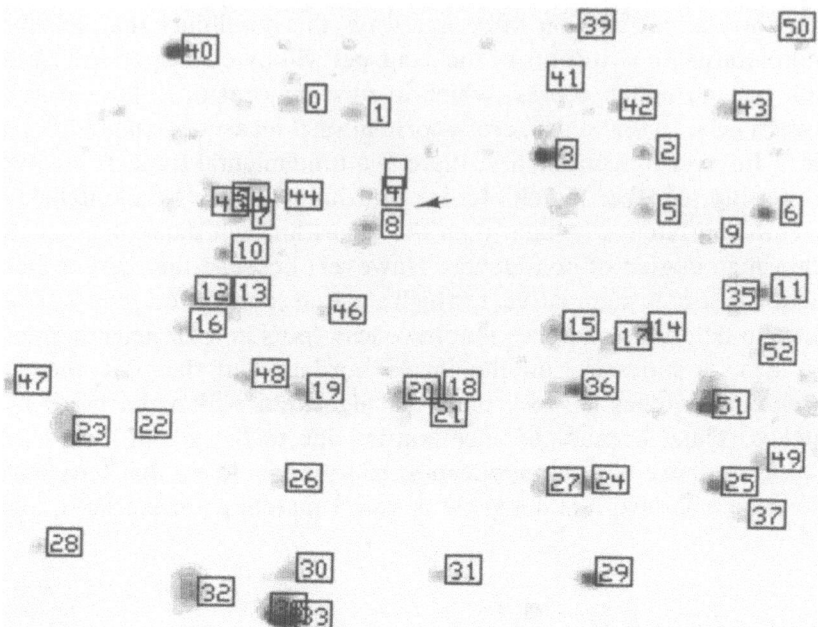

Fig. 18. Mother's match graph, with position of inconsistent match again indicated as for Fig. 17.

is the more general issue of the robustness of the algorithm under different parameter settings. That is, it is desirable to understand how changes in parameter settings affect performance. The robustness of the algorithm will be examined more closely in the section on Validation of the Current Algorithm, but for now it would be useful to consider Figs. 17–19, which show, respectively, some match graphs derived from the lysate gels from the father, mother, and child analyzed in this section. These comparison graphs were generated under parameter settings identical with those that produced the previous comparison (used to explain the algorithm), with the exception that the previous comparison examined the 30 most intense spots on each gel, while the current comparison examined the 40 most intense spots. This change in parameters increases the density of spots in the regions being compared. The performance of the algorithm at the higher density is comparable to the previous comparison except in the regions indicated by the arrows drawn on the figures. Match number 4 is a clear mismatch: on the child it is below match number 8, while on the parents it is above match number 8. Thus, in order to assure robustness

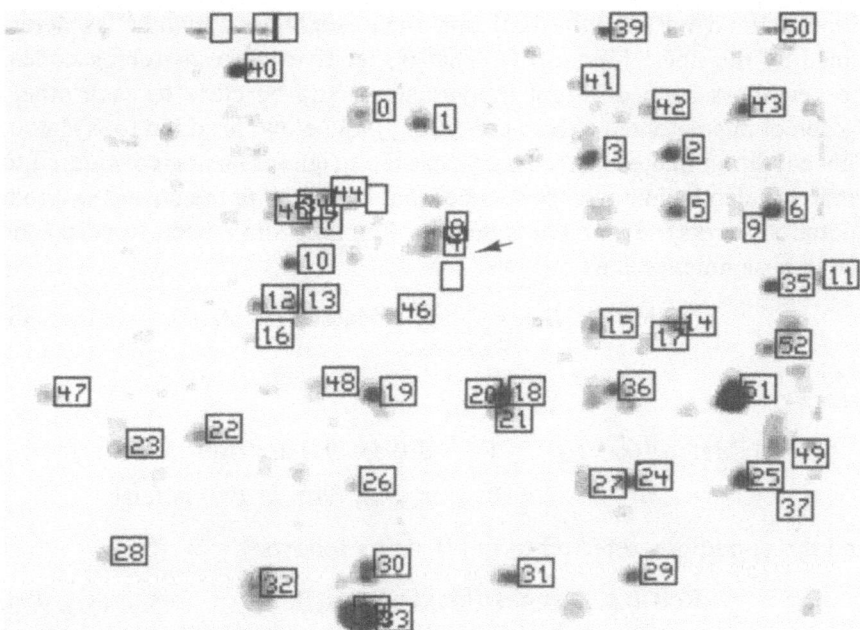

Fig. 19.   Child's match graph, with position of inconsistent match again indicated as for Fig. 17.

under different parameter settings, it is desirable to find and recover from errors in match assignments.

There are a variety of ways in which the comparison algorithm might detect mismatches, or, in other words, determine the accuracy of its match assignments. Our current method of checking accuracy will be described in this section. An advantage of the method to be presented is that it uses slightly modified versions of the functions (subroutines) used to determine the original matches. A more general discussion of possible algorithms for checking accuracy will be found in the section on Improving the Accuracy of the Algorithm. Accuracy checking is accomplished by reconsidering each match and recomputing the match score for the nodes in the match. Consider how the nth match consisting of nodes i_F, j_M, and k_C is verified. In terms of our notation, MatchState[i_F], MatchState[j_M], and MatchState[k_C] are all equal to n. The match score is recomputed based upon the pairwise comparison function Sim, which in turn depends upon the function NMatch used to determine whether neighboring nodes "match." In order for nodes to match it was necessary [under the condition defined by formula (6a)] that their neighbors "match" as determined by the noise function Ω. That is, relative to the matching nodes, the neighbors from different individuals should be close to each other. To detect mismatches, a third condition, (9c) below, is added to NMatch. This condition makes it necessary that the neighbors being considered to "match" also be in correspondence; that is, match in the strong (without quotation marks) sense. The similarity function SimV used to verify the match assignments is as follows:

$$\text{SimV}(i_F, j_M) = \sum_{r_F} \sum_{s_M} \text{NMatchV}(r_F, s_M) \tag{8}$$

where

$$\text{NMatchV}(r_F, s_M) = 1 \quad \text{if (9a)–(9c) are true} \tag{9}$$
$$= 0 \quad \text{if (9a), (9b), or (9c) is false}$$

and the conditions referred to in (9) are as follows:

$$\text{RelD}(r_F, s_M) < \Omega(\text{MaxD}(r_F, s_M)) \tag{9a}$$

$$\text{RelD}(r_F, s_M) < \text{RelD}(r'_F, s_M)$$

for all $r'_F \in \text{Nhbrs}[i_F]$ such that $r'_F \neq r_F$

and $\tag{9b}$

$$\text{RelD}(r_F, s_M) < \text{RelD}(r_F, s'_M)$$

for all $s'_M \in \text{Nhbrs}[j_M]$ such that $s'_M \neq s_M$

$$\text{MatchState}[r_F] = \text{MatchState}[s_M] \neq \text{Null} \tag{9c}$$

Thus, a new match score is recomputed for each match where NMatchV adds to the count of "matching" neighbors only if the neighbors did in fact match. If the recomputed match score falls below the match score threshold AccepNumMatches, then the match is considered to be a mismatch and is removed. In this fashion, the algorithm was able to detect the mismatch in the fourth match of Figs. 17–19. In addition, any virtual nodes created due to the mismatch are removed: such virtual nodes can be seen as empty boxes surrounding the fourth match on Figs. 17–19. This scheme ensures more global consistency between the initially independent match determinations, a notion examined further in the section on Improving the Accuracy of the Algorithm.

After the removal of any detected mismatches, the algorithm then

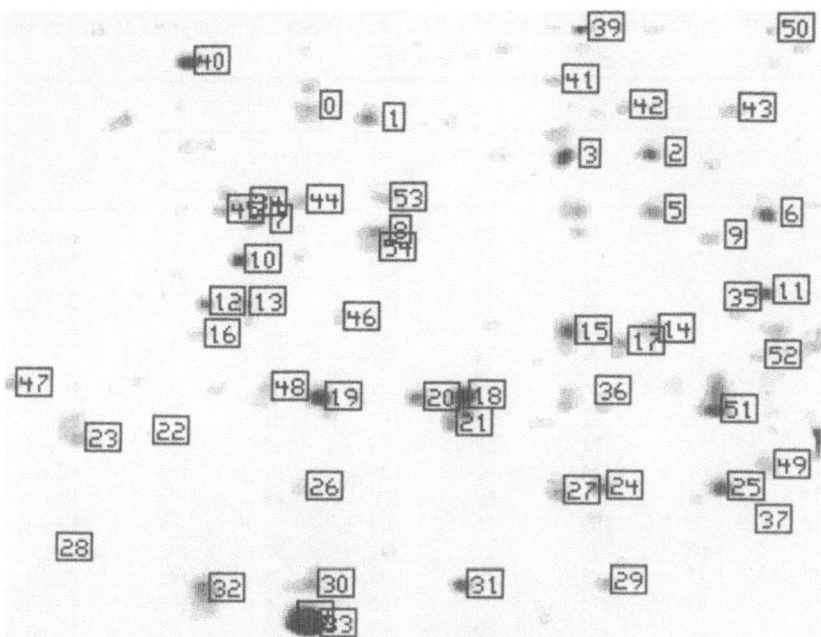

Fig. 20.   The father's match graph, after the inconsistent match shown on Fig. 17 has been rectified.

searches for a correct match involving the same spots. This is accomplished by reexamining all unmatched nodes with the verifying match score function [given by condition (9c)]. In addition, the match score threshold AccepNumMatches is lowered (by two-thirds of its original value) so that nodes at the boundaries of the images have a better chance of being matched. It is reasonable to lower the threshold, because the match score function is now more highly constrained as to what it accepts as a "match." Figures 20–22 show the removed mismatch and corrected matches (involving match numbers 53 and 54), that result from the verification pass of the comparison algorithm. Table III gives the match categories of the match graphs of Figs. 20–22.

There is one more additional difference between the matching procedure during the verification pass and the matching procedure used in the nonverification pass. In the search for below-threshold spots prior to the verification stage, the neighboring spots that determined the search coordinates were required to be the nearest neighbors of the matched spots. This was necessary in order to minimize the effects of increases

TABLE III. Match Status Information for Gel Trio Illustrated in Figures 20–22 (40 Most Intense Spots)

| Match number | Father | | Mother | | Child | | Match type |
	Node number	Inten	Node number	Inten	Node number	Inten	
0	25	83	20	83	24	94	Family
1	28	107	26	100	27	128	Family
2	35	116	33	107	35	131	Family
3	37	120	38	139	37	127	Family
5	48	87	51	92	52	95	Family
6	51	112	52	131	54	114	Family
7	53	70	53	74	58	83	Family
8	56	92	55	107	61	96	Family
9	57	72	59	75	62	70	Family
10	61	126	62	105	67	122	Family
11	64	107	69	107	68	82	Family
12	67	109	71	102	71	99	Family
13	68	93	72	91	72	103	Family
14	73	73	78	93	75	103	Family
15	75	113	77	110	76	108	Family
16	76	77	79	93	79	56	Family
17	77	89	81	91	80	60	Family
18	91	129	93	105	92	142	Family
19	92	128	96	95	91	117	Family
20	93	95	97	92	123	0	Childless
21	99	87	143	0	124	0	Bachelor
22	103	30	103	38	98	85	Family
23	105	92	104	98	101	78	Family
24	112	118	113	117	106	128	Family
25	113	129	114	135	107	129	Family
26	114	70	117	71	108	70	Family
27	116	105	119	102	109	91	Family
28	121	40	129	85	113	86	Family
29	125	99	134	137	115	131	Family
30	126	87	132	86	114	97	Family
31	127	132	133	103	116	128	Family
32	128	87	136	96	117	72	Family
33	132	145	140	154	121	120	Family
34	134	0	46	75	49	65	Fatherless
35	135	0	142	0	70	118	Orphan
36	136	0	88	105	87	94	Fatherless
37	137	0	123	74	126	0	Spinster
38	138	0	144	0	120	111	Orphan
39	3	98	2	87	6	104	Family
40	16	125	11	156	14	142	Family
41	17	67	15	31	16	63	Family
42	23	51	22	75	22	71	Family

TABLE III. (*continued*)

Match number	Father Node number	Inten	Mother Node number	Inten	Child Node number	Inten	Match type
43	26	73	23	90	19	113	Family
44	44	88	44	66	46	91	Family
45	50	78	47	61	55	63	Family
46	70	66	74	66	73	82	Family
47	83	67	90	82	90	82	Family
48	85	62	86	76	84	62	Family
49	107	75	106	93	125	0	Childless
50	6	40	4	64	7	87	Family
51	96	64	99	98	89	129	Family
52	79	30	82	30	81	85	Family
53	43	66	42	73	47	67	Family
54	139	0	145	0	64	102	Orphan

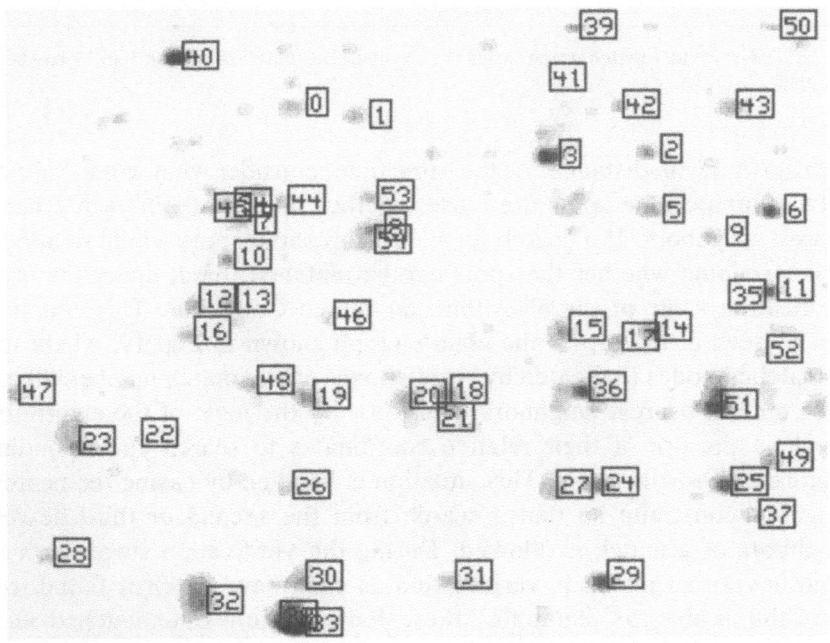

Fig. 21.   The mother's match graph, after the inconsistent match shown on Fig. 18 has been rectified.

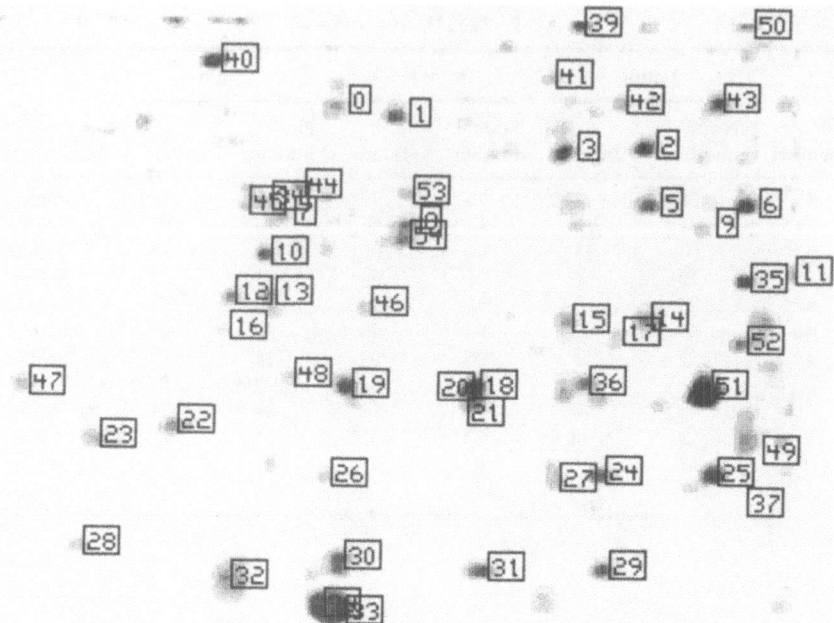

Fig. 22.   The child's match graph, after the inconsistent match shown on Fig. 19 has been rectified.

in distortion with distance. At the same time, consider what would happen if two unmatchable spots are close together, making them each other's nearest neighbors. If a search for below-threshold spots would be useful in determining whether the spots can be matched, then, under the non-verification stage of the algorithm, no search can occur. This situation can be seen at the top of the child's graph shown in Fig. 19, where the unmatched nodes (indicated by empty boxes above match number 40) are each other's nearest neighbors, and thus, by the logic of the algorithm, preclude the use of their relative coordinates to search corresponding regions on the other gels. This situation is handled by easing the nearest neighbor constraint so that a search from the second or third nearest neighbors of a match is allowed. During the verification stage, both as each unverified match is verified and as each new match is found, the algorithm is able to "penetrate" these denser regions of unmatched nearest neighbors. In particular, prior to the verification stage (to return to Fig. 19), the algorithm (from the "perspective" of match number 40) could not penetrate the regions corresponding to the neighboring unmatched nodes above it. Under the loosened constraints of the verification stage of the algorithm, the relative coordinates of these neighbors are available and are used to determine that potential corresponding spots on other images would be outside the boundaries of the other images and thus these neighbors should be removed (as shown in Fig. 22), since they could never be matched.

In summary, the check for accuracy [given in condition (9c)] constrains the match process to be more consistent, effectively countering the myopia of a cross-correlational measure of neighborhood similarity. This consistency check compensates for the uncertainty inherent in a match score threshold and increases the robustness of the comparison algorithm under different parameter settings. Because the addition of the accuracy check increases the constraints on the "match" function, other constraints within the algorithm can be eased. Thus, the match score threshold can be lowered to ease the search process on image boundaries and the nearest neighbor search restriction can be removed.

What the Algorithm Does Not Do

It is important at this juncture to state clearly what this algorithm does not do. Although the output contains a great deal of information concerning the occurrence of genetic variation, this algorithm was not developed for the study of genetic variation *per se*. In principle, any spot that the algorithm characterizes as spinster, bachelor, childless, motherless, or fatherless is potentially a segregating variant. However, the output of the algorithm provides no clue as to the "standard" spot of which this is a variant. Currently, this can only be determined by visual inspection. Furthermore, the designation of a spot as "family" does not preclude genetic variation; in our system of nomenclature this appellation would be applied to a variant spot present in all three of the individuals being compared, on the basis of either homozygosity or heterozygosity of the allele encoding for the variant spot in question.

VALIDATION OF THE CURRENT ALGORITHM

This section examines the performance of the two-dimensional gel comparison algorithm in terms of accuracy, evaluated in terms of how well the results of the algorithm correspond to analyses performed by humans. The performance of the feature-measurement algorithms will also be examined, especially in terms of the effect on the performance of the comparison algorithm. It will be apparent that although much has been accomplished in automating the reading of these gels, much remains to be done.

Initially, we will consider two types of errors, corresponding to whether the algorithm fails to detect a mutation or creates one because of failure to identify an appropriate match of a spot in a child's gel with one in either or both parents. The first type of error, failure to detect a mutation, is referred to as a "false negative," since the algorithm is *falsely* stating that there *is no* mutation. In the context of the current algorithm, this type of error occurs when a noncorresponding spot on a child (which should be categorized as an "orphan") is falsely determined to be in correspondence (i.e., belonging to a "family," "motherless," or "fatherless" match). The second type of error is referred to as a "false positive," since the algorithm is *falsely* stating that there *is* a mutation. In the context of the current algorithm, this type of error appears when a spot on a child's gel is falsely categorized as an "orphan" when it should have been matched with some combination of spots from the father's and mother's gels; i.e., as a "family," "motherless," or "fatherless" match.

From the perspective of comparing two-dimensional gels in order to estimate the rate of mutation, the most damaging error is the false negative. There must be a high degree of confidence that when a mutation occurs it will be detected. Since mutations are estimated to occur with a frequency on the order of between 10^{-5} and 10^{-6}, even a very low false-negative error rate can cause a large increase in the number of events that have to be examined if the research design includes some arbitrary statistical endpoint. As opposed to the false-negative error, the false-positive error is less damaging. Each "orphan" spot will be verified by a visual analysis. It is better that the laboratory must check out some (as we shall see, relatively small) number of polypeptides falsely labeled as "orphans" than that the algorithm fail to identify the true "orphans"; i.e., mutations. Estimating the rate of mutation involves determining the ratio of the number of mutations to the total number of observations. The estimate by the comparison algorithm of the number of nonmutations corresponds to the number of match categorizations describing events consistent with inheritance (i.e., all match categorizations except "orphan").

While the categorization of errors into false negatives and false positives is of fundamental importance, it does not capture the nuances of the ways in which the algorithm can make mistakes. For example, consider some of the ways in which a "family" match categorization can be wrong. Assume that the spot from the child's gel involved in the "family" categorization is a spot that is incorrectly matched with spots from the father and mother (both of which are correctly matched). Assume further that there exists a spot on the child's gel that should have been matched with a spot in the father's and mother's gels; i.e., the specific spot in the father's and mother's gels does in fact (according to visual inspection) match another spot on the child's gel, and these particular spots of the father and mother should have been classified as a "family" with some other spot from the child's gel. Next, consider two (out of many possible) ways in which this situation can occur. First, the child's spot, which was incorrectly matched with the father's and mother's spot, may actually be a mutational event; i.e., the child's spot should have been categorized as an "orphan." The result is a false-negative error. Second, the child's spot corresponds to some other spot (or spots) on the father's or mother's gels; i.e., the child's spot should have been categorized within a "family"; "motherless," or "fatherless" match. The latter result is neither a false-negative nor a false-positive error. Rather, this second case represents the more general category of error involving some form of mismatch— no mutation was missed or incorrectly reported. For present purposes, false-negative and false-positive errors are defined solely with repect to the question of mutation.

Algorithm Performance on Artificially Constructed Gels

Early in our efforts at validation we created a number of artificial gel images which varied in a highly controlled manner, i.e., we had complete knowledge of the positional noise characteristics of the images. For the first test, a family trio of 17 cm^2 gel images, each with 49 spots well distributed over the gel, was created in which there were no positional distortions between corresponding spots; i.e., the images were in perfect registration. Examples of all the types of genetic variation listed in Table I were incorporated into the images. The algorithm correctly determined all match categorizations. For the second test, another artificial family was constructed. The gels of the trio were out of registration only in terms of being shifted with respect to each other; i.e., a two-dimensional vector (different in orientation for each gel in the trio but having the same magnitude of 6 mm) was added to the coordinates of each spot on a gel. Thus, the images were shifted relative to each other, but were in perfect registration relative to the shifts. The performance of the algorithm was again perfect. Finally, for a third test, we introduced into the images the type of nonregistration between homologous spots that may result from localized pH gradient shifts in these gels (the nonregistration amounted to 3–5 mm.) Corresponding spots were thus subjected to differing amounts of distortion. Using the same $\Omega(d)$ shown in Fig. 27, the algorithm was again able to perform correctly all match categorizations.

Although in this limited set of tests the performance of the algorithm was flawless, one could of course construct test families where the spot placement and distortion were such that the algorithm would be compromised. Such tests would be useful in the development of a more analytical model of algorithm performance, since the noise properties of the images are under experimental control. To date, however, our efforts have been directed more toward examining the performance of the algorithm on real data, to which we now turn our attention.

Algorithm Performance on Real Gels

In order to evaluate the performance of the algorithm on actual gels, we must consider further the nature of mismatches. Mismatches can be thought of as arising from inadequacies in the positional noise function Ω, inadequacies in the sense that $\Omega(d)$ is either being underestimated or overestimated for a given value of d. Consider what would happen if $\Omega(d)$ is being underestimated. In this case, relative neighbors (of the match candidates) that should be determined to "match" by Ω will be found not to "match," since the underestimated noise radius of $\Omega(d)$ will be too small to permit the relative neighbors to be "matched." Besides resulting in a failure to contribute to the match score, the relative neighbors may become involved in a search for a below-threshold spot, which, in turn, may sometimes result in the creation of a virtual node that should not exist. Such virtual nodes may result in incorrect match categorizations. In sum, an underestimated Ω results in the detection of image differences where none exist. These "bogus" image differences may sometimes have very little effect on the accuracy of the algorithm, but also may result in a mismatch. (In particular, if the "bogus" image differences result in the false creation of an "orphan" match categorization, then the result is a false-positive error.)

Consider next what would happen if $\Omega(d)$ is being overestimated. In this case, relative neighbors that should not be determined to "match" by Ω will be found to "match," since the overestimated noise radius of $\Omega(d)$ will be large enough to allow the relative neighbors to be falsely "matched." Besides incorrectly increasing the match score (of the match candidates), the relative neighbors will not be seen as different and thus will not become involved in below-threshold searches. The relative neighbors will not be used to generate associated virtual nodes. The result of an overestimated Ω is a failure to detect image differences. As above, the failure to detect image differences may have very little effect on the accuracy of the algorithm or may result in a mismatch. In particular, if the missed image differences involve a missed mutation, then the result is a false-negative error.

It is useful to divide the examination of accuracy into an analysis of whether the errors occurred because Ω is being underestimated or overestimated, but it would be an oversimplification to assume that this exhausts all the possible reasons for mismatches. Two points are worth mentioning in this regard. First, only relatively small ("high-frequency") positional variations are meant to be embodied within Ω. For example, Ω is not intended to compensate for technical imperfections in the gels. Thus, while it may be useful to think of Ω as underestimating or overestimating the "true" distance between "matching" relative neighbors, it does not follow that Ω could be set to compensate for all kinds of positional variations. Further, while the first-order effects of an inaccurate Ω may result in either a missed or an "invented" difference, the second- and third-order effects of an inaccurate Ω are not as easily described. For example, consistent underestimation of Ω may be implicated in the creation of virtual nodes that eventually become matched. It is then possible, if these incorrect matches are not detected, that other spots that should not have been matched will become matched. Thus, the first-order effect of an underestimation of Ω may be the "invention" of an image difference, based upon the creation of an inappropriate virtual spot. If the error is not corrected, it may propagate other types of errors, a second-order effect.

We will now examine in greater detail some of the match categorizations realized in the family of gel images used to describe the comparison algorithm. Consider Figs. 20–22 in conjunction with the resulting match categorizations given in Table III. Summary information for this family is also shown on the *first* line of Table IV (family number 1). Table IV divides the total set of matches (55 of them, as indicated in the second column) into a set of correct matches and a set of mismatches. A further breakdown is made into "family" (FAM) versus "nonfamily" (NFAM) match categorizations. Consider first the "family" categorizations. Out of the 46 "family" categorizations, we have determined that five "family" categorizations were mismatches. [While visual inspection is a reasonable way to validate the algorithm's accuracy, there is the reasonable concern about any subjectivity that an observer brings to the inspection. This issue is addressed in greater detail in Skolnick (1984).] The match numbers corresponding to these mismatches are 11, 30, 32, 44, and 51 (refer to Figs. 20–22 and Table III).

Consider match 32, where the father's and childs's spots are correctly matched (as the upper spots of two vertically oriented spots that are near each other), while the mothers's match corresponds to the lower spot. In this case the feature-measurement algorithm failed to detect the lower spots on the father's and childs's gels (since they form shoulders on other spots, without individual maxima of their own). If the feature-measurement algorithms had detected the shoulder spots, then the correct family matches would have been made. Additionally, however, the comparison algorithm was not sufficiently sensitive to the positional differences; this resulted in the creation of virtual nodes both with reference to the lower spot of the child and the upper spots of the father and mother.

Consider match 30, a mismatch that is very similar to that of match 32. In this case, the father's and mother's spots (in this case, the two lower spots) are correctly matched, while the child's spot (the upper spot) is incorrectly matched with the father's and mother's spots. Figure 23 shows the relative neighborhood surrounding the mismatched spots of match 30. (The "matching" relative neighbors are enclosed in circles.) Since the distance between the mismatched spots is relatively small, there is a uniform, but small, shift in the positions of the relative neighbors with regard to each other. All the relative neighbors of the child's (match candidate) spot appear shifted downward (a small distance) from the relative neighbors of the father and mother. The values of $\Omega(d)$ operating at the distances d of these relative neighbors were accurate and did not overestimate the appropriate noise radii. Ω is intended to compensate for the small variations in relative distances of the relative neighbors. It is not intended to compensate for some consistent pattern over the entire neigh-

TABLE IV. Results of Comparison of 15 Mother–Father–Child Trios of Two-Dimensional Gels

Number	Number of matches	Correct matches			Mismatches			Causes			
		FAM	NFAM	Total	FAM	NFAM	Total	NF	FM	GEN	FPOS
Five American lysate gels											
1	55	41(76%)	4(7%)	45(83%)	5(8%)	5(9%)	10(17%)	7(12%)	3(5%)	2(4%)	3(5%)
2	60	45(75%)	10(17%)	55(92%)	2(3%)	3(5%)	5(8%)	5(8%)	0(0%)	2(3%)	1(2%)
3	59	38(64%)	9(15%)	47(80%)	5(8%)	7(12%)	12(20%)	12(20%)	0(0%)	5(8%)	3(5%)
4	51	42(82%)	3(6%)	45(88%)	4(8%)	2(4%)	6(12%)	6(12%)	0(0%)	3(6%)	1(2%)
5	54	28(52%)	7(13%)	35(65%)	7(13%)	12(22%)	19(35%)	17(31%)	2(3%)	8(15%)	0(0%)
	279	194(70%)	33(12%)	227(81%)	23(8%)	29(11%)	52(19%)	47(17%)	5(2%)	20(7%)	8(3%)
Five Japanese lysate gels											
6	58	44(76%)	5(9%)	49(85%)	2(3%)	7(12%)	9(15%)	6(10%)	3(5%)	5(9%)	0(0%)
7	57	44(77%)	4(7%)	48(84%)	3(5%)	6(11%)	9(16%)	4(7%)	5(9%)	6(11%)	0(0%)
8	50	43(86%)	1(2%)	44(88%)	0(0%)	6(12%)	6(12%)	1(2%)	5(10%)	2(4%)	0(0%)
9	53	35(66%)	2(4%)	37(70%)	4(8%)	12(22%)	16(30%)	11(21%)	5(9%)	8(15%)	1(2%)
10	52	36(69%)	1(2%)	37(71%)	7(13%)	8(16%)	15(29%)	12(23%)	3(6%)	9(17%)	1(2%)
	270	202(75%)	13(5%)	215(80%)	16(6%)	39(14%)	55(20%)	34(13%)	21(7%)	30(11%)	2(1%)
Five French platelet gels											
11	56	42(75%)	1(2%)	43(77%)	3(5%)	10(18%)	13(23%)	8(14%)	5(9%)	4(7%)	2(4%)
12	54	41(76%)	0(0%)	41(76%)	3(6%)	10(18%)	13(24%)	10(18%)	3(6%)	6(11%)	2(4%)
13	49	46(94%)	0(0%)	46(94%)	1(2%)	2(4%)	3(6%)	1(2%)	2(4%)	1(2%)	0(0%)
14	56	39(70%)	1(1%)	40(71%)	5(9%)	11(20%)	16(29%)	11(20%)	5(9%)	7(13%)	2(4%)
15	55	45(82%)	1(2%)	46(84%)	5(9%)	4(7%)	9(16%)	7(13%)	2(3%)	7(13%)	0(0%)
	270	213(79%)	3(1%)	216(80%)	17(6%)	37(14%)	54(20%)	37(14%)	17(6%)	25(9%)	6(2%)
	819	609(74%)	49(6%)	658(80%)	56(7%)	105(13%)	161(20%)	115(14%)	43(6%)	75(9%)	16(2%0)

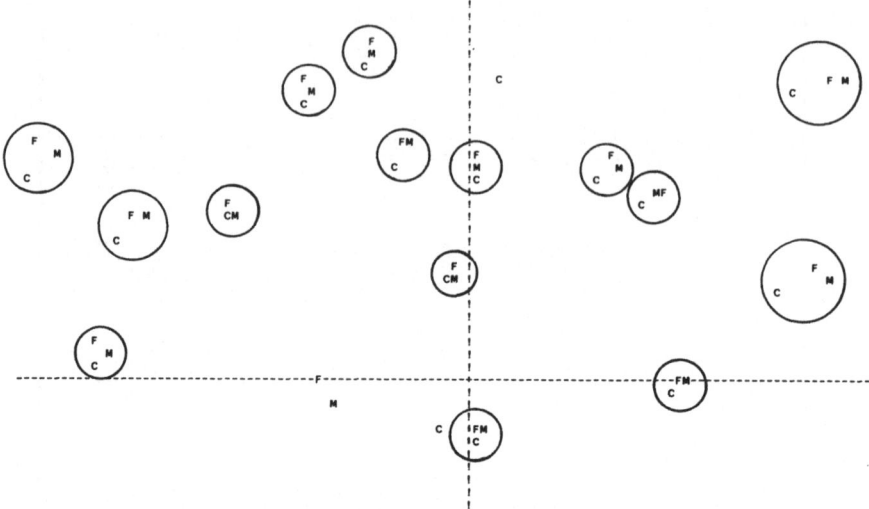

Fig. 23. Relative neighborhood of the mismatched spots of match 30, described in the text and illustrated in Figs. 20–22. The circles indicate "matching" relative neighbors. Note the characteristic pattern of a downward shift of the child's relative neighbors as compared with the relative neighbors of the father and mother.

borhood; e.g., involving a small (but uniform) shift downward in the relative neighbors of the child relative to those of the father and mother. In order to compensate for such patterns and thus detect the mismatches under consideration, the algorithm must be provided with more complex computational mechanisms; i.e., more complex procedures for maintaining accuracy, capable of detecting contextual patterns (like a uniform but small shift over the entire relative neighborhood). This will be a subject of the section on Improving the Accuracy of the Algorithm.

In the context of a search for mutation, what is critical is that a spot in the child be correctly identified as inherited if that is the case. Thus one can tolerate errors where a "family" categorization is incorrectly read but the participating spot from the child is correctly matched with one of the spots from either parent. The pattern of inheritance is detected in such a case, albeit not completely. For example, match 32 correctly matched the father's spot with that of the child (despite the fact that the mother's spot was not correctly matched). It represents a valid (but not quite accurately described) observation of a pattern of inheritance. On the other hand, match 30 correctly matched the father's and mother's spots, but failed to correctly match the child's spot. It represent a failure to observe a familial pattern. If the accuracy of the algorithm is assessed from the standpoint of how accurately image similarities and differences are detected, then these two mismatches represent two failures. On the other hand, if we approach this issue from the standpoint of estimating the rate of mutation, then only match 30 represents a failure.

Our statistics on the accuracy of the algorithm will reflect (and distinguish between) these two viewpoints. In Table IV all entries (except the second to last column) reflect the accuracy of the algorithm in terms of the broader issue of image comparison. The second to last column (labeled GEN) gives the number of mismatches that (from our genetic standpoint) represent valid observations of the inherited nature of the spot. Match number 32 is an example of a mismatched "family" categorization that preserved the inherited nature of the spot. It is also possible to have incorrect "fatherless" and "motherless" categorizations that preserve a genetic pattern; e.g., when a "fatherless" match missed the correct spot on the father's gel (creating a virtual spot on the father) but correctly matched the spots from the mother and child. Thus, while all mismatches involving "family," "fatherless," and "motherless" categorizations are counted in all but the GEN column of Table IV, those mismatches in these categories that correctly preserve a genetic pattern are counted in the GEN column. Out of the mismatches examined in the family under consideration, two matches (32 and 34) fall into this (more tolerable) class of mismatches. (We of course recognize the rare possibility of nongenetic reasons for familial polypeptides.)

In each of the five instances of family mismatches, it is a "lack of sensitivity" on the part of Ω that is the reason for the mismatch. Either Ω is insensitive because it is overestimated or it is encountering phenomena that it is not designed to accommodate (e.g., the small shifts throughout the neighborhood of mismatch number 30, discussed above). In Table IV, the number of mismatches due to insensitivity in Ω are counted in "Causes" column under NF, for "noise function." Five NF mismatches involving "family" categorizations have been accounted for up to this point. The remaining 2 NF mismatches involve instances were Ω is underestimated (resulting in incorrect non-"family" categorizations) and will be examined below. Thus, the results of the visual inspection to this point can be summarized as follows: out of the 46 "family" categorizations for this trio of gels, 41 were correct and five were mismatches. Mismatches involving incorrect categorizations of spots as "family" are always classified as NF errors.

We now consider the remaining nine nonfamily categorizations. Four matches (corresponding to match numbers 20, 21, 36, and 37) are confirmed by visual screening (and are entered into the fourth column of Table IV). Three matches (corresponding to match numbers 34, 38, and 54) are due to errors in the feature-measurement algorithms. That is, virtual nodes had to be created due to lack of robustness in the feature-measurement algorithms. These errors are indicated in the column labeled FM in Table IV. The two remaining nonfamily matches (corresponding to match numbers 35 and 49) are NF-related errors. Match number 49 is a result of underestimated values for Ω, resulting in the spurious creation of a virtual node in the child's gel. Match number 35 is actually a second-order effect of the mismatch in match 11; that is, match 11 put into correspondence a spot from the child with spots from the father and mother that did not match the child's; this resulted in spurious virtual nodes being created in the father and mother that eventually were matched to the "orphan" mismatch of match 35. These two NF errors are added to the five NF errors involving "family" categorizations, giving a total of seven NF errors.

We now consider the performance of the algorithm over a set of 15 family trios: five involved lysate gels prepared in our (American) laboratory; five involved lysate gels prepared by collaborators in Japan, and the last five involved gels prepared from platelets harvested by collaborators in France. (We thank Prof. G. Siest of the University of Nancy for his cooperation.) The output was compared with a visual analysis and classified according to the categories described above and is summarized in Table IV. Over all three groups, the range of correct matches varied between 65 and 94%, with an average of 80% correct matches. Of this average, 74% were family categorizations and 6% were nonfamily categorizations. On the other hand, 20% of the matches were mismatches. The percentage breakdown of the reasons for the mismatches is as follows: 14% were due to insensitivities related to the positional noise function (NF) and 6% were due to errors in the feature-measurement algorithms (FM). Considered in a different light, the 20% breaks down into 7% incorrectly categorized as "family" spots and 13% incorrectly categorized as nonfamily spots. At the same time, as mentioned above in terms of mismatches that correctly reflect the pattern of inheritance (e.g., "fatherless/"bachelor" mismatches), not all of the mismatches represent difficulties in the detection of mutations. Out of the 20% of mismatches, 9% did recognize that the spot detected in the child was familial. Thus, from the point of view of validating the algorithm for the study of mutation, 89% were correct and 11% were incorrect.

What do these figures mean? Basically, a little more than two-thirds of the mismatches are related to insensitivities in Ω and the remaining one-third are due mainly to errors originating in the feature-measurement algorithms. Thus, improvements to Ω should substantially reduce the error rate. At the same time, as mentioned above, there will always remain positional variations that cannot be embodied within Ω. These positional variations must be dealt with through improvements in the procedures for maintaining accuracy, a topic to be covered below (as well as improved standardization of the gels). The remaining one-third of the errors can be addressed through improvements to the feature-measurement algorithms (to be considered in future publications).

It is important to emphasize that as presently implemented, our algorithms are attempting to analyze all spots above a certain intensity. Often these are crowded together in "busy" regions of the gel, violating the conditions we introduced earlier as essential to accurate scoring. Altering the algorithm to eliminate such regions from consideration, as will be discussed later, would undoubtedly improve the performance of the algorithm.

It is of interest to consider how well the performance of our comparison algorithm compares with that of other algorithms. Here, the comparison is in terms of mismatches and not in terms of correct detection of inheritance patterns, since other algorithms are not concerned with the specific question of mutation. In general, the present accuracy of our comparison algorithm (on the average, 80%) is within the range reported by those investigators who provide measures of accuracy. For example, Miller *et al.* (1982) report that their semiautomatic comparison algorithm "is generally successful in matching 80–90% of the matchable spots" (p. 869). (Note that our analysis considered all spots to be "matchable.") Lemkin and Lipkin (1981*b*) report an accuracy measure "in the range of 70 to 85% depending upon the artifactual noise of the gels" (p. 373). The reasons for mismatches are generally described as involving such phenomena as spots on the borders of gels, regions of low spot density, and regions of overlapping or highly crowded spots. There is commonality both in the accuracy of our algorithm compared with other approaches and in the reasons given for inaccuracies. At the same time, it is worth keeping in mind that our approach is completely automatic. No set of initial matches ("landmarks" of "perfect reliability") are provided to the algorithm. In addition, some approaches (Garrels, 1984) permit the flagging of especially problematic spots, effectively removing them from the matching process. From the perspective of genetic monitoring, these operator interventions are costly and should be eliminated, or at least minimized. Finally, in this comparison of the relative accuracies of the various approaches, it should be kept in mind that whereas other investigators are comparing *two* images (often where one image is a "smoothed prototypic" image and the other an experimental run), we are comparing *three* images (all experimental runs). It is our impression that the mismatch rate is a complex nonlinear function of the number of gels compared; i.e., an error rate of 20% for three-way matches corresponds to a much lower rate for two-way matches. This impression is confirmed by the fact that the error rate is lowered to 11% when considering the (subset of) pairwise matches that preserve the pattern of inheritance.

It is worth reiterating that, because we are using two-dimensional gels for the particular purpose of studying mutation, an 80% accuracy in match categorizations is not as problematic as may initially appear. We have seen how the fact that a spot is an inherited trait can be correctly detected even in the presence of mismatches, effectively increasing the accuracy in our context to 89%. In addition, as indicated in the FPOS column of Table IV, only 2% of the mismatches were false positives (or false "orphan" categorizations). Of these entries, most were easily disposed of by visual inspection of a digitized image such as Fig. 2, but three (0.4% of total) required further study. Returning to the image files and expanding the resolution of the associated regions of the gels, we could demonstrate that two of the three "orphans" were due to unusually large differences in spot intensity between the child's spot and those of the parents. The remaining "orphan," which involves a complex change, is currently being analyzed further.

In our proposals for future improvements to the algorithm we will indicate steps which should substantially reduce the frequency of false orphans, to perhaps 1%. It would not be unreasonable to require an operator to check on this frequency of "orphan" categorizations.

Algorithm Performance on Simulated Mutations

Since the most troublesome error, from the point of view of studying mutation, is the false negative (failing to detect a "real orphan"), we next tested the system (including both the feature-measurement and image-comparison algorithms) by randomly placing an orphan spot within a digitized image of a child's gel. The two-dimensional gel trio used earlier to illustrate the comparison algorithm provided the framework for the experiment. The assumption was made that the 30 most heavily stained spots of each family member were being tested for the occurrence of a mutational event. As discussed earlier, a charge-change mutation in one of these 30 most intense spots (presumably representing the product of two alleles) can be expected to result in two spots, each with about half the intensity of the original spot. In order to test the ability of the system to detect such a mutational event, the threshold in the analysis was set at half the intensity of the least heavily stained of the 30 most heavily stained spots. A "typical" spot was selected from a digitized gel image and scaled down to correspond to the intensity set by that threshold. Then, a pair of x and y coordinates were generated by a random number generator and a mutant spot was added to the original digitized image at these coordinates. The corresponding gel trio was then subjected to the feature-measurement algorithms, followed by the comparison algorithm. (Since the test involves going to a threshold at half the intensity of the lowest of 30 spots, it became necessary to have the algorithm examine the 70 most intense spots on the gel images, resulting in a much denser pattern of spots. It then became clear that the form of Ω used to process the gels at a threshold of 30 spots was not adequate. Thus, we altered Ω to a more appropriate set of values, essentially decreasing the noise radii to compensate for the additional crowding.) This was repeated 100 times, each time using new randomly generated coordinates. Out of the 100 tests of the algorithm on the randomly placed "mutant" child spot, 70 of the orphans were correctly detected. Figure 24 shows the locations where each of the 100 mutant spots were placed on the child's gel. A location marked by a circle indicates a location where the mutant spot was detected.

We now consider the causes for the remaining 30 false-negative errors. Five of these errors resulted from the mutant spot being placed too close to the image borders for effective comparison with other members of the gel trio, since searching for corresponding spots on the father's or mother's images would have involved going beyond the image boundaries. The human eye would encounter the same problem. For each of these five errors the comparison algorithm removed the mutant, flagging it as not being suitable for comparison. These five errors are of little signifi-

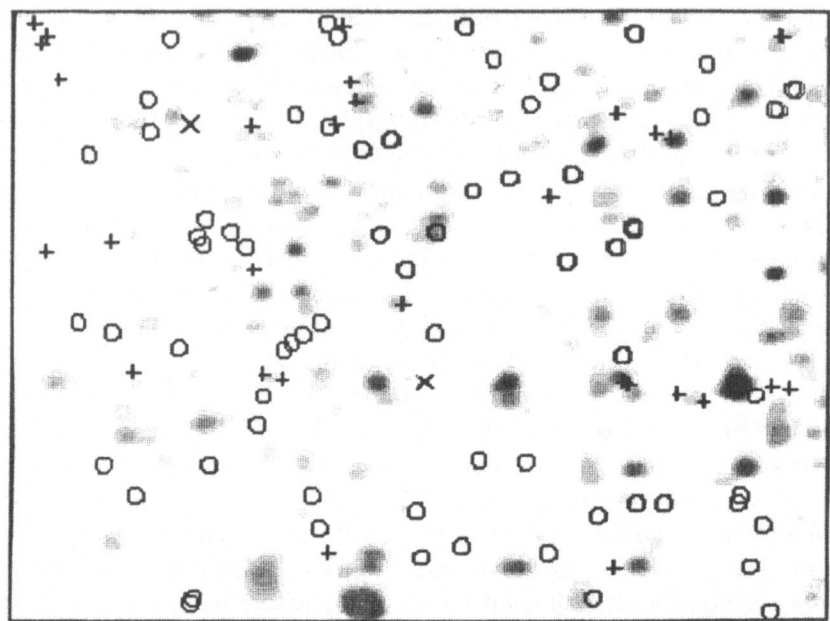

Fig. 24.   The locations in the child's gel of the randomly placed spots simulating a consequence of mutation. The circles represent detected mutations, the plus signs represent
missed mutations due to inadequacies in the feature measurement algorithms, and the crosses
represent missed mutations due to inadequacies in the comparison algorithm.

cance, since they would not have occurred if we were digitizing entire
gels or (assuming subsections of gels were being scored) if we allowed
the border spots to guide searches for matches onto other neighboring
sections of the digitized gels. These "border" errors represent technical
limitations of our current procedures that could easily be changed; e.g.,
by using a higher resolution digitizing camera.

   Eleven of the false-negative errors occurred due to inadequacies in
the feature-measurement algorithms. As indicated in the previous section,
substantial improvements to the feature-measurement algorithms are
needed. Twelve of the false-negative errors occurred because the mutant
spot was completely or partially superimposed on a preexisting spot, resulting only in a quantitative difference. It is doubtful whether visual
analysis would detect such events. The locations of the mutant spots
comprising these 28 errors ("border," "feature measurement," and "quantitative") are indicated by the crosses on Fig. 24. Of special interest in

our examination of the accuracy of the comparison algorithm are the remaining two errors, indicated by "X"'s on Fig. 24. These two errors fall into the category of failures in the sensitivity of the positional noise function. They were the result either of an inaccurate noise function or of a positional noise effect for which the noise function is not designed to compensate. Thus, of the 83 detectable orphans (i.e., after the elimination of the two sources of undetectable events), the algorithm detected 70, resulting in an 84% accuracy. While 16% is an undesirably high error rate, even now the algorithm could be applied to the study of mutation, since the proportion of mutations detected would be the same for the children of controls and of a presumptively mutagenized population. In the section on Improving the Accuracy of the Algorithm we will consider how the comparison algorithm could be modified to achieve a substantially lower rate of false-negative errors.

IMPROVING THE SYSTEM: NECESSARY DEVELOPMENTS IN THE ALGORITHM

In this section we consider some possibilities for improvement in the performance of the comparison algorithm.

A More Rigorous Treatment of the Noise Function

In general, little or no *a priori* knowledge exists about the characteristics of the positional noise in the images being compared. In this section, we consider a plausible scheme by which, as the comparison algorithm runs, statistics are gathered which are useful in generating an accurate estimate of Ω. Some of the ideas in this section have been implemented in a preliminary fashion and the results will be examined. The assumptions made in the effort to arrive at a more accurate estimate of Ω are at best oversimplified (and at worst are wrong), but at least are useful in quickly arriving at the heart of the matter. Inadequacies in the assumptions will be considered at the end of the section.

Consider how NMatch determines whether two relative neighbors "match" (see Fig. 8). A necessary condition for a "match" between relative neighbors r_F and s_M is that their relative distance $\text{RelD}(r_F, s_M)$ be less than the positional noise radius $\Omega(\text{MaxD}(r_F, s_M))$. [For the sake of conciseness we denote MaxD(r_F, s_M) as MaxD, and RelD(r_F, s_M) as RelD.] The positional noise radius Ω(MaxD) is an upper bound on the amount of positional distortion allowable at a given distance MaxD from the match candidates. At the same time, the actual relative distance RelD between the relative neighbors is a data point from the distribution of positional distortions within MaxD. This suggests that, if these data points are saved, they will provide information relevant to performing a statistical analysis of the positional noise distribution. After all matching has been completed, these data points can be used to estimate a more accurate Ω. (In order to ensure as accurate an estimate as possible, the RelD data points should only be collected during the validation pass of the comparison algorithm.)

The current image comparison algorithm can be used to gather these statistics and, in turn, these statistics can be used to determine the form of Ω used to compare the images presented in this work. In order to use the comparison algorithm to gather these statistics it is necessary to have some *a priori* estimate of Ω, since the comparison algorithm requires Ω to run. Accordingly, and somewhat arbitrarily, we have explored the consequences of initially setting $\Omega(d) = d/4$. The comparison algorithm was then run on a single family with this initial noise function and, as NMatch determined that two relative neighbors "matched," the distribution was obtained of the actual relative distance RelD associated with the distance MaxD from the match candidates. (While MaxD and RelD are real numbers, they were truncated in order to reduce the statistics to integer values.) The three histograms shown in Fig. 25 correspond, respectively, to the distribution of the RelD values sampled at MaxD distances (from the match candidates) equal to 25, 50, and 75. For example, in the histogram of Fig. 25a, a relative distance of 2 was recorded seven times between relative neighbors (where the maximally distant relative neighbor was a distance of 25 from the match candidates). There was only a single event characterized by a relative distance equal to 4 and no such events beyond 4. As MaxD increases, the distribution covers ever increasing values, confirming the basic intuition that Ω should be a nondecreasing function.

The next step was to estimate from each distribution the appropriate value of the new Ω. Despite the fact that the histograms are constructed from RelD values collected during the validation pass of the algorithm, spurious RelD values (not representative of the true distribution) may still contribute to the observed distribution. One reason for this, as we have seen, is that matches are not completely accurate and gels are occasionally

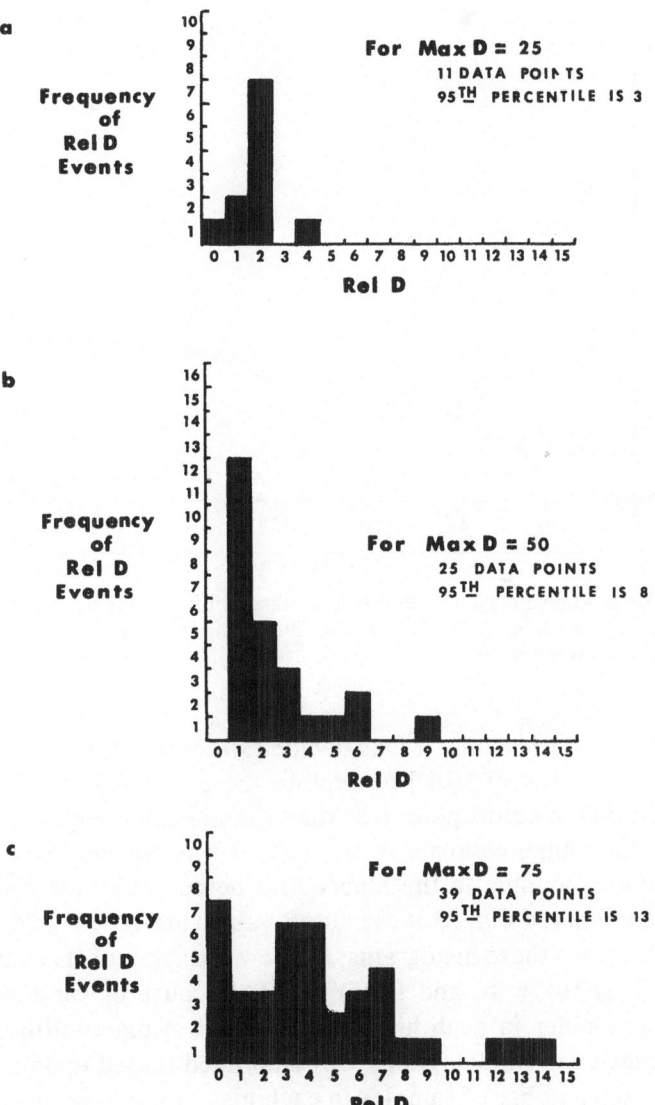

Fig. 25. Three histograms representing distributions useful in estimating Ω. Further explanation in the text.

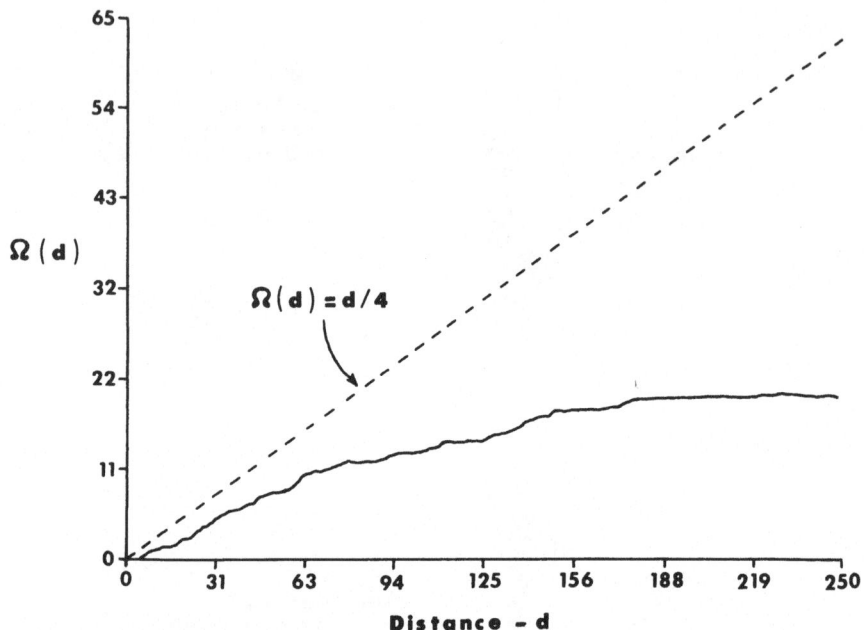

Fig. 26.   The positional noise function Ω as estimated by (—) the comparison algorithm and (– –) an *a priori* form of Ω, $\Omega(d) = d/4$, initially used by the comparison algorithm. Further explanation in the text.

flawed. For these reasons, it was decided [in order to determine the appropriate new value of $\Omega(d)$] to explore the consequences of choosing, for each MaxD, a cutoff point less than the maximum entry in each distribution. The initial estimate of the new Ω was equated to the relative distance corresponding to the ninety-fifth percentile of the distribution. In the histograms of Fig. 25 these cutoff values are at 3, 8, and 13. Thus, based solely upon these histograms, the new estimates of Ω are as follows: $\Omega(25) = 3$, $\Omega(50) = 8$, and $\Omega(75) = 13$. Because of variations in the number of samples in each histogram, the set of ninety-fifth percentile cutoff values over all histograms was smoothed (based upon a weighted average of the number of samples in each histogram) to produce the new estimated Ω shown in Fig. 26 (as compared with the initial *a priori* form of Ω).

When Ω as estimated by this procedure was used to compare gels, there were fewer errors than when the *a priori* form of Ω, $\Omega(d) = d/4$, was used. Nevertheless, the estimated form of Ω resulted in too many

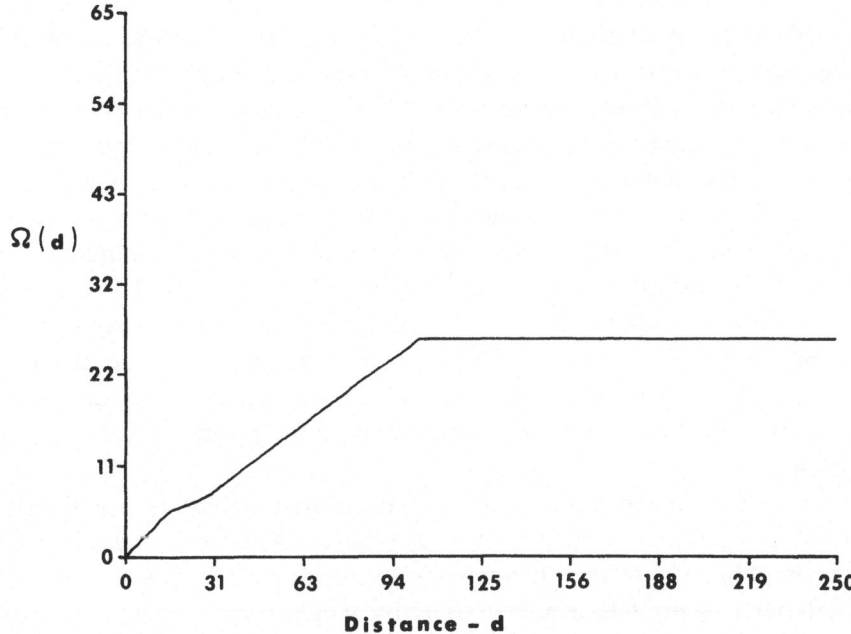

Fig. 27.   The form of Ω used to process images.

errors (in our opinion), making it clear that the procedures outlined above overly simplify a complex situation. Accordingly, the automatically estimated form of Ω (shown in Fig. 26) was altered (by hand) in order to provide comparison results more consistent with visual criteria. This was done based upon the idea, presented above, that Ω can either underestimate or overestimate the true positional noise radius. For example, if we noticed that within a given set of MaxD values the comparison algorithm was generating spurious virtual nodes, then this meant that Ω was being underestimated (for the given set of MaxD values); the associated values of Ω were then increased some small amount (by hand). The new form of Ω would then be tested to see if the spurious virtal nodes disappeared, the procedure being repeated if necessary. Likewise, if it was apparent that a specific value of Ω was placing noncorresponding nodes into correspondence, then the value of Ω was decreased. Using this procedure to iteratively "tune" Ω, we arrived at the function shown in Fig. 27; it is the form of Ω used to process the images presented in this chapter.

There are many reasons why the current procedure for estimating Ω is inadequate. Most obvious is that the current form of Ω was estimated from statistics restricted to a single gel type in a single family and no allowance is made for the possibly differing characteristics of various types of two-dimensional gels (e.g., nucleated white blood cells versus non-nucleated platelets). A more fundamental issue involves how to detect RelD values that skew the distributions because they result from distortions (such as stretches in the fragile gels or pH discontinuities in the first dimension) that should not be embodied within Ω. The use of a ninety-fifth percentile cutoff is obviously inadequate for this purpose. In the next section we will consider how the algorithm could be made to detect such distortions and, in turn, exclude the statistics associated with the distortions from the process of estimating the positional noise distribution.

Another problem with the current procedure involves the use of RelD as the basic sample unit. The use of relative distances is certainly an oversimplification of the phenomenon of positional noise. Recall that Ω is intended to provide a noise radius by which relative neighhbors are judged to "match" and that the concept of a "noise radius" is restricted to the distance between points on the plane. No attention is paid to the vertical and horizontal axes individually. In the two-dimensional gel problem, considering the relevant distances on each axis separately might be important, since the physical processes used to generate each axis depend on different attributes (molecular weight, isoelectric point). Thus, it is likely that the noise characteristics of the two dimensions are not the same. This suggests that RelD-based statistics might profitably be decomposed into vertical and horizontal components to be studied independently, resulting in the decomposition of Ω into vertical and horizontal components. In addition, we have found that the positional noise characteristics vary systematically depending upon the region of a gel; e.g., high-molecular weight proteins are subject to less positional variations than low-molecular weight proteins. These considerations all point to the need to make both Ω and the statistical procedures for estimating Ω more complex. In any case, regardless of the complexity of Ω or the associated estimation procedure, the fact remains that the comparison algorithm can be used to estimate a "parameter" Ω fundamental to the comparison process.

Improving the Accuracy of the Algorithm

While a more accurate form of Ω would render the task of maintaining accuracy easier, one encounters positional variations in two-dimensional gels that cannot be embodied in Ω. The detection and management of these other types of positional variations will be the focus of this section. A more elaborate class of routines must be added to the current comparison algorithm to deal with these other classes of positional variation, especially if we are to approach the degree of confidence required in the application of the comparison algorithm to the detection of mutations. It is worth bearing in mind that, for less demanding applications, less complex procedures for maintaining accuracy are necessary. The mechanisms we suggest are intended to indicate how the comparison algorithm would have to deal with the (more general) accuracy problem as it presents itself in this genetic application. For other applications, various subsets of the proposed accuracy maintenance procedures would suffice.

Besides increasing the power of the algorithm, the improvements in achieving accuracy will clarify the nature of the image comparison problem. Accuracy of the output involves being able to distinguish between various classes of variation in images. Every increase in the type of variation that the algorithm must consider increases the need for sophisticated routines to ensure accuracy. We will show how these more complex procedures give rise to more "intelligent" behavior from the algorithm. It becomes feasible to have the algorithm "reason" about the inconsistencies is encounters. For example, some pattern of events may alert the algorithm to the possibility of a mismatch; then, the algorithm would be able to determine whether there is any (contextual) evidence that confirms the initial hypothesis of mismatch.

Analysis of Current Procedures for Maintaining Accuracy

We begin our discussion of possible improvements in the maintenance of accuracy by examining how the cross-correlational measure of similarity can give rise to mismatches. Recall that the cross-correlational measure for determining the similarity of relative neighborhoods is defined by the Sim function. In turn, Sim makes use of judgments concerning which, if any, of the relative neighbors are close enough to be considered "matching," judgments performed by the NMatch function and based upon Ω. Thus, the dependence upon Ω to determine whether two relative neighbors "match" (in conjunction either with inaccuracies in Ω or in the inability of Ω to embody all types of noise) is at the heart of inaccuracy. This dependence of the similarity measure on an Ω which accurately embodies the noise characteristics of the visual environment has implications for how accuracy of the output can be ensured. Basically, the measures used in ensuring accuracy must not directly use Ω, since any errors introduced in the similarity measure by Ω will be repeated if the checks for accuracy use Ω. Rather, as we will see, one approach to maintaining accuracy should involve determining the consistency with which Ω is applied.

Consider how mismatches are detected by the current comparison algorithm. In NMatchV [the version of NMatch given in formula (9) with an accuracy check], the added condition for achieving accuracy requires that, when relative neighbors are considered to be "*matching*" by Ω, they must also have the same *match* state. Thus, if one of the "matching" relative neighbors has been matched, then the other relative neighbor must be matched and have the same match number. From the standpoints of NMatch and the noise function, two relative neighbors may be seen as "*matching*" based upon their proximity. At the same time, the similarity measure of the two relative neighbors (in the role of match candidates) may result in a *match*. The check for equality of match states in NMatchV is a way to detect inconsistencies between two different "perspectives" on the relative neighbors: that of the relative neighbors as "viewed" by some other match candidates versus that of the relative neighbors themselves as match candidates. We will refer to these inconsistencies as "match"/match inconsistencies. Detection of such inconsistencies provides a mechanism for checking accuracy which is independent of Ω, in the sense that the mechanism focuses on the consistency with which Ω is applied and does not directly use Ω.

Once inconsistencies are detected, action must be taken to correct them. In the current spot comparison algorithm, inconsistent relative neighbors are not counted as "matching"; i.e., NMatchV returns a value of zero. This action—not to count the relative neighbors as "matching"— leads to the removal of inconsistent matches by decreasing the similarity measure to the point where it falls below threshold. Removing inconsistent matches frees spots for new, and presumably correct, match assignments. In addition, NMatchV (besides removing inconsistent matches) requires that any new matches also not contain inconsistencies. This helps ensure that the new matches will be correct. (Since NMatchV is constrained in this manner, it is possible to loosen the constraints on the similarity measure threshold AccepNumMatches, as is done in the match verification pass of the current algorithm.) At the same time, failure to score relative neighbors as "matching" is a limited action based upon limited information. The action is not based upon any knowledge concerning how the inconsistencies arise and no attention is given to the pattern of the "match"/match inconsistencies. The only information to which NMatchV has access (from the "perspective" of the match candidates) is that the relative neighbors are not matching, contradicting the indication by Ω that the relative neighbors are "matching." The issue of ensuring accuracy concerns the types of information relevant both to the detection of mismatches and to the determination of actions to be taken. The current comparison algorithm is limited in both of these regards.

Patterns of Inaccuracy Involving Contextual Information

More complex information about the patterns of inconsistencies can be incorporated into the comparison algorithm. As in much of the analysis in this work, we start with Ω. Ω can either overestimate or underestimate the "true" noise radius. It is important to consider what it means to have an inaccurate estimate of the "true" noise function. Since Ω may be applied in particular situations (e.g., gel imperfections) where the positional noise encountered is not the high-frequency noise for which Ω is intended, no correct setting for Ω may exist in the particular situation (which is consistent with the embodiment within Ω of high-frequency noise). In other words, if Ω is not estimating the "true" noise radius, it does not necessarily follow that Ω should be changed. At the same time, in all situations in which Ω is applied, it is useful to consider some "true" noise radius to exist (whether or not that noise radius could be produced by Ω).

Overestimating or underestimating the "true" noise radius results in well-defined discrete "patterns," which the algorithm is capable of detecting. The patterns are based upon the ways in which "match"/match inconsistencies can occur. These patterns can alert the algorithm to potential problems. The algorithm then can allocate additional computational resources to investigate the reasons for these problems. One possible reason is that Ω is not correctly "tuned" to the noise characteristics; i.e., the noise radius specified by Ω should be changed. On the other hand, Ω may be correctly "tuned" but the algorithm is encountering noise where the noise radius provided by Ω is, in principle, incapable of estimating the "true" noise radius. In what follows, when we refer to underestimates or overestimates in Ω we are referring to Ω as not providing the "true" noise radius. There is no implication that Ω should be modified, even though this is one of many possibilities.

With respect to overestimates in Ω, it is possible to view the decision by NMatch as to whether two relative neighbors "match" as having some degree of uncertainty. To whatever extent it is possible that Ω is overestimating positional noise, the decision that the relative neighbors "match" is uncertain. When a "match" is determined to exist there is a sense in which NMatch is making an implicit "prediction," namely, that the relative neighbors will match some time in the future. Suppose that the comparison algorithm were to save information about the predicted match. If the relative neighbors eventually become matched, then the decision of NMatch would be supported. On the other hand, if the relative neighbors did not match, then the decision of NMatch would not be supported. In the current version of the comparison algorithm, NMatchV can be thought of as determining whether the relative neighbors that were "matched" during the nonverification stage of the algorithm were indeed correctly matched. In a sense NMatchV verifies the "predictions" made by NMatch during the nonverifying stage. Our discussion is intended to show how one could make "predictions" and verify them in a more flexible manner; i.e., without separating the algorithm into two different stages of nonverification (using NMatch) followed by verification (using NMatch V).

A "match" prediction that is not confirmed is evidence that Ω has overestimated the "true" noise radius. Under what circumstances can this happen? One possibility is that the match candidates (from which the "match" prediction is made) are incorrectly matched. Another possibility is that the match candidates are correctly matched, but the current match of the relative neighbors is incorrect. A further possibility is that both the match candidates and the relative neighbors may be matched correctly, but there may be a flaw in the gels (unrelated to any inaccuracies in Ω), causing the prediction to fail. It is also possible that the noise radius provided by Ω is overestimating the (high-frequency) positional noise characteristic; in other words, the noise radius should be decreased, resulting in a better "tuned" form of Ω. Finally, if we think of Ω as performing a threshold operation (based upon some cutoff on the distribution of positional noise variations), then it may be that the cutoff overestimates the "true" noise radius. Viewed as a threshold operation, Ω is subject to the same kinds of variations about a threshold that have been mentioned in other contexts.

Underestimating the "true" noise radius results in NMatch determining that neighbors are not "matching" when, in fact, they should be "matching." As above, a non-"match" determination functions as a prediction, with an associated uncertainty rooted in the possibility that the "true" noise radius is being underestimated. Consider what happens when a relative neighbor is not "matched." On the one hand, the neighbor may be used to provide constraints in a search for a missing below-threshold spot. Such a search results in the addition of either a below-threshold or virtual node. On the other hand, the neighbor may be too distant from the match candidates to induce a below-threshold search. In either case, when no "match" is determined to exist, NMatch can be thought of as making an implicit prediction about matches at some future point in time. When a below-threshold node is found or a virtual node is created, then the "prediction" is that a node will eventually be found to match the "nonmatching" neighbor that guided the search. On the other hand, if the neighbor is too distant to induce a search, there is (at the very least) the "prediction" that it should not be found later to "match" with some other near (but outside the noise radius) relative neighbor. As above, a failed non-"match" prediction can have many different causes. If the prediction fails, it may be that Ω should be changed; e.g., by increasing the noise radius provided by Ω. On the other hand, it may be that some other form of noise, not associated with the high-frequency variety embodied in Ω, is being encountered.

The failure of a "match" (or non-"match") prediction can be interpreted as resulting from an overestimation (or underestimation) by Ω of the "true" noise radius. At the same time, there are many possible causes for a failed prediction; e.g., Ω may be providing the wrong noise radius, the algorithm may be encountering positional variations for which Ω is not intended, the algorithm may be involved in a mismatch, etc. This ambiguity as to the cause of a failed prediction is a result of the fact that the prediction only concerns how the match candidates "view" the relative neighbors. There is no information concerning how the relative neighbors "view" the match candidates nor about how other neighbors "view" the relative neighbors and match candidates. Thus, in order to get a clear resolution of the reason for the failed prediction, it would seem that if a "match" or non-"match" prediction fails, then the algorithm must investigate the reason for the failure. This involves getting more information concerning how other neighbors "view" the situation. In other words, it involves incorporating more contextual information into the decision-making process of the comparison algorithm.

Let us consider in more concrete terms how the algorithm could be developed to use the contextual information we have been discussing. Suppose that at some point in time the algorithm detects a "match"/match inconsistency. For example, from the perspective of two match candidates some relative neighbors are detected that do not match but, at the same time, are determined to "match" by Ω. The procedure within the comparison algorithm that evaluates the match score of the match candidates could send a "message" to the procedure within the comparison algorithm responsible for maintaining accuracy. The message would contain information about "who" saw it (the match candidates), what was the pattern detected (a "match" prediction that was not confirmed), and "who" was involved in the pattern (the particular relative neighbors). The accuracy maintenance procedure, upon receipt of this message, could check if it has received any other messages that might confirm (or deny) the following hypotheses (among others): a gel distortion in the image; an inadequacy in Ω; a possible mutational event; nothing of importance. The procedure responsible for maintaining accuracy may be programmed to pospone actions until further information is obtained; e.g., in investigating the possibility of a localized gel distortion, the algorithm could see if other matches in the immediate vicinity encounter patterns that confirm that possibility.

The development discussed above, which would be responsible for integrating all this contextual information (arriving in the form of messages), is in effect building a "model" of the gel "environment." In other words, the system integrates the messages by attempting to form an interpretation that is consistent with the vast majority of messages. At some point in time, enough information would be accrued to take either "real" or "informational" actions; e.g., removing a mismatch ("real") or alerting other procedures that a gel distortion has been detected ("informational"). The "match"/match inconsistencies can be thought of as "primitive" inconsistency hypotheses. These hypotheses serve to draw the "attention" of the algorithm to potential problem areas. The algorithm, once alerted, can devote additional computational resources to understanding the causes of the primitive inconsistency hypothesis. This can eventually result in the removal of inconsistent matches and the building of a model of the match and distortion process. As we continue our discussion, we will describe further patterns of inconsistencies (useful in generating primitive inconsistency hypotheses) and how they lead to the generation of a more sophisticated model of the images being compared. Recent work in artificial intelligence provides a useful computational framework for implementing this kind of system. In particular, the programming language "Prolog" (Clocksin and Mellish, 1981)—an integral part of the Japanese fifth generation of computers—is a useful tool for implementing the kind of (message passing) system being proposed. In addition, the type of system under consideration can be implemented as a "production system" (Davis and King, 1976) using the programming language OPS5 (Brownston, *et al.*, 1985).

Up to this point, our considerations of more complex procedures for ensuring accuracy have been based upon a failed prediction which occurs over *time*. For example, "match"/match inconsistencies occur when, at a given point in time, the algorithm detects an inconsistency between the *current* "match" decision (involving relative neighbors and based upon Ω) and a *previous* decision concerning whether the relative neighbors match (where the relative neighbors were considered to be match candidates). We will now consider how certain match patterns over *space* are worthy of attention. The first match pattern to be considered is useful in the detection and resolution of mismatches caused by an underestimated Ω. If Ω is underestimated, then "matches" that should have been made will be missed, resulting in the spurious creation of virtual nodes. What pattern might such errors create? Consider the gel matches shown on Figs. 28–30 and, in particular, match numbers 22, 3, and 30. There are two spots in each individual that participated in the three matches. That is, match number 22 is an orphan, match number 3 is a family, and match number 30 is childless. Based upon visual examination, it seems that the six spots should have been matched into two "family" categorizations, as opposed to have been "divided" among three matches. What happened in this case was that virtual nodes were falsely created from match number 25 (the nearest neighboring match), where match number 25 is a false orphan; i.e., virtual nodes have been falsely created because of the relative isolation of the spot pairs, the distortions affecting the

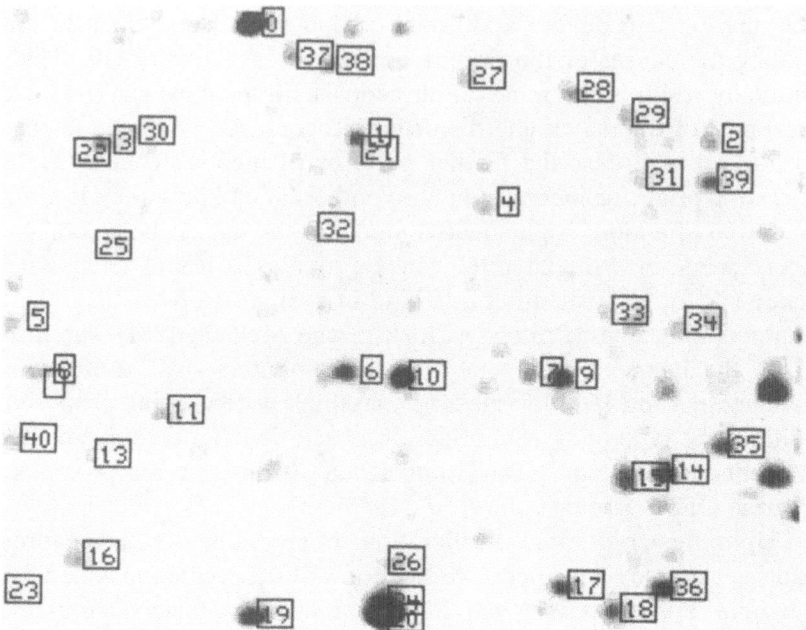

Fig. 28.   Father's match graph illustrating orphan/family/childless error pattern. See text.

position of their distant neighbors, inadequacies in Ω, and possibly other, even more complex reasons. These falsely created virtual nodes give rise to the pattern of orphan/family/childless as one moves upward from match 22, through match 3, to match 30. The observed (nonvirtual) child spot in match 22 should have been paired with spots of the mother and father, resulting in a family categorization in match 3. In turn, the child spot that was observed in match 3 should have been matched with the observed mother and father spots of match 30. It would seem then that the match category pattern of orphan/family/childless would be a useful pattern to look for in the search for spurious virtual nodes. More generally, any pattern which could result from the misalignment of two spots would also be useful, for example, fatherless/family/bachelor and motherless/family/ spinster. As above, it is important to realize that these patterns occur where errors *may* have occurred and represent primitive inconsistency hypotheses. Thus, their detection may only be the beginning of a search for further information to determine the true situation (in this case, causing match number 25 to be reconsidered).

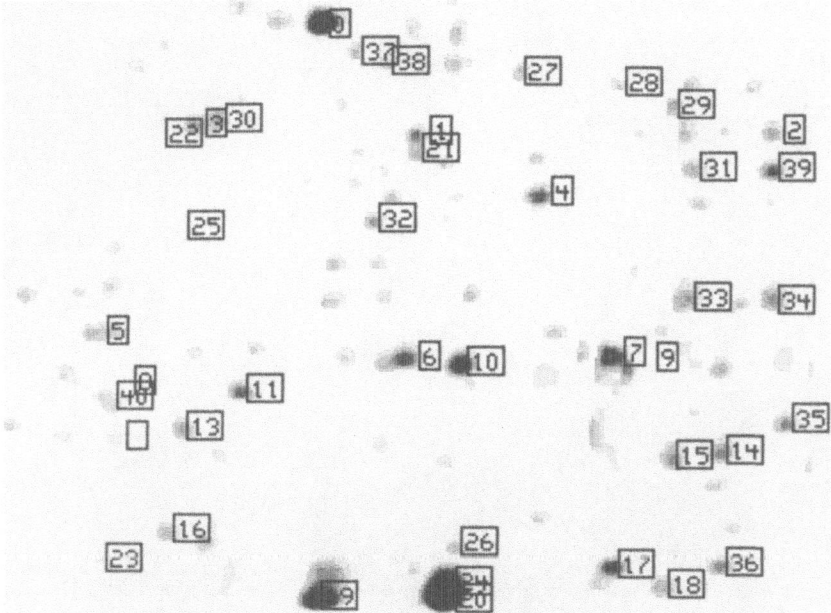

Fig. 29.   Mother's match graph illustrating orphan/family/childless error pattern. See text.

Other match patterns are of use in the maintenance of accuracy and in the development by the algorithm of an appropriate model of environmental noise. Consider the spatial pattern of relative neighbors in Fig. 9. As one moves from the origin to the left, there is an increase in distortion in the gels of the father and mother relative to the child. Assume that such distortions could be detected by the algorithm and in turn be confirmed from the perspective of other match candidates. Again, there is the possibility of building a more sophisticated model of noise. For example, if the pattern in Fig. 9 arises from distortions in the two-dimensional gels and if other match candidates, vertically aligned with the match candidates of Fig. 9, showed the same (or a consistent) distortion pattern, then the algorithm would be justified in concluding that the indicated region is subject to some distortion. This information might then be fed back into the matching procedures so that their "decisions" (e.g., as embodied in NMatch) reflect this new information. This gives rise to a more sophisticated model of noise in the sense that such distortions might be distinguished from the "normal" positional distortions intended to be

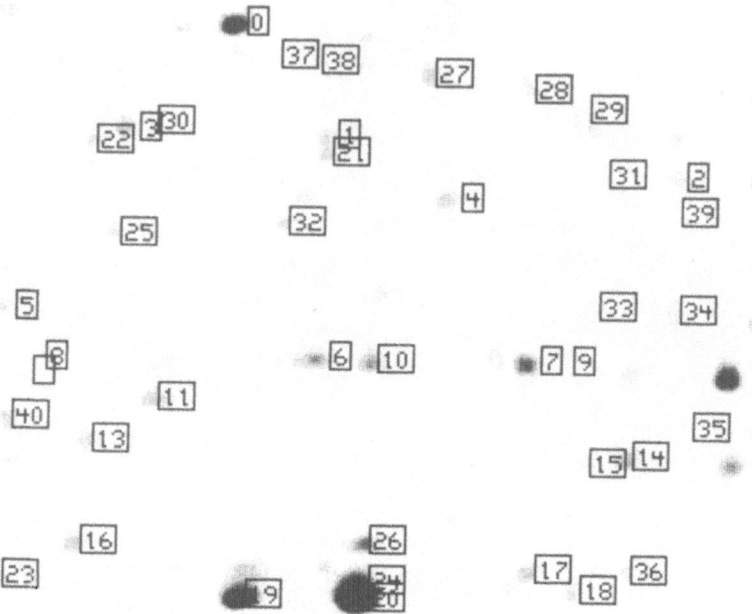

Fig. 30.   Child's match graph illustrating orphan/family/childless error pattern. See text.

modeled by Ω. Besides aiding accuracy, such models would allow for a better estimation of the statistics for determining a more accurate Ω.

Still another match pattern involves the spatial pattern of unmatched nodes (indicated by empty boxes on the gel figures). These are nodes that, despite all attempts by the algorithm, cannot be matched. Consider Figs. 28–30, where there is an inconsistency (not detected by the current procedures) involving match numbers 40 and 8. Match number 40 looks correct, but match number 8 looks incorrect. In this case, the mismatch began from match number 5. That is, match number 5 on the gel of the mother should be the spot immediately above the matched spot. Because the relative neighbors of match number 5 extended far into the image and Ω overestimated the proper noise radius, the error in match number 5 was not detected. This resulted in the "crowding" of match number 8 and the spurious creation of virtual nodes. An improved algorithm could use the occurrence of such unmatched nodes as a clue to a likely region for reinvestigation. In this way, the original error of match number 5 might be detected, in turn leading to the correction of match number 8.

Inherent Difficulties in Achieving Complete Accuracy

In the foregoing, we have attempted to provide imagery concerning patterns of events over space and time that are relevant to improving the accuracy of the output. The patterns over time involve discrepancies between "match" and match predictions. The patterns over space involve configurations of match categorizations that can be the result of match errors. These patterns should be easily detected by the algorithm. At the same time, these patterns result in hypotheses that must be termed "primitive," in the sense that they are ambiguous as to cause. The ambiguity resides in the fact that the hypotheses incorporate only a minimal amount of contextual information. In order to resolve the underlying causes of these primitive hypotheses, an improved algorithm could integrate the set of hypotheses into a consistent interpretation of what is happening; i.e., a model of the images being compared. The additional complexity in the proposed algorithm for maintaining accuracy results from the complexities involved in using more contextual information.

To a large extent, the proposed mechanisms for ensuring accuracy are intended to compensate for some of the basic inadequacies of the cross-correlational measure of similarity. Basically, cross-correlation can only consider the similarity in the spatial pattern of the relative neighbors of match candidates. When certain relative neighbors are determined to "match," the similarity measure is increased. At the same time, one would expect that if the similarity measure were applied to the relative neighbors, it would confirm the similarity measure of the match candidates. A basic problem of cross-correlational measures is that it is impossible, when the cross-correlation is measuring the similarity of relative neighborhood patterns surrounding match candidates, to incorporate *simultaneously* information about the spatial similarity of the neighborhoods surrounding the relative neighbors. In other words, the cross-correlation function cannot, as it evaluates the similarity pattern from a given pair of match candidates, simultaneously incorporate information about the similarity measures of the relative neighbors, and of the relative neighbors of the relative neighbors, and so on. It is in this sense that cross-correlation remains a myopic measure and one must consider ways to integrate the multiple perspectives of these measures as they are distributed in space. Embedding a check for consistency in the match label assignments of relative neighbors is one way of compensating for the inability of cross-correlational measures to consider higher order effects, such as whether the similarity measure of match candidates is consistent with that of their relative neighbors, and of the neighbors' neighbors, and so on.

There exists another mechanism, different from those already proposed, for integrating the multiple perspectives of the cross-correlation. This mechanism is specified by a class of relaxation algorithms (Rosenfeld, 1978; Rosenfeld *et al.*, 1976; Davis and Rosenfeld, 1981). Relaxation algorithms, when applied to the general image comparison problem (Kahl *et al.*, 1980; Ranade and Rosenfeld, 1980; Barnard and Thompson, 1980), start with a cross-correlational measure of the spatial pattern of relative neighbors. The measure is translated into the probability that the match candidates match. The initial probabilities for all match candidates are then altered by measuring the *average* amount of discontinuity between the similarity measures of the match candidates and the similarity measures of their relative neighbors. If the similarity measures of the match candidates and their relative neighbors are close, then the probability of the match candidates being a match is increased. Conversely, to the extent that there is a difference between the similarity measures, then the probability is decreased. A single "step" of a relaxation algorithm can be thought of as involving a recomputation (in parallel) of all of the match probabilities, based upon the the degree of discontinuity between "neighboring" probabilities. The entire relaxation algorithm iterates some number of these "steps" until the probabilities cease to show much change. At each iteration the network of probable match assignments is altered to be *minimally distorting* in relation to the relative neighbors. Information about relative neighbors ever more distant from the match candidates is (at each iteration) incorporated into the probabilities that the match candidates match. After a period of time, the network of probability assignments converges to a set of assignments upon which the algorithm cannot improve.

It is interesting to consider how the proposed comparison algorithm differs from a relaxation algorithm. Basically, the difference lies in the way in which accuracy is maintained or, in other words, the way in which the myopia of a cross-correlational similarity measure is overcome. With relaxation the match state is consistent with neighboring match states if its similarity measure is close to the similarity measure of its neighbors. In other words, there is a basic identification of *inconsistency* with *discontinuity*. This, in turn, is a reflection of the fact that relaxation focuses on the image correspondences that are minimally distorting with respect to perfect registration. Relaxation algorithms were developed for image comparison problems where differences between images can justifiably be treated as noise: stereopsis (Barnard and Fischler, 1982) and motion detection (Ullman, 1979). In contrast, the problem of comparing two-dimensional gels focuses on differences between images just as much as on correspondences. While the cross-correlation measure is justifiably biased toward minimizing distortion, the two-dimensional gel comparison problem requires that we be concerned with those relatively few situations where assumptions that minimize distortion lead to incorrect determinations of the similarities and differences between images.

Comparison of Approaches to Maintaining Accuracy

We are now in a better position to consider other approaches to the comparison of two-dimensional gels. Common to all approaches is the use of some criterion of distortion minimization in the procedures for determining spot correspondences. In our algorithm, the criterion of minimization appears in the way in which NMatch determines "matches"; i.e., based upon the relative neighbors being a minimal distance apart (in addition to falling within the bounds of Ω). Lemkin and Lipkin (1981b) use a similar minimization criterion (in conjunction with a simpler positional noise function) that allows their algorithm to determine spot matches. Miller et al. (1982), Taylor et al. (1981), and Garrels et al. (1984) estimate a linear transformation to put spots into correspondence (followed by matches based upon nearest neighbors). Insofar as a linear transformation is a first approximation to the actual distortions operative within a region, it, too, can be viewed as a procedure that minimizes distortion. It is worth reiterating that, for the most part, the minimization of distortion produces the "correct" results, the term "correct" having different meanings according to the context of the analysis. Errors currently have a frequency of 11–20% with our algorithm, 10–20% with Miller's, and 15–30% with Lemkin's. (Note that the percentage of errors for our algorithm is not directly comparable to those of the other investigators, since their approaches require a certain amount of "editing" of the gels by operator interaction. In addition, as noted above, our figures represent the errors from a comparison of three gel images, whereas the other investigators are concerned with pairwise comparisons.) In fact, it is only because the minimization criterion works so well that the algorithms are capable of detecting mismatches, mismatches that result from situations where the distortion minimization assumption is invalid.

A fundamental difference between gel comparison algorithms is in how the issue of consistency maintenance is addressed. Lemkin and Lipkin (1981*b*), Miller *et al.* (1982), Taylor *et al.* (1982), and Garrels *et al.* (1984) all rely on some form of operator intervention to identify an initial set of "landmark spot" matches, which then provide the initial set of matches from which their algorithms determine the remaining set of matches. In terms of detecting errors in the remaining matches, all of these systems make use of operator intervention to remove any subsequent errors introduced by their comparison programs. While this is most certainly useful, it has removed the pressure on their algorithms to have complex mechanisms for assuring accuracy. Since our comparison algorithm was designed with the intent of as little operator intervention as possible (due to the large number of gels to be examined in the measurement of the rate of mutation), we have had to confront the accuracy issue in a more detailed fashion. Where these other comparison algorithms do attempt to deal with the issue of accuracy, there are certain commonalities of approach to ours. Thus, both Garrels *et al.* (1984) and Lemkin and Lipkin (1981*b*) utilize multiple passes over the unmatched spots, attempting to classify spots within each pass as to the certainty of their matches. The initial passes are constrained to match only those spots that either (according to some heuristics based upon a set of parameters) are better candidates for matches (Garrels *et al.*, 1984) or are participating in more certain matches (Lemkin and Lipkin, 1981*b*). This introduces the more certain matches early in the analysis, which matches then can be used as a basis for resolving the more difficult matches. At the same time, the commonalities to our approach exist only at a surface level. We have tried to suggest that the best way to ensure accuracy involves the construction of a model of the images being compared, by developing algorithms that systematically incorporate contextual information into the matching process. Only through these higher levels of "reasoning" can we achieve the performance necessary for the application of two dimensional gels to the detection of mutational events.

Increasing the Speed of Execution

We restrict our discussion of speed of execution to the comparison algorithm. The time complexity of the feature-measurement algorithms is negligible in this context, given the existence of specialized hardware. The feature-measurement algorithms process images on the scale of seconds, while the comparison algorithm operates on the scale of minutes.

There are two operations of interest in terms of a time complexity analysis of the comparison algorithm. The first operation measures the computation needed to determine the neighbors of a spot; i.e., the computation of the generalized Gabriel graph. The second operation measures the computation needed to determine the match score of spots on father, mother and child images. Basically, the first operation measures the graph construction component of the algorithm, while the second operation measures the comparison component. We will make the simplifying assumption that there are n spots on the gels of the three individuals being compared. Despite the fact that more (virtual and below-threshold) spots will be added as the comparison algorithm proceeds, this is a reasonable assumption, since the ratio of new spots added to the initial number n will be small.

The time to compute the generalized Gabriel graph of n nodes is $O(n^3)$, since there are n^2 potential edges and for each edge the other n spots may require examination (to determine if the edge construction criterion is violated). The time complexity of the comparison component can be estimated by considering the number of times the similarity function Sim is computed. For each of the n spots on the father's gel, Sim is used to calculate the similarity measure with spots on the mother's gel [in a restricted region specified by the MaxDistortion parameter in Eq. (7)]. Let the number of such spots in the mother be a maximum of k, where k is much smaller than n. Thus, the number of times the match score is computed between the father and mother is nk. Similarly, for each mother's node found to have an acceptable score, Sim will be computed with spots from a similar region on the child's gel. If we assume that the child will also have a maximum of k spots, then the total complexity of the comparison component of the algorithm is nk^2. Furthermore, by making the simplifying assumption that k equals the square root of n, the comparison component takes on an $O(n^2)$ complexity. (This assumption is based upon the fact that the MaxDistortion parameter is an order of magnitude less than the dimensions of the images. Thus, k should be roughly an order of magnitude less than n.)

This analysis is confirmed from data collected on the actual run time behavior of the algorithm. The data consist of the number of times the subroutines corresponding to the graph construction and comparison op-

TABLE V. Number of Graph Construction and Comparison
Operations As a Function of Number of Spots

Number of spots n	Number of operations	
	Comparison (Sim)	Construction (GabrielG)
40	1189	163,261
60	2241	461,709
80	3350	1,021,740
100	5276	1,915,405
Approximately equal to	$n^2/2$	$2n^3$
Order of complexity	n^2	n^3

erations are called. The subroutine "GabrielG" is responsible for checking the edge construction criterion and the subroutine "Sim" is responsible for calculating the similarity measure between two spots on different
individuals. Table V shows the number of times GabrielG and Sim were
called for different values of n, where n varies over the set {40, 60, 80,
100}. Notice that the number of times each subroutine is called corresponds to the order of complexity determined above; the abstract analysis
of the computational complexity is a valid simplification of the actual
behavior of the algorithm.

The time complexity analysis and data indicate that the dominant
task in the comparison algorithm is the determination of spot neighborhoods through the process of graph construction. In other words, the
$O(n^3)$ process will dominate any lower order process; e.g., $O(n^2)$. At the
same time, it is important to realize that the complexity analysis only
deals with the number of times a given operation is performed and ignores
the complexity of the operation itself. Thus, if substantial improvements
can be made in the complexity of the graph construction operation, it is
possible to reduce significantly its effect on the total complexity of the
algorithm.

To this end, consider the subroutine (GabrielG) that determines
whether a given node (NodeK) violates the edge construction criterion
between two other nodes (NodeI and NodeJ). To make the decision,
GabrielG measures the distance between NodeK and NodeI and between
NodeK and NodeJ. This gives rise to a fundamental issue concerning the

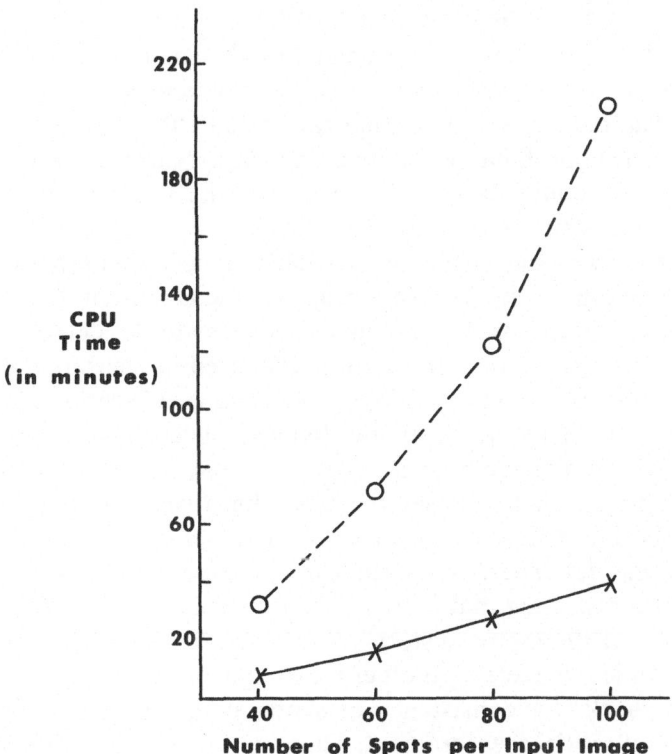

Fig. 31.　Graph contrasting run time with (- -) a Euclidean versus (——) a non-Euclidean metric. The *x* axis measures the number of spots per input image and the *y* axis measures the CPU minutes for the comparison algorithm to run on a VAX 11/780.

metric to be used to compute distance. The most intuitive metric is Euclidean, but it is computationally costly, since it uses floating point operations and numerical approximation routines for the square root function. Other metrics can be used, which distort Euclidean space but have the advantage of being computationally efficient. For example, the maximum metric takes the maximum of the coordinates of a point to measure the distance of the point from the origin (as opposed to the square root of the sum of the individually squared coordinates, as in the Euclidean metric). A number of experiments were performed in order to compare the relative efficiencies of the Euclidean and maximum metrics. Figure 31 shows the run times, under input sizes of *n* varying over the set {40, 60, 80, 100}, of the comparison algorithm using the two metrics. The

Euclidean-based run times are indicated by the dashed line and the non-Euclidean-based run times are indicated by the solid line. The algorithm was run on a VAX 11/780 under UNIX and the time is measured in CPU minutes. The comparison algorithm ran in 204 CPU min under the Euclidean metric (a prohibitive run time for a large-scale study), while it ran in 40 CPU min under the non-Euclidean metric. Dramatic time savings were achieved with the maximum metric.

In the above experiment, the Euclidean metric was replaced by the non-Euclidean maximum metric throughout the algorithm. Not only was the maximum metric used to compute distances in the determination of the relative neighbors of a spot, but it was used in measuring distances in the match score and in determining the locations of searches for below-threshold spots. This brings up an obvious concern about possible distortions which may have been introduced. It may at first seem surprising that over the set of test cases the algorithm (using the non-Euclidean metric) introduced less than 1% new mismatches (as compared with the Euclidean metric). There are a number of reasons for this robustness in the face of a distorting (but more efficient) metric. Most immediately, to the extent that the metric distorts all measurements equally, the effects of distortion are canceled. Another reason for this robustness is that the algorithm checks for consistency of match assignments in a manner independent of spatial measurement. Thus, even if a non-Euclidean metric were to introduce mismatches, these matches must have neighbors consistent in terms of their match labelings. The match labelings, in turn, are judged to be consistent if the labelings are identical, and not based upon the closeness in relative coordinate space, no matter what metric is used. As we have seen, consistency maintenance requires examining the consistency with which the positional noise function is applied. An independence from the noise function is achieved, which, in turn, ensures independence from a potentially distorting non-Euclidean metric (the metric being a basic part of the noise measurement process).

A compromise position, in terms of the choice between nondistortion and efficiency, is possible. Assume that the non-Euclidean metric was used only to generate neighborhoods, with the Euclidean metric being retained in the comparison process. Distortions introduced by the non-Euclidean metric would result only in differences in the relative neighborhoods of matching spots. At the same time, differences in relative neighborhoods of matching spots are reconciled through the below-threshold search mechanisms. That is, if a relative neighbor fails to appear in the neighborhoood of a match (due to the distorting effects of a non-Euclidean metric) and its "matching" relative neighbor on another individual is determined to be in the neighborhood, then the latter relative neighbor will guide a search for the former relative neighbor. The ability to search for below-threshold spots allows the algorithm to compensate for noise-related variations in the appearance and disappearance of neighboring spots. Up to this point, such variations were due to the fundamental uncertainty involved in a feature—measure threshold. Now, for the sake of efficiency, the same below-threshold search mechanism can also compensate for variations due to the distorting effect of a non-Euclidean metric. The above "compromise" position should still provide the kinds of improvement in run time illustrated in Fig. 31.

A run time requiring 40 CPU min (for the comparison of three individuals, for each of whom 100 spots are scored) is in our opinion still undesirably long. Two steps are being taken to make the computer operation more efficient. On the one hand, there are many more ways to increase the efficiency of the algorithm. For example, it may be possible to replace the computations that are currrently based on real numbers (represented as floating point values on a computer) entirely with integer-valued computations. For example, given the speculations (presented in the section on A More Rigorous Treatment of the Noise Function, p. 123) concerning the decomposition of the positional noise function into separate x and y comoponents, it may be possible to decompose distance measurements into separate one-dimensional components (involving the absolute values of integers). We are also considering other less computationally costly means for determining the neighborhood of a spot. On the other hand, we are in the process of bringing all the routines of the current system, beginning with the digitizing, up on a dedicated computer (a Motorola 68000 CPU with specialized hardware for the feature-measurement algorithms). We anticipate that the total time to analyze a trio can be reduced to 20 min. on the 68000 computer. (Even this improved run time is probably more than that required for visual scoring of the same gels. The gain is in the fact that the computer does not tire and the technician is relieved for other tasks.) We see this latter system as a first step toward greater efficiency. Improvements in run time by a factor of three or four should be achieved if the system is implemented on a more powerful dedicated computer.

Introduction of a Priori Knowledge

The current comparison algorithm is designed to compare automatically gel family trios without the benefit of any prior knowledge about the gels. This is a fundamental capability of the algorithm in the sense that it is being used to detect events about which no prior information exists; i.e., mutations. At the same time, the introduction of *a priori* information into the algorithm is desirable for the development of a truly sophisticated system for monitoring mutation.

One of the primary limitations of the current comparison algorithm involves the inability to compare and tabulate the results of family comparisons across families automatically. For each family trio of gels the final output of the current comparison algorithm consists of a labeling of the matched spots (some of which may be virtual spots) on each gel image. Each match has an associated match number. Across two arbitrary family trios of gels, the match numbers of matching spots within families need not be the same. In order to tabulate the comparison results across different families, an operator is currently required to examine visually the comparison output so as to record the results in terms of the individual spots undergoing screening, each such spot bearing an arbitrary designation (Neel *et al.*, 1984). (In time these arbitrary designations will be replaced by a biologically meaningful nomenclature, comparable to the evolution of a biological nomenclature for the abnormal hemoglobins.)

A mechanism for the automatic tabulation of corresponding information across families can be provided by introducing *a priori* information into the comparison algorithm. Once the completely automatic algorithm is run on an initial sample of families for the various gel preparations, then those spots to be screened (based upon the criteria of intensity and isolation, as mentioned above) will be determined, along with characteristic "constellations" of neighboring spots which surround the spots being screened. The characteristic constellations for each spot to be screened can be stored on a disk file. This amounts to developing a reference file. A modified version of the current comparison algorithm can then be run on new family gel trios, with the difference that as the algorithm matches spots it will determine whether there is a constellation of neighboring spots (associated with a disk file) which matches the neighborhood patterns of new spots being matched. If a newly confirmed match has a similar neighborhood pattern as a neighborhood pattern on one of the disk files, then the comparison algorithm can automatically tabulate the comparison results for the spot associated with the saved neighborhood pattern. The current comparison algorithm can be easily modified to use the *a priori* information saved on the disk files, since the match score used to match new spots can just as easily be used to match these new spots with the spot pattern saved on a disk file. *A priori* information about characteristic constellations of spots allows the algorithm to restrict its sampling to a subset of spots having desirable properties for our purposes (isolation and size, as mentioned above). This can result not only in more accurate results, but in increased efficiency in the algorithm (since the algorithm need not compare all spots above a given threshold on the gels, as is currently done).

The *a priori* information to be incorporated into the algorithm could also include (improved) data on spot quantity. Since the total amount of protein in the sample used to load a given gel will always be subjected to some sampling variations, the integrated volumes of the spots (assuming that they are accurately measured by the feature-measurement algorithms) need to be normalized in order to be useful in cross-gel comparisons. Using *a priori* constellations of spots, the algorithm could identify (on different gels) some set of "normalizing" spots. Their measured intensities would form the basis of a normalizing process: the normalized intensity of a spot would be the ratio of its measured intensity to the sum of the measured intensities of the set of "normalizing" spots.

The ability to normalize spot intensity measurements could greatly increase the accuracy of the comparison algorithm. Consider how on two-dimensional gels it is generally reasonable to expect the differences between the amount of polypeptide in matching spots to be small. This means that (normalized) spot size would be a useful feature in determining "matches." For example, if two relative neighbors are determined to "match" by Ω based upon their locations relative to each other, then they should be similar in amount. The current comparison algorithm computes a match score involving the cross-correlation of a two-dimensional pattern of points in the plane (i.e., the coordinates of the relative neighbors). If the algorithm had available a normalized measure of spot quantity, then the cross-correlational measure could be generalized to a third dimension. This additional dimension would increase the certainty of the cross-correlational measure. The generalization of the current algorithm to the use of such multidimensional feature information is considered in greater detail in Skolnick (1984).

If there are gel regions that may exhibit characteristic forms of distortion, then *a priori* knowledge about such regions would allow the algorithm to identify and adopt special procedures for interpreting them. *A priori* information can also be used to detect more general classes of "events" that are relevant to the accuracy of the output. While it is generally true (as mentioned above) that matching spots should be quantitatively similar, there is one infrequent situation when matching spots may not be the same size. One result of certain types of mutation is that the protein product associated with the normal allele should be halved in quantity relative to matching spots on other individuals. Thus, a very important event such as a mutation will violate the general rule that intensities of matching spots should be comparable. The algorithm can be programmed to detect unusual events such as halved intensities. Such events are rare and should result in the algorithm "entertaining the hypothesis" that a mutational event has occurred.

In the section on Improving the Accuracy of the Algorithm, production systems (Davis and King, 1976) were mentioned as appropriate computational structures for future enhancements to the algorithm. In recent years, there has been much research in computer science devoted to incorporating *a priori* information into such a computational framework, a research area commonly referred to as "expert systems" (Hayes-Roth *et al.*, 1983; Brownston *et al.*, 1985). All of the suggestions that we have entertained for incorporating *a priori* information into the comparison algorithm can be viewed as a proposal for incorporating "expert system" mechanisms into the algorithm. Some of the "expert" knowledge corresponds to knowledge about specific spots. Other "expert" knowledge provides constraints specific to the use of two-dimensional gels in the study of mutation; e.g., knowledge about mutations resulting in a halving of spot size. Still other "expert" knowledge involves more general procedures for ensuring accuracy; e.g., the match patterns over space and time.

IMPROVING THE SYSTEM: NECESSARY DEVELOPMENTS IN TWO-DIMENSIONAL GELS

Two developments can be visualized with reference to two-dimensional gels, which would contribute greatly to the effectiveness of the approach we are advocating:

1. *Greater standardization of the gel technology.* Two-dimensional

elecrophoresis is a very demanding technology, still, given its introduction in 1975, in its infancy. Under close scrutiny, even after allowance for segregating genetic variation, in no two gels will the pattern of spots be found to be completely superimposable. Much of this can currently be explained by minor day-to-day variations in the casting of both first- and second-dimension gels, by minor temperature variations at various steps in the procedures, by variations in the polypeptide content of the gel inoculum, by discontinuities (perceptible and imperceptible) in the first-dimension "noodle," by variations in reagents from manufacturer's batch to batch, etc. The need for standardization of the ampholytes used in the gels is especially acute. In the context of our needs, the impact of these sources of variability can and is being minimized by strict attention to detail and by running gels on the members of a trio simultaneously, but this does not meet the problem of the noise in the comparison of gels run at intervals of several months or in different laboratories. One obvious, highly desirable development would be commercially available, highly standardized, precast gels. The silver-staining procedures continue to improve (Tollaksen et al., 1984); a further possible development would be greater reproducibility in the ability of some silver-based stains to impart various colors to the polypeptides; i.e., to introduce reliable color coding to the procedures. Finally, more attention needs to be addressed to the study of enzyme activities in gels run under less denaturing conditions than are current (Manabe et al., 1979); the judicious use of enzyme substrates coupled with dye reduction techniques offers a further opportunity for "color coding" of potential use in studies of mutation.

It may well be that even after all possible steps have been taken, there will remain subtle gel-to-gel variations. Polypeptides are after all complex, amphoteric compounds, some with specific binding functions, which may be fulfilled to variable degrees from individual to individual. Each gel may have its own Gestalt and the possibility of familial Gestalts cannot be excluded, and indeed, from preliminary data, seems quite likely (Neel et al., 1984).

2. *Simple and effective procedures for fractionating suspensions of proteins.* A silver-stained gel based on an erythrocyte, platelet, or lymphocyte lysate presents an embarrassment of riches. It is difficult to identify, out of the hundreds of spots present, a subset of more than 40 or 50 that approach the ideal criteria for scoring mentioned earlier. Increasing the size of the gels is a step in the right direction, but since the migrational distance of variants from the polypeptide of origin is also increased, this

does not solve the problem of superimposed spots. One needs to fractionate the polypeptides in a sample by some criterion unrelated to molecular size or charge, such as hydrophobicity. Any efforts in this direction must bear in mind that the primary criteria in using two-dimensional gels for monitoring for mutation is efficiency. Thus, if separation of a suspension into two fractions on the basis of hydrophobicity of the polypeptides doubled the time involved in an analysis but only resulted in a 40% increase in the amount of information, it would not be an effective procedure in a screening mode (although it might be in other contexts).

EXPERIMENTAL VALIDATION OF THIS APPROACH

Although the ability of one-dimensional electrophoresis to detect very probable mutations in both humans (Satoh et al., 1982) and experimental mammals (Soares, 1979; Johnson et al., 1981; Johnson and Lewis, 1981, 1983) is well established, a similar empirical demonstration of the potential of the technically more demanding two-dimensional methodology for genetic monitoring is highly desirable. Two "approaches", which could be combined within a single experiment, present themselves. Male mice should be treated either with high (approximately 500 rem) doses of radiation or a potent chemical mutagen and mated to females of the same inbred strain. (It would be desirable to conduct experiments with both forms of treatment in parallel, since the extent to which radiation induces mutations resulting in electrophoretic variants is unknown.) Appropriate controls should of course be examined. The use of inbred strains will minimize background genetic noise in the experiment, and presumably permit the use of the same "mother" and "father" gel for all the F_1 of a particular experiment, although appropriate checks are indicated. To avoid results unduly influenced by the idiosyncrasies of a particular strain it would be desirable to replicate the experiment in three or four different lines. Because the protein indicators of mutation will be "standard equipment," no time-consuming synthesis of special strains is necessary for the experiment. The male offspring of treated animals should be mated to several females (to preserve their gene pool) and then sacrificed, and multiple tissues examined by two-dimensional gels (liver, kidney, skin, erythrocytes, etc.). In the event of an unusual finding in these F_1, it can be followed up in the F_2; otherwise the F_2 can be discarded at birth.

The various two-dimensional preparations from each F_1 should be scored both visually and by the improved version of the current algorithm we have been discussing. In addition to this primary validation procedure, a secondary validation can be embedded in the design. The data on detected orphan spots can be managed by two different approaches, one "orthodox," the other "unorthodox." The orthodox approach involves the examination of each gel of each F_1 for orphan spots and, in the event one is detected, an effort to relate the spot to a preselected group of near-ideal reference spots. Orphan spots will be scored as mutations only if by the criteria of intensity, proximity, whatever color clues are available, and, where possible, chemical characterization they can be related to the reference spots. Breeding experiments will be performed to validate the genetic nature of each orphan. Mutation rates will be calculated as frequency of orphan spots/total locus tests. This is a conservative approach.

If with respect to each of the preparations the image reflected the genetic state of several hundred loci encoding for polypeptides, which, were they to occur in a mutant form, would usually be recognizable as an orphan spot, then only a minority of mutations could be related to the "ideal" spots mentioned above, and considerable information would be sacrificed. An unorthodox procedure is to score each orphan as a mutation, after verification by appropriate breeding experiments. An opinion concerning the mutagenicity of a treatment would be based on a comparison of the numbers of (genetically transmitted) orphan spots occurring in identical numbers of gels from treated and untreated animals. Approximate mutation rates could be obtained by estimating the number of polypeptides in each gel whose intensity, at the threshold chosen for the analysis, was such that a mutant product of roughly half that intensity would be detectable. With either the orthodox or unorthodox approach some adjustment in the observed mutation rates would be necessary because of mutation resulting in polypeptides superimposed on preexisting polypeptides and so undetectable. The mutation simulation experiments described earlier should be useful in this respect.

SOME ISSUES IN DATA MANAGEMENT

A principal thrust of this presentation is that a combination of developments is making it possible to search for smaller increases in mutation rates in both experimental and human populations than was previously feasible. This development, however, raises some major questions in data management. As noted earlier, given the rarity of mutations, an appropriate study will require millions of observations, the exact number depending on the populations under study and the desired accuracy. How should a data file of this magnitude be managed, especially for a heterogeneous (highly heterozygous) human population? At one extreme, one can visualize a file with separate entries with reference to each polypeptide scored, these entries including information on associated variants, nature of variant, integrated density of spot, etc. Only the results on polypeptides meeting rather rigid criteria for scoring would be admitted into the data bank, and only mutations that can definitely be related to these polypeptides would be scored. Other possible mutations would be ignored. This would result in relatively "clean" numerators and denominators. At the other extreme, one can visualize a data base in which the entry for each gel is simply the number of *properly verified* orphan spots and the number (estimated or counted) of spots scored, the computer output (see Table III) being filed separately. In either event, a separate file would be established for the results of the special studies necessary to characterize orphan spots, and negatives should be preserved of all scored gels.

The former type of procedure would result, in addition to the information on mutation, in a vast body of information on human qualitative and quantitative variation, as well as coordinate variation, but at a very major expense in computer and technical time. The latter procedure would be much less demanding, but informative only with reference to the specific matter of mutation.

The issue of the moment, as documented in the introductory section, is mutation, not the study of genetic variation. The authors would thus hope that the murine experiment just described would also include an effort to validate the latter procedure for data management, with the proviso that the gel information be stored on high-quality negatives rather than as a digitized image on tape or disk. This is in the belief that with current technology for digitizing images, it will be less expensive to redigitize a negative when needed than to maintain an extensive file of digitized images.

SUMMARY

An algorithm dedicated to the detection of presumed mutational events involving the polypeptides displayed with two-dimensional polyacrylamide gel electrophoresis has been described. Because of the large number of gels necessary in most studies of mutation, the algorithm has been designed to minimize operator intervention in its execution. The basic principle involves a comparison of the graph structures of the gels of a father, mother, and one or more children, searching for protein spots in the child not found in either parent. These so-called "orphan" spots are considered a probable manifestation of mutation only after other possible causes of such an isolated event have been excluded as rigorously as possible.

At present, the analysis of gels prepared from a platelet or erythrocyte lysate yields about 2% "false-positive" findings, i.e., results in the incorrect designation of a unique spot in a child. These errors can be disposed of by technician intervention. In an experiment designed to simulate the occurrence of mutational events, the algorithm operated with 70% accuracy. Most of the "errors" ("false negatives") occurred when the position of the simulated mutant polypeptide coincided in whole or part with that of a preexisting polypeptide, resulting in a class of mutation not detectable by the eye either. With correction for this fact, the accuracy was 84%.

Possible improvements in the algorithm which would substantially increase accuracy have been discussed at some length, as have some ideas as to how to manage the large body of data resulting from the operation of the algorithm. A murine experiment designed to validate the approach has been outlined.

RECENT DEVELOPMENTS

During the period in which this paper has been written there have been several noteworthy developments. The gel comparison algorithm has been implemented on a dedicated Motorolla 68000-based system with special purpose image processing hardware. A trio of gel sections can now be compared in approximately ten minutes (including the time to digitize and perform feature measurements). Since the 68000 CPU is a microcomputer with restricted computational power, the system is limited in the sophistication of its procedures for maintaining accuracy (as compared with the "reasoning" capabilities outlined in this paper). Thus, extensive viewing and editing facilities have been added so that the user can modify any incorrect matches made by the algorithm. The 68000-

based system will be used in our initial examination of the two-dimensional gels and should also be useful to the larger community of two-dimensional gel researchers.

Simultaneously, a more powerful A.I.-based system is being developed to implement a completely automatic algorithm with the capabilities for maintaining accuracy outlined in this paper. The A.I.-based system will utilize a Symbolics 3600 Lisp computer attached to the special purpose image processing hardware of the 68000-based machine. It is our intention to use this system for the automatic analysis of the large number of gel trios (with the high degree of accuracy) required in the estimation of the rate of mutation.

ACKNOWLEDGMENTS.   The original investigations described in this chapter were supported by National Cancer Institute grant CA-26803 and Department of Energy contract ER-60089.

REFERENCES

Aasakawa, J., Takahashi, N., Neel, J. V., and Rosenblum, B. B., 1985, Two-dimensional gel studies of genetic variation in the plasma proteins of Amerindians and Japanese, *Human Genetics* **70**:222–230.
Ames, B. N., 1983, Dietary carcinogens and anticarcinogens, *Science* **221**:1256–1264.
Anderson, L., and Anderson, N. G., 1977, High resolution two-dimensional electrophoresis of human plasma proteins, *Proc. Natl. Acad. Sci. USA* **74**:5421–5425.
Anderson, N. L., Taylor, J., Scandora, A. E., Coulter, B. P., and Anderson, N. G., 1981, The TYCHO system for computer analysis of two-dimensional gel electrophoresis patterns, *Clin. Chem.* **27**:1807–1820.
Baird, H. S., and Steiglitz, K., 1982, A linear programming approach to noisy template matching, in: *Proceedings IEEE Conference on Pattern Recognition and Image Processing*, pp. 50–57, IEEE Computer Society Press, New York.
Barnard, S. T., and Fischler, M. A., 1982, Computational stereo, *ACM Computing Surv.* **14**(4):553–572.
Barnard, S. T., and Thompson, W. B., 1980, Disparity analysis of images, *IEEE Trans. Pattern Anal. Machine Intell.* **2**:333–340.
Barrow, H. G., Tenenbaum, J. M., and Bolles, H. C., 1977, Parametric correspondences and chamfer matching: Two new techniques for image matching, *Proc. IJCAI* **77**:659–663.
Bossinger, J., Miller, M. J., Vo, K. P., Geiduschek, E. P., and Xuong, N. H., 1979, Quantitative analysis of two-dimensional electrophoretograms, *J. Biol. Chem.* **254**:7986–7998.
Burks, A. W. (ed.), 1970, *Essays on Cellular Automata*, University of Illinois Press.
Brownston, L., Farrell, R., Kant, E., and Martin, N., 1985, *Programming Expert Systems in OPS5: An Introduction to Rule Board Programming*, Addison-Wesley, Reading, Massachusetts.

Burr, D. J., 1981, A dynamic model for image registration, *Comput. Graph. Image Proc.* **15**:102–112.

Celis, J. E., and Bravo, R. (eds.), 1984, *Two-dimensional Gel Electrophoresis of Proteins*, pp. xvi and 487, Academic Press, New York.

Clocksin, W. F., and Mellish, C. S., 1981, *Programming in Prolog*, Springer-Verlag, New York.

Comings, D. E., 1982, Two-dimensional gel electrophoresis of human brain proteins. III. Genetic and non-genetic variation in 145 brains, *Clin. Chem.* **28**:798–804.

Davis, R., and King, J., 1976, An Overview of Production Systems, in: *Machine Intelligence 8* (E. W. Elcock and D. Mitchie, eds.), pp. 300–332, Wiley, New York.

Davis, L. S., and Rosenfeld, A., 1981, Cooperating processes for low-level vision: A survey, *Artif. Intell.* **17**:245–263.

Denniston, C., 1982, Low level radiation and genetic risk estimation in man, *Annu. Rev. Genet.* **16**:329–355.

Dunn, M. J., and Burghes, A. H. M., 1983, High resolution two-dimensional polyacrylamide gel electrophoresis, I and II, *Electrophoresis* **4**:97–116, 173–189.

Eastman Kodak Co., 1983, Kodavue electrophoresis visualization kit, Trade Brochure.

Gabriel, K. R., and Sokal, R. R., 1969, A new statistical approach to geographic variation analysis, *Syst. Zool.* **18**:259–270.

Garrels, J. I., Farrar, J. T., and Burwell, C. B., 1984, The QUEST system for computer-analyzed two-dimensional electrophoresis of proteins, in: *Methods and Applications of Two Dimensional Gel Electrophoresis of Proteins* (J. E. Celis and R. Bravo, eds.), pp. 38–92, Academic Press, New York.

Goldman, D., and Merril, C. R., 1983, Human lymphocyte polymorphisms detected by quantitative two-dimensional electrophoresis, *Am. J. Hum. Genet.* **35**:827–837.

Hamaguchi, H., Ohta, A., Mukai, R., Yabe, E., and Yamada M., 1981, Genetic analysis of human lymphocyte proteins by two-dimensional gel electrophoresis. I. Detection of genetic variant polypeptides in PHA-stimulated peripheral blood lymphocytes, *Hum. Genet.* **59**:215–220.

Hamaguchi, H., Yamada, M., Noguchi, A., Fujii, K., Shibasaki, M., Mukai, R., Yabe, T., and Kondo, I., 1982a, Genetic analysis of human lymphocyte proteins by two-dimensional gel electrophoresis: 2. Genetic polymorphism of lymphocyte cytosol 64K polypeptide, *Hum. Genet.* **60**:176–180.

Hamaguchi, H., Yamada, M., Shibasaki, M., Mukai, R., Yabe, T., and Kondo, I., 1982b, Genetic analysis of human lymphocyte proteins by two-dimensional gel electrophoresis, *Hum. Genet.* **62**:142–147.

Hanash, S. M., Tubergen, D. G., Heyn, R. M., Neel, J. V., Sandy, L., Stevens, G. S., Rosenblum, B. B., and Krzesicki, R. F., 1982, Two-dimensional gel electrophoresis of cell proteins in childhood leukemia, with silver staining: A preliminary report, *Clin. Chem.* **28**:1026–1030.

Hanash, S. M., Neel, J. V., Baier, L. J., Rosenblum, B. B., Niezgoda, W., and Markel, D., 1986, Genetic analysis of thirty-three platelet polypeptides detected in two-dimensional polyacrylamide gels. *Am. J. Hum. Genet.* (in press).

Hayes-Roth, F., Waterman, D. A., and Lenat, D. B., 1983, *Building Expert Systems*, Addison-Wesley, Reading, Massachusetts.

Johnson, F. M., and Lewis, S. E., 1981, Electrophoretically detected germinal mutations induced in the mouse by ethylnitrosourea, *Proc. Natl. Acad. Sci. USA* **78**:3138–3141.

Johnson, F. M., and Lewis, S. E., 1983, The detection of ENU-induced mutants in mice by electrophoresis and the problem of evaluating the mutation rate increase, in: *Utilization of Mammalian Specific Locus Studies in Hazard Evaluation and Estimation of*

Genetic Risk (F. J. deSerres and W. Sheridan, ed.), pp. 95–108, Plenum Press, New York.

Johnson, F. M., Roberts, G. T., Sharma, R. K. Chasalow, F., Zweidinger, R., Morgan, A., Hendren, R. W., and Lewis, S. E., 1981, The detection of mutants in mice by electrophoresis: Results of a model induction experiment with procarbazine, *Genetics* 97:113–124.

Kahl, D. J., Rosenfeld, A., and Danker, A., 1980, Some experiments in point pattern matching, *IEEE Trans. Syst. Man Cybernet.* 10:105–116.

Klose, J., 1975, Protein mapping by combined isoelectric focusing and electrophoresis of mouse tissue. A novel approach to testing for induced point mutations in mammals, *Humangenetik* 26:231–243.

Kohn, H. I., 1983, Radiation genetics: The mouse's view, *Radiat. Res.* 94:1–9.

Lemkin, P. F., and Lipkin, L. E., 1981a, GELLAB: A computer system for 2D gel electrophoresis analysis. I. Segmentation and system preliminaries, *Comput. Biomed. Res.* 14:272–294.

Lemkin, P. F., and Lipkin, L. E., 1981b, GELLAB: A computer system for 2D gel electrophoresis analysis. II. Pairing spots, *Comput. Biomed. Res.* 14:355–380.

Lemkin, P. F., Lipkin, L. E., and Lester, E. P., 1982, Some extensions to the GELLAB two-dimensional electrophoretic gel analysis system, *Clin. Chem.* 28:840–849.

Lutin, W. A., Kyle, C. F., and Freeman, J. A., 1979, Quantitation of brain proteins by computer analyzed two-dimensional electrophoresis, in: *Electrophoresis '78* (N. Catsimpoolas, ed.), pp. 93–106, Elsevier/North-Holland, Amsterdam.

Lyon, M. F., 1983, Problems in extrapolation of animal data to humans, in: *Utilization of Mammalian Specific Locus Studies in Hazard Evaluation and Estimation of Genetic Risk* (F. J. de Serres and W. Sheridan, eds.), pp. 289–305, Plenum Press, New York.

Manabe, T., Tachi, K., Kojima, K., and Okuyama, T., 1979, Two-dimensional electrophoresis of plasma proteins without denaturing agents, *J. Biochem.* 85:649–659.

Marshall, E., 1984, Juarez: An unprecedented radiation accident, *Science* 223:1152–1154.

McConkey, E. H., Taylor, B. J., and Phan, D., 1979, Human heterozygosity: A new estimate, *Proc. Natl. Acad. Sci. USA* 76:6500–6504.

Merril, C. R., Goldman, D., Sedman, S. A., and Ebert, M. H., 1981, Ultrasensitive stain for proteins in polyacrylamide gels show regional variation in cerebrospinal fluid proteins, *Science* 211:1437–1438.

Miller, M. J., Vo, P. K., Nielsen, C., Geiduschek, E. P., and Xuong, N. G., 1982, Computer analysis of two-dimensional gels: Semi-automatic matching, *Clin. Chem.* 28:867–875.

Miller, M. J., Olson, A. D., and Thorgeirsson, S. S. 1984, Computer analysis of two-dimensional gels: Automatic matching, *Electrophoresis* 5:297–303.

Neel, J. V., 1971, The detection of increased mutation rates in human populations, *Perspect. Biol.* 14:522–537.

Neel, J. V., 1981, Genetic effects of atomic bombs, *Science* 213:1205.

Neel, J. V., 1983, Frequency of spontaneous and induced "point" mutations in higher eukaryotes, *J. Hered.* 74:2–15.

Neel, J. V., and Schull, W. J., 1956, *The Effect of Exposure to the Atomic Bombs on Pregnancy Termination in Hiroshima and Nagasaki*, Publication No. 461, National Academy of Sciences–National Research Council, Washington, D.C.

Neel, J. V., 1986, Strategy and results to date of follow-up studies on the genetic effect of the atomic bombs, in: *Proceedings, World Health Organization Workshop on the Prevention of Mutational Disease* (in press).

Neel, J. V., Satoh, C., Hamilton, H. B., Otake, M., Goriki, K., Kageoka, T., Fujita, M., Neriishi, S., and Asakawa, J., 1980a, Search for mutations affecting protein structure in children of atomic bomb survivors: Preliminary report, *Proc. Natl. Acad. Sci. USA* 77:4221–4225.

Neel, J. V., Mohrenweiser, H. W., and Meisler, M. M., 1980*b*, Rate of spontaneous mutation of human loci encoding protein structure, *Proc. Natl. Acad. Sci. USA* 77:6037–6041.

Neel, J. V., Mohrenweiser, H., Hanash, S., Rosenblum, B. B., Sternberg, S., Wurzinger, K., Rothman, E., Satoh, C., Goriki, K., Krasteff, T., Long, M., Skolnick, M., and Krzesicki, R., 1983, Biochemical approaches to monitoring human populations for germinal mutation rates. I. Electrophoresis, in: *Utilization of Mammalian Specific Locus Studies in Hazard Evaluation and Estimation of Genetic Risk*, (F. J. deSerres, and W. Sheridan, eds.), pp. 71–93, Plenum Press, New York.

Neel, J. V., Rosenblum, B. B., Sing, C. F., Skolnick, M. M., Hanash, S. M., and Sternberg, S., 1984, Adapting two-dimensional gel electrophoresis to the study of human germline mutation rates, in: *Methods and Applications of Two Dimensional Gel Electrophoresis of Proteins* (J. E. Celis and R. Bravo, eds.), pp. 259–306, Academic Press, New York.

O'Farrell, P. H., 1975, High resolution two-dimensional electrophoresis of proteins, *J. Biol. Chem.* 250:4007–4021.

Radiation Effects Research Foundation, 1983, *U.S.–Japan Joint Workshop for Reassessment of Atomic Bomb Radiation Dosimetry in Hiroshima and Nagasaki*, Radiation Effects Research Foundation, Hiroshima.

Radiation Effects Research Foundation, 1984, *Second U.S.–Japan Joint Workshop for Reassessment of Atomic Bomb Radiation Dosimetry in Hiroshima and Nagasaki*, Radiation Effects Research Foundation, Hiroshima.

Ranade, S., and Rosenfeld, A., 1980, Point pattern matching by relaxation, *Pattern Recog.* 12:260–275.

Rosenblum, B. B., Neel, J. V., and Hanash, S. M., 1983, Two-dimensional electrophoresis of plasma polypeptides reveals "high" heterozygosity indices, *Proc. Natl. Acad. Sci. USA* 80:5002–5006.

Rosenblum, B. B., Neel, J. V., Hanash, S. M., Joseph, J. L., and Yew, N., 1984, Identification of genetic variants in erythrocyte lysate by two-dimensional gel electrophoresis, *Am. J. Hum. Genet.* 36:181–187.

Rosenfeld, A., 1978, Iterative methods in image analysis, *Pattern Recog.* 10:181–187.

Rosenfeld, A., Hummel, R. A., and Zucker, S. W., 1976, Scene labeling by relaxation operators, *IEEE Trans. Syst. Man Cybernet.* 6:420–433.

Rothman, E. D., Neel, J. V., and Hoppe F. M., 1981, Assigning a probability for paternity in apparent cases of mutation, *Am. J. Hum. Genet.* 33:617–628.

Sammons, D. W., Adams, L. D., and Nishizawa, E. E., 1981, A silver-based color development system for staining of polypeptides in polyacrylamide gels, *Electrophoresis* 2:135–141.

Satoh, C., Awa, A. A., Neel, J. V., Schull, W. J., Kato, H., Hamilton, H. B., Otake, M., and Goriki, K., 1982, Genetic effects of atomic bombs, in: *Human Genetics, Part A* (B. Bonné-Tamir, ed.), pp. 267–276, Alan R. Liss, New York.

Scheele, G., 1975, Two-dimensional gel analysis of soluble proteins. Characterization of guinea pig exocrine pancreatic proteins, *J. Biol. Chem.* 250:5375–5385.

Schull, W. J., Otake, M., and Neel, J. V., 1981, A reappraisal of the genetic effects of the atomic bombs: Summary of a thirty-four year study, *Science* 213:1220–1227.

Serra, J. P., 1982, *Image Analysis and Mathematical Morphology*, Academic Press, London.

Serra, J. P., 1986, Morphological algorithms for binary images, *Comput. Vision Graph. Image Proc.* (in press).

Skolnick, M. M., 1982, An approach to completely automatic comparison of two-dimensional electrophoresis gels, *Clin. Chem.* 28:979–986.

Skolnick, M. M., 1984, Automated Comparison of Image Similarities and Differences, PhD Dissertation, University of Michigan, Ann Arbor, Michigan.

Skolnick, M. M., 1986, Morphological algorithms for the automatic analysis of 2-D electrophoretograms, *Comput. Vision Graph. Image Proc.*, in press.

Skolnick, M. M., Sternberg, S. R., and Neel, J. V., 1982, Computer programs for adapting two-dimensional gels to the study of mutation, *Clin. Chem.* **28**:969–978.

Smith, C. R., Racine, R. R., and Langley, C. H., 1981, Lack of genic variation in the abundant proteins of human kidney, *Genetics* **96**:967–974.

Soares, E. R., 1979, TEM-induced gene mutations at enzyme loci in the mouse, *Environ. Mutat.* **1**:19–25.

Special Issue, 1982, Two-dimensional gel electrophoresis, *Clin. Chem.* **28**:737–1092.

Sternberg, S. R., 1981, Language and architecture for parallel image processing, in: *Proceedings of Conference on Pattern Recognition in Practice* (L. N. Kanal and E. S. Gelsema, eds.), pp. 35–44, Elsevier/North-Holland, New York.

Sternberg, S. R., 1983, Biomedical image processing, *Computer* **16**(1):22–34.

Sternberg, S. R., 1986, Morphological algorithms for grey-scale images, *Comput. Vision Graph. Image Proc.* (in press).

Taylor, J., Anderson, N. L., and Coulter, B. P., 1980, Estimation of two-dimensional spot intensities and positions by modeling, in: *Electrophoresis '79* (B. Radola, ed.),pp. 383–400, deGruyter, New York.

Taylor, J., Anderson, N. L., and Anderson, N. G., 1981, A computerized system for matching and stretching two-dimensional gel patterns represented by parameter lists, in: *Electrophoresis '81* (R. Allen and P. Arnaud, eds.), pp. 383–400, deGruyter, New York.

Tollaksen, S., Anderson, N. L., and Anderson, N. G., 1984, Operation of the Iso-dalt System. Seventh Addition, Argonne National Library, Argonne, Illinois, ANL-BIM-84-1, pp. vi and 66.

Toussaint, G. T., 1980, Pattern recognition and geometrical complexity, in: *Proceedings 5th International Conference on Pattern Recognition*, pps. 1324–1347, IEEE Computer Society Press, New York.

Ullman, S., 1979, *The Interpretation of Visual Motion*, MIT Press, Cambridge.

Walton, K. E., Styer, D., and Guenstein, E. I., 1979, Genetic polymorphism in normal human fibroblasts as analyzed by two-dimensional polyacrylamide gel electrophoresis, *J. Biol. Chem.* **254**:7951–7960.

Wanner, L. A., Neel, J. V., Meisler, M. H., 1982, Separation of allelic variants by two-dimensional electrophoresis, *Am. J. Hum. Genet.* **34**:209–215.

Wray, W., Boulikas, T., Wray, V. P., and Hancock, R., 1981, Silver staining of proteins in polyacrylamide gels, *Anal. Biochem.* **118**:197–203.

Yamasaki, E., and Ames, B. N., 1977, Concentration of mutagens from urine by absorption with the nonpolar resin XAD-2: Cigarette smokers have mutagenic urine, *Proc. Natl. Acad. Sci. USA* **74**:3555–3559.

Chapter 3

The Human Argininosuccinate Synthetase Locus and Citrullinemia

Arthur L. Beaudet
Departments of Pediatrics and Cell Biology
Baylor College of Medicine
Houston, Texas 77030

William E. O'Brien
Department of Pediatrics and Biochemistry
Baylor College of Medicine
Houston, Texas 77030

Hans-Georg O. Bock, Svend O. Freytag, and Tsung-Sheng Su*
Department of Pediatrics
Baylor College of Medicine
Houston, Texas 77030

INTRODUCTION

Argininosuccinate synthetase is an enzyme which functions in the urea cycle in ureotelic animals, and genetic deficiency of the enzyme in man causes an inborn error of metabolism, citrullinemia. The purpose of this chapter is to summarize recent developments in the molecular analysis of the human argininosuccinate synthetase locus and to relate this information to available clinical, metabolic, enzymatic, and genetic information. We also will discuss the opportunities to study gene regulation in tissue culture using this locus.

The molecular analysis of argininosuccinate synthetase has not been reviewed previously. The Krebs–Henseleit urea cycle and the associated

* *Present addresses*: for H.-G. O., University of Mississippi Medical Center, Jackson, Mississippi 39216; for S. O. F., University of Michigan Medical School, Ann Arbor, Michigan 48109; for T.-S. S., Veterans General Hospital, Taipei, Taiwan.

human diseases have been the subject of two international symposia within the last decade (Grisolia *et al.*, 1976; Lowenthal *et al.*, 1982). The enzymology of argininosuccinate synthetase was reviewed by Ratner (1976). The clinical and metabolic aspects of the disease citrullinemia are reviewed periodically in the various editions of *The Metabolic Basis of Inherited Disease*, most recently by Walser (1983).

HISTORICAL ASPECTS

In the early 1930s, Sir Hans Krebs began to investigate the mechanisms for urea synthesis, using liver tissue slices. With the aid of a medical student, Kurt Henseleit, he demonstrated that high rates of urea synthesis occurred when both ornithine and ammonium ions were added to the perfusion medium. Based on ideas developed from paper chemistry, Krebs used the liver slice method to examine the effect of citrulline, which recently had been isolated both from watermelons and as a product of bacterial degradation of arginine. Rapid synthesis of urea occurred in the presence of citrulline and ammonium salts, leading to the suggestion of a metabolic cycle for urea synthesis. A simplified urea cycle was proposed, with the formation of urea from carbon dioxide and ammonium, with citrulline, arginine, and ornithine as intermediates. The history of the early events in the development of the concept of the urea cycle was reviewed by Krebs (1952, 1976).

The exact role of citrulline in the urea cycle remained unclear until the late 1940s. Borsook and Dubnoff (1941) demonstrated that either aspartic acid or glutamic acid, but not ammonia, could contribute nitrogen for the conversion of citrulline to arginine. Cohen and Hayano (1946) demonstrated arginine synthesis in respiring liver homogenates, and this led to a reexamination of the mechanism for conversion of citrulline to arginine. Sarah Ratner demonstrated that citrulline combined with aspartate in the presence of ATP to form argininosuccinate in a first step. A second step was required for the hydrolysis of argininosuccinate to yield arginine and fumarate (Ratner 1947, 1954). The formation of argininosuccinate is catalyzed by the enzyme argininosuccinate synthetase, which is the subject of this review. Genetic deficiency of this enzyme in humans was first reported by McMurray *et al.* (1962).

TABLE I. Biological Aspects of Argininosuccinate Synthetase

1. Arginine biosynthetic enzyme in lower organisms
2. Urea cycle enzyme in ureotelic organisms such as man
3. High enzyme activity in liver and low but detectable in other tissues
4. Positive correlation of hepatic enzyme activity with dietary protein intake
5. Repression of enzyme activity by arginine in some tissue culture cells
6. Canavanine-resistant tissue culture cells overproduce enzyme and are not repressible
7. Genetic deficiency of the enzyme causes citrullinemia in man
8. Some rodent tissue culture cell lines do not express the enzyme
9. Modest hormonal effects on expression in animals and in hepatocyte cultures

BIOLOGY OF THE ARGININOSUCCINATE SYNTHETASE LOCUS

The enzyme reactions for argininosuccinate synthetase and argininosuccinate lyase are, respectively,

citrulline + aspartate + MgATP

$\rightleftharpoons$ argininosuccinate + AMP + magnesium pyrophosphate   (1)

argininosuccinate $\rightleftharpoons$ fumarate + arginine   (2)

These two reactions can function in sequence to convert citrulline to arginine, representing the terminal steps for arginine biosynthesis. For urea production, arginine is hydrolyzed to yield ornithine and urea.

Some biological aspects of the argininosuccinate synthetase locus are summarized in Table I. Argininosuccinate synthetase functions in the biosynthetic pathway for arginine in many lower organisms. The structural gene for this enzyme is designated *arg*G in *Escherichia coli* (Bachman and Low, 1980) and *arg*1 in *Saccharomyces cerevisiae* (Mortimer and Schild, 1980). Carbamoyl phosphate synthetase, ornithine transcarbamoylase, argininosuccinate synthetase, and argininosuccinate lyase are all enzymes which function in arginine biosynthesis in lower organisms and have undergone evolutionary adaptation to function in the urea cycle in ureotelic organisms. The findings in lower organisms will be discussed further in the context of gene regulation below.

In man, argininosuccinate synthetase carries out an essential step in the urea cycle, which functions primarily in the liver. Argininosuccinate synthetase activity in normal human liver is 3.5–16 mU/mg protein. One

TABLE II. Argininosuccinate Synthetase Activity in Human Cells

Source	Activity, nmole/min per mg protein	References
Liver	3.5–16	Walser (1983)
Kidney	3.3 ± 1.5	Saheki *et al.* (1982*b*)
Brain	0.19 ± 0.06	Saheki *et al.* (1982*b*)
Erythrocytes, leukocytes	<0.02	Present work[a]
Cultured skin fibroblasts	1.0–4.0	Su *et al.* (1982)
Lymphoblasts		Irr and Jacob (1978), Jacoby
Arginine medium	0.002–0.11	(1978)
Citrulline medium	0.25–0.57	
Canavanine-resistant	0.82–4.30	
RPMI-2650 cell line		Su *et al.* (1981*a*)
Arginine medium	0.14	
Citrulline medium	0.86	
Canavanine-resistant	4.7–25.1	

[a] A. L. Beaudet, W. E. O'Brien, H.-G. O. Bock, S. O. Freytag, and T.-S. Su (unpublished results).

mU is the ability to produce 1 nmole of product per minute. The level of activity in other tissues is substantially lower, as summarized in Table II. Enzyme activity is detectable in cultured skin fibroblasts and in Epstein–Barr virus-transformed lymphoblast cultures. All of the urea cycle enzymes show increased activity in liver after the time of birth, as reviewed by Räihä (1976). In the rat and the human, argininosuccinate synthetase activity during fetal life ranges from 2 to 20% of the adult value. Argininosuccinate synthetase activity is particularly low in the prenatal rat and increases abruptly at birth.

Certain aspects of the regulation of argininosuccinate synthetase have been studied in intact mammals. Schimke (1962*a*) demonstrated three- to fivefold increases in activity of all urea cycle enzymes when rats were fed a high-protein diet as compared to a low-protein diet. Nuzum and Snodgrass (1971) made similar observations in monkeys. Schimke (1962*b*) observed increased enzyme activity in response to fasting. Urea cycle enzymes also are subject to coordinate regulation by hormones. Administration of physiological doses of glucagon induces the five urea cycle enzymes, and there is evidence that glucagon plays a role in the induction of the enzymes by protein feeding (Snodgrass *et al.*, 1978). Glucagon also causes an acute stimulation of hepatic citrulline formation in rats, in a manner too rapid to be explained by enzyme induction (Yamazaki and

Graetz, 1977; Rabier *et al.*, 1982). Activity of the urea cycle enzymes is increased by pharmacological doses of corticosteroids (Schimke 1963) and is reduced by adrenalectomy (McLean and Gurney, 1963). Aebi (1976) reviewed the coordinate effects of dietary protein and hormone variation on urea cycle enzymes. Increased expression of urea cycle enzymes in response to glucocorticoids and glucagon also has been reported for some hepatoma cell lines (Haggerty *et al.*, 1982) and for primary hepatocyte cultures (Gebhardt and Mecke, 1979; Lin *et al.*, 1982). The preferential expression of urea cycle enzymes in hepatic tissue and the coordinate regulation in response to protein intake suggest some degree of shared regulatory mechanisms involving the urea cycle enzymes.

The role of argininosuccinate synthetase in mammals can be considered in the context of the overall metabolism of arginine in the intact animal. Since both argininosuccinate synthetase and argininosuccinate lyase are expressed in most peripheral tissues, they could combine to synthesize arginine from citrulline, but it is unlikely that this is a quantitatively significant pathway. There is evidence that intestine is the principal source of circulating citrulline, and that the majority of this citrulline is taken up by the kidney (Windmueller and Spaeth, 1981). In rats and man, arginine is essential for normal growth, but dietary arginine is not required in the adult. Net synthesis of arginine can occur by conversion of glutamate to ornithine, which can then proceed through the urea cycle. However, genetic deficiency of ornithine aminotransferase, which blocks the interconversion of ornithine and glutamate, leads to accumulation of ornithine, suggesting that the usual net flux is from ornithine toward glutamate with usual dietary protein intake (Valle and Simell, 1983). Arginine is required as an intermediate in the urea cycle in addition to the requirement for protein synthesis. Cats are unusually susceptible to ammonia intoxication due to dietary arginine deficiency (Morris and Rogers, 1978). Low concentrations of hepatic ornithine probably contribute to this susceptibility in cats (Stewart *et al.*, 1981). Premature infants experience higher concentrations of blood ammonia, which can be reduced by addition of arginine to the diet (Batshaw and Brusilow, 1978). Although argininosuccinate synthetase may be considered as part of a biosynthetic pathway for arginine in mammals, this pathway is not sufficient to prevent arginine deficiency under all circumstances.

Expression of argininosuccinate synthetase in tissue culture cells is subject to metabolite regulation. Schimke (1964) first reported higher activity for both argininosuccinate synthetase and argininosuccinate lyase when human HeLa cells or KB cells or mouse L cells were grown in medium with a low arginine concentration or with citrulline substituted for arginine. Since the simultaneous addition of high concentrations of citrulline and arginine resulted in decreased enzyme activity, this was considered to be a form of repression by arginine. Similar results were reported for argininosuccinate synthetase using cultured human lymphoblasts (Irr and Jacoby, 1978) and cultured human epithelial cells (Su *et al.*, 1981a). These later studies of lymphoblasts and epithelial cells did not demonstrate repression of argininosuccinate lyase by arginine, and the reason for this lack of repression of the lyase as compared to Schimke's (1964) results is unclear. Not all human tissue culture cells demonstrate repression of the synthetase by arginine in our experience. Human skin fibroblasts are not affected significantly by changes in arginine concentration in the medium. There is a wide range of expression of argininosuccinate synthetase in different tissue culture cell types, as exemplified in Table II. Expression is so low as to be nearly undetectable in many cultured human lymphoblasts, but these cells express increased enzyme activity when adapted to growth in medium with citrulline substituted for arginine (Jacoby, 1974; Lockridge *et al.*, 1977; Irr and Jacoby, 1978). It may be significant that cells such as lymphoblasts with low enzyme activity tend to demonstrate metabolite regulation, while cells with higher enzyme activity such as fibroblasts do not appear to be as readily subject to metabolite regulation. We and others (Hudson *et al.*, 1980; Jacoby *et al.*, 1981) have observed higher enzyme activity when tissue culture cells are grown at higher density.

It is curious that many of the widely used Chinese hamster tissue culture cell lines do not express argininosuccinate synthetase activity (Naylor *et al.*, 1976; Sun *et al*, 1979). These tissue culture cells die in medium with citrulline substituted for arginine. The cells do express argininosuccinate lyase, and they can be used to select for the synthetase activity. These cells have been useful in selecting for expression of the synthetase in somatic cell hybrids (Carritt *et al.*, 1977) and in chromosome-mediated (Hudson *et al.*, 1980) or DNA-mediated (Su *et al.*, 1984b) gene transfer experiments. The Chinese hamster cells may be valuable reagents for analysis of regulation of the argininosuccinate synthetase gene in mammalian cells.

Jacoby (1978) was the first to isolate canavanine-resistant (Can[r]) human cells, and she demonstrated that these cells overproduce argininosuccinate synthetase. Canavanine is an analogue of arginine, and it is known to be incorporated into protein in place of arginine. Can^r cells had been isolated in *E. coli* and yeast, with an alteration in arginine transport being the basis for the phenotype in many instances (Maas, 1972; Whelan *et al.*, 1979). Initial observations with human Can^r cells indicated increased accumulation of enzyme, which was indistinguishable from the normal form (Kimball and Jacoby, 1980; Su *et al.*, 1981a). Measurement of arginyl-tRNA synthetase did not indicate any major abnormality (Jacoby, 1978). Can^r cells were not subject to repression by arginine, and the phenotype of enzyme overproduction was stable when cells were grown for long periods in medium containing high concentrations of arginine. It is unclear if Can^r cells represent some stable type of epigenetic event, or whether these represent true mutants; i.e., a change in the DNA sequence of the genome. Can^r cells will be discussed in greater detail below.

Genetic deficiency of argininosuccinate synthetase has been known for many years to cause citrullinemia. This condition results in hyperammonemia with secondary neurological manifestations. Abnormal kinetic properties of the mutant enzyme have indicated that at least some, and perhaps all, citrullinemia patients have defects in the structural gene for the enzyme (Tedesco and Mellman, 1967; Walser, 1983). A suggestion of a "regulatory" form of citrullinemia has been described in Japan (Saheki *et al.*, 1982a). These patients are reported to have qualitatively normal enzyme, but there is decreased enzyme activity in the liver.

BIOCHEMISTRY OF THE ENZYME

Argininosuccinate synthetase (EC 6.3.4.5) catalyzes the synthesis of argininosuccinate from citrulline, aspartate, and ATP as described above. The enzyme is located in the cytosol and is present in all body tissues examined, except that activity is not readily detected in erythrocytes or leukocytes. The enzyme has been purified from numerous animal species, including humans (O'Brien, 1979; Kimball and Jacoby, 1980; Saheki *et al.*, 1983a) rats (Saheki *et al.*, 1975), and cattle (Ratner 1976, 1982). In all species examined, the enzyme is a homotetramer with a subunit molecular weight of about 46,000.

The kinetic mechanism has been studied extensively using the beef liver and human liver enzymes. There is an ordered addition of MgATP, citrulline, and aspartate, followed by the ordered release of argininosuc-

TABLE III. Amino Acid Composition of
Bovine and Human Argininosuccinate
Synthetase

	Bovine[a]	Human[b]
Aspartic acid	}34	16}32
Asparagine		16
Threonine	17	18
Serine	23	24
Glutamic acid	}53	35}52
Glutamine		17
Proline	23	21
Glycine	33	31
Alanine	29	28
Valine	29	30
Cysteine	3	5
Methionine	8	9
Isoleucine	25	27
Leucine	34	35
Tyrosine	19	19
Phenylalanine	17	14
Tryptophan	4	4
Lysine	31	33
Histidine	10	9
Arginine	21	21
Total	413	412

[a] Bovine data are based on amino acid composition and were taken from Ratner (1982).
[b] Human data are based on cDNA sequence and were taken from Bock *et al.* (1983).

cinate, MgPPi, and AMP. There is also a reactive intermediate, citrulline-adenylate, that is firmly bound to the enzyme (Rochovansky and Ratner, 1967). Rochovansky *et al.* (1977) observed nonlinear double reciprocal plots for all substrate combinations, but Raushel and Seiglie (1983) were not able to confirm these results. No evidence for nonlinearity was observed with the enzyme from human liver by O'Brien (1979), but Saheki *et al.* (1983a) demonstrated slight negative cooperativity for MgATP binding. It is not known if these *in vitro* observations are of any significance for the *in vivo* regulation of this enzyme. The amino acid compositions for the bovine and human enzymes are compared in Table III, showing a remarkable similarity. The amino acid sequence for the human enzyme was derived from the cloned cDNA (Bock *et al.*, 1983) as discussed below.

The monomer contains 412 amino acids, counting the initiator methionine, and the mature subunit is predicted to have a molecular weight of 46,301. The enzymology of argininosuccinate synthetase was reviewed in greater detail by Ratner (1976).

CLONING OF HUMAN ARGININOSUCCINATE SYNTHETASE GENE

The report by Jacoby (1978) that Can^r human lymphoblasts over-produced argininosuccinate synthetase provided the impetus to attempt cloning of the cDNA for this enzyme. Since Can^r cells overproduced apparently normal enzyme as described above, the amount of mRNA for the enzyme might be expected to be increased. Increased translatable mRNA for the enzyme was demonstrated in Can^r cells isolated from the human epithelial cell line RPMI-2650 (Su et al., 1981a). Su et al. (1981b) used RNA isolated from these Can^r cells and differential filter hybridization to isolate a cDNA clone for argininosuccinate synthetase. The cDNA was used to analyze RNA and DNA from tissue culture cells. When RNA isolated from wild-type cells grown in arginine, from wild-type cells grown in citrulline, and from Can^r cells was analyzed by nucleic acid hybridization, the relative amounts of mRNA for argininosuccinate synthetase were 1, 7, and 180, respectively. This represented a good correlation of the relative amounts of mRNA with enzyme activity. Similar results were obtained with Can^r lymphoblasts (Amos et al., 1984). Initial analysis of genomic DNA from human cells using the cDNA probe indicated a large number of argininosuccinate synthetase-related sequences in the human genome. However, there was no indication that the patterns of DNA fragments from normal cells and from Can^r cells differed in any way. The data indicated that gene amplification was not the mechanism for overproduction of argininosuccinate synthetase.

The nucleotide sequence for a nearly full-length cDNA for argininosuccinate synthetase was determined (Bock et al., 1983). In addition to the coding region described above, three tandem arginine codons were found in the 5'-untranslated region of the cDNA. The tandem arginine codons occur in exon 2, which is subject to alternative splicing and is not present in the predominant mature mRNA in human cells. This finding is of unknown biological significance, although it is of interest, since this gene is thought to be repressed by arginine.

Splicing pattern A

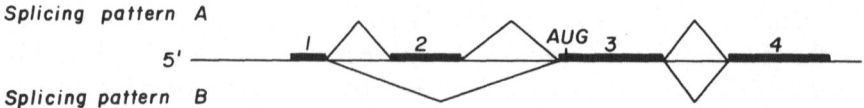

Splicing pattern B

Fig. 1. Alternative splicing patterns for argininosuccinate synthetase mRNA. Exons are designated by the heavy bars. AUG indicates the site for initiation of translation. Splicing pattern A is predominant in baboon liver, while splicing pattern B is predominant in human cells. [From Freytag *et al.* (1984*b*), by permission.]

Analysis of genomic DNA clones indicated the presence of multiple processed dispersed pseudogenes and a single large expressed gene for argininosuccinate synthetase (Freytag *et al.*, 1984*a,b*; Jinno *et al.*, 1984). Analysis of rodent–human somatic cell hybrids indicated that the DNA fragments from the expressed gene map to human chromosome 9q34–qter (Su *et al.*, 1984*a*), consistent with the previous assignment of enzyme activity to this region (Carritt and Povey, 1979). The expressed gene was characterized by isolation of a series of overlapping genomic DNA clones. The gene spans 63 kb and is composed of at least 14 exons. Multiple exons have been sequenced, including the 5′-most and 3′-most exons. Examination of mRNA from various sources using S1 nuclease analysis indicated two alternative splicing patterns (Fig. 1) (Freytag *et al.*, 1984*b*). One form of the mRNA contains all of the exons, with the initiator AUG codon occurring in exon 3. The other form of RNA is exactly missing the sequences included in exon 2. In normal human liver and cultured fibroblasts, the predominant mature argininosuccinate synthetase mRNA lacks sequences encoded by exon 2. In contrast, the predominant argininosuccinate synthetase mRNA in baboon liver contains exon 2 sequences. The biological significance, if any, of this alternative splicing pattern is unknown.

ARGININOSUCCINATE SYNTHETASE PSEUDOGENES

When the human cDNA was used as a probe for Southern blotting analysis of human genomic DNA, a large number (15–30) of hybridizing fragments were observed with all restriction enzymes. Solution hybridization analysis also indicated the presence of multiple copies of homologous sequences in the genome. Since argininosuccinate synthetase deficiency occurs as an autosomal recessive enzyme defect, it was unlikely that multiple genes were active. Screening of a human genomic DNA library resulted in isolation of many of these argininosuccinate synthetase-related sequences. Many genomic DNA clones contained different processed dispersed pseudogenes (Freytag *et al.*, 1984*a*). Seven different clones characterized in some detail had lost all intervening sequences. Sequence analysis of three of the pseudogenes indicated an 89–93% homology. Freytag *et al.* (1984*a*) estimated that the pseudogenes arose over the last 10–20 million years. Southern blotting analysis indicated the presence of virtually all the same pseudogenes in chimpanzee DNA (Daiger and Hoffman, 1983). Therefore, these pseudogenes arose prior to the evolutionary divergence of the great apes and hominids. There is no clear explanation for the large number of dispersed processed pseudogenes for argininosuccinate synthetase. There are a variety of possible explana-

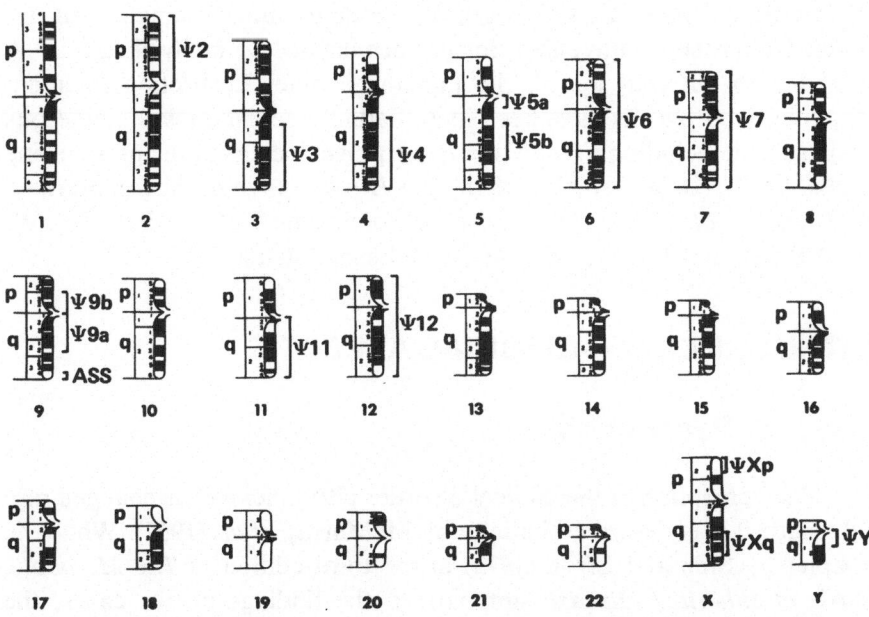

Fig. 2. Chromosome mapping assignments for human argininosuccinate synthetase sequences. The site for the expressed gene at 9q34–qter is designated ASS. Sites for pseudogenes are designated ψ followed by chromosome number and chromosome arm or arbitrary a or b assignments as appropriate. Assignments are based on data from Su *et al.* (1984*a*) and Carlock *et al.* (1985). We proposed that the pseudogenes be designated ASSψC2, ASSψC3, ASSψC5a, etc., with the symbol ψ for pseudogene followed by C for chromosome followed by the designations in this figure.

tions, some of which could involve common intermediates in the formation of the pseudogenes, as discussed in more detail by Freytag *et al.* (1984*a*).

The human cDNA was used as a probe for Southern blotting analysis of genomic DNA from rodent–human somatic cell hybrids. DNA sequences closely homologous to argininosuccinate synthetase were found to be present on multiple human chromosomes, including sites on chromosomes 6, 9, and X (Beaudet *et al.*, 1982). Comparison of DNA from male and female individuals identified argininosuccinate synthetase-like sequences on the human X and Y chromosomes (Daiger *et al.*, 1982). Further mapping studies identified 14 separate pseudogene loci mapped to 11 different chromosomes (Fig. 2) (Su *et al.*, 1984*a*; Carlock *et al*, 1985). The existence of a large number of highly homologous but dispersed sequences in the human genome facilitates certain applications with the cDNA probe. The probe is useful for analyzing the presence or absence of 11 different human chromosomes in rodent–human somatic cell hybrids. The probe is convenient for performing dosage analysis at a DNA level for 15 different loci in the human genome. Restriction fragment length polymorphisms have been identified in association with numerous of these loci, including a *Hind*III polymorphism located at the pseudogene on 9q11–q22 (Daiger *et al.*, 1984). The *Hind*II polymorphism described by Daiger *et al.* (1984) is located on chromosome 7 (A. L. Beaudet, W. E. O'Brien, and D. H. Ledbetter, unpublished data).

CITRULLINEMIA—CLINICAL ASPECTS

General Description

The perception of the clinical disorder citrullinemia has changed rapidly since it was described initially by McMurray *et al.* (1962). While the chapter by Shih and Efron (1972) in the third edition of *The Metabolic Basis of Inherited Disease* summarized the findings in two cases, the chapter by Walser (1983) in the fifth edition tabulated 53 published cases. Certainly tens of additional unpublished cases are known, and most of these are affected with the neonatal form of disease. The incidence of the disease is unknown, but we believe that the majority of cases still die undiagnosed. Initial reports of the disease described milder forms associated with prolonged survival. Improved neonatal care, better availability of quantitative serum amino acid analysis, and increased awareness of hyperammonemia in neonates have led to the recognition that the most common form of the disease presents in the neonatal period with hyperammonemia. This form of citrullinemia presents with subtle symptoms often beginning at 24–36 hr of age and severe symptoms occurring on the second, third, or fourth day of life. Early symptoms such as poor feeding or lethargy progress to vomiting, further impairment of consciousness, tachypnea, and sometimes apnea or seizures. If the condition is unrecognized, infants usually will become comatose and die in the first few days of life. Early recognition depends upon a high level of awareness on the part of the neonatologist and upon a willingness to measure blood ammonia in infants with mild, nonspecific symptoms.

Children with a later presentation are described as having a subacute form of citrullinemia. These children may present with mental retardation and other neurological findings, such as ataxia. They also may present with episodic vomiting and hyperammonemia in association with minor illnesses or other catabolic episodes. The clinical heterogeneity may represent a spectrum of severity correlating with residual *in vivo* enzyme activity rather than distinct neonatal and subacute forms. The time of presentation in patients with some residual enzyme function is influenced substantially by the extent of protein catabolism occurring in the neonatal period and by subsequent minor illnesses. Presumably, patients with 10–50% of residual enzyme activity could have increased susceptibility to hyperammonemia with unusual catabolic stress or in the presence of some unrelated liver disease.

Reports of a late onset form of citrullinemia and possible relationships to a regulatory form of citrullinemia described in Japan deserve special comment. Walser (1983) lists 24 reported cases in the late onset category. Some of these patients show abnormal enzyme kinetics, and it is likely that a substantial portion represent mutations in the structural gene for argininosuccinate synthetase. In these instances, the late onset presumably is due to the presence of residual enzyme activity, and factors such as growth rate, diet, catabolic episodes, and incidental liver disease interact to affect the clinical presentation. However, a significant proportion of these patients are from Japan, and it has been suggested that these patients may have a disorder which involves a tissue-specific defect in the regulation of argininosuccinate synthetase activity with decreased expression of enzyme activity in the liver (Saheki *et al.*, 1981, 1982a). Evidence of decreased enzyme activity in the liver with normal activity

in cultured skin fibroblasts is intriguing in this regard. Immunohistochemical analysis of argininosuccinate synthetase in liver from these patients demonstrated two patterns, some with homogeneous distribution
of enzyme and some with nodules of increased enzyme activity (Saheki
et al., 1983*b*). These patients experience a late onset of neurological and
psychiatric symptoms with elevations of blood citrulline and ammonia.
Walser's (1983) review of the reports of these patients, including publications in Japanese, states that the pathological findings include fatty liver
in all cases and additional changes in some instances. Although there is
limited genetic information, and it is not possible to draw a conclusive
interpretation regarding a regulatory form of citrullinemia, the findings
are of great interest.

Differential Diagnosis

Hyperammonemia in the neonatal period requires thorough evaluation of amino acid and organic acid metabolism, and reviews of the clinical
approach are available (Donn and Banagale, 1984; Batshaw, 1984). When
neonatal hyperammonemia is recognized, quantitative serum amino acid
analysis should be performed on an emergency basis. A blood citrulline
value of >500 μM, with the absence of argininosuccinic acid in the analysis, is virtually diagnostic of citrullinemia. Blood citrulline is low or
undetectable with proximal defects in the urea cycle, such as carbamoyl
phosphate synthetase deficiency or ornithine transcarbamoylase deficiency. Argininosuccinic aciduria is usually associated with a moderate
elevation of citrulline in the range of 100–500 μM, but the presence of
argininosuccinic acid and its anhydrides in the analysis is diagnostic. Py-
ruvate carboxylase deficiency and transient hyperammonemia of the newborn also can give moderate citrulline elevations, but these are usually
below the values seen with citrullinemia. Infants with citrullinemia are
usually normal in the first few hours of life, while infants with transient
hyperammonemia usually are premature and have respiratory illness. Hyperammonemia associated with organic acidemia results in more normal
concentrations of blood citrulline. Despite the relative ease of diagnosis,
many errors occur due to failure to resolve citrulline from other amino
acids in the chromatogram, failure to detect argininosuccinic acid, and
misinterpretation of available data.

Definitive diagnosis of citrullinemia depends on enzyme assay, which
should always be carried out. In infants who do well, the diagnosis should

be confirmed by enzyme assay of cultured skin fibroblasts. There is no need for liver biopsy in usual cases. Many neonates still die with citrullinemia, and enzyme measurements can be carried out in those instances using autopsy liver and/or cultured skin fiboblasts. Despite reports that leukocytes can be used to measure enzyme activity (Wolfe and Gatfield, 1975), we do not find leukocytes or erythrocytes to be adequate for enzyme assay. Although spectrophotometric assays have been used in the past (Schimke, 1962a; Nuzum and Snodgrass, 1976; O'Brien, 1976), radioisotopic enzyme assays now offer greater sensitivity and specificity (Kato *et al.*, 1976; Su *et al.*, 1981a; Ratner, 1983). Abnormal kinetic properties have been observed in the case of mutant enzyme from a number of patients, as tabulated by Walser (1983). Measurement of incorporation of radioactive citrulline into acid-precipitable protein by intact fibroblasts provides a useful adjunct in assessing the relative enzyme activity within intact cells (Kennaway and Curtis, 1981; Jacoby *et al.*, 1981; Su *et al.*, 1982 Fleisher *et al.*, 1983). There is a general correlation of a milder phenotype with the presence of detectable residual enzyme activity (Walser, 1983), but this cannot be expected to be an exact correlation, because of discrepancies in the properties of mutant enzymes *in vivo* and *in vitro*.

Definitive diagnosis in the late onset group of patients is particularly difficult. A few of the patients seem to have clear abnormalities involving the synthetase gene, including patients where the enzyme displays abnormal kinetics or where the enzyme activity is very low in both fibroblasts and liver. The more challenging situation is that where low levels of enzyme activity are observed in liver but normal levels of enzyme activity are found in fibroblasts. Definitive diagnosis and characterization of these patients awaits better understanding of the basis for a "regulatory" form of citrullinemia with identification of the exact molecular basis for this phenomenon. Unlike uncomplicated neonatal cases, the diagnosis of this group of patients requires liver biopsy with evaluation of all the urea cycle enzyme activities, including kinetic analysis of the synthetase, and requires comparative analysis of the enzyme activity in fibroblasts.

Therapy

Until relatively recently, dietary therapy for urea cycle disorders and specifically for citrullinemia was disappointing. Restriction of protein intake to a minimal amount necessary for growth in children offered some improvement, but patients with severe defects did not survive. A number of important advances have occurred. The use of α-keto analogues of essential amino acids improves the ability to achieve the very low protein intake without risking essential amino acid deficiency (Batshaw *et al.*, 1975; Thoene *et al.*, 1977; Walser *et al.*, 1977; Batshaw *et al.*, 1981*a*), but this adjunct has largely been abandoned in citrullinemia. It was recognized earlier that arginine deficiency might be important in some urea cycle disorders (Danks *et al.*, 1974), and in time it became clearer that arginine administration was of major benefit in citrullinemia and in argininosuccinic aciduria (Batshaw *et al.*, 1981*b*). For these two diseases, the arginine can traverse the urea cycle, causing a decrease in blood ammonia and increased accumulation of citrulline or argininosuccinic acid. Citrulline and argininosuccinic acid are less toxic than ammonia and eventually are cleared by the kidney. On arginine supplementation, citrullinemia patients experience extremely high blood citrulline values, but they appear to grow and develop well. In addition, the group of investigators from Baltimore (Brusilow *et al.*, 1979, 1980; Batshaw *et al.*, 1982) has demonstrated the benefit of sodium benzoate and phenylacetate administration to provide an alternative pathway for nitrogen excretion. Sodium benzoate is more readily available and does not have the unpleasant odor of phenylacetate. However, these investigators currently recommend that both phenylacetate and sodium benzoate be administered in the treatment of neonatal citrullinemia (Msall *et al.*, 1984). They recommend a protein intake of 1.2–1.5 g/kg per day with addition of 0.4–0.7 g/day of arginine and 0.25 g/day of both sodium benzoate and sodium phenylacetate. There is evidence that phenylacetate is more effective than sodium benzoate in promoting waste nitrogen excretion (Brusilow, 1984). We are managing multiple patients with neonatal citrullinemia with arginine and sodium benzoate without the use of phenylacetate. An odor-free derivative of phenylacetate would be desirable.

Treatment of citrullinemia can be broken down into multiple phases. The first is management of acute neonatal hyperammonemia. By far the most critical variable in this process is early diagnosis. Once hyperammonemia is detected, it should be possible in major medical centers to make a specific diagnosis in a few hours using quantitative serum amino acid analysis. It then becomes possible to use specific intravenous therapy with arginine, adding sodium benzoate and phenylacetate if necessary. Prior to clarifying the exact etiology of the hyperammonemia, more general supportive measures can be used. These include administration of high-dose intravenous glucose accompanied by insulin as necessary to suppress protein catabolism. In the face of life-threatening coma, exchange transfusions, peritoneal dialysis, and hemodialysis all have been employed (Donn *et al.*, 1979; Wiegand *et al.*, 1980; Batshaw and Brusilow, 1980; Brusilow *et al.*, 1984). Hemodialysis is probably the most effective but least available therapeutic procedure in neonates. Exchange transfusion is the most readily available but least effective procedure, and peritoneal dialysis may represent a frequent compromise. If a specific diagnosis is established very rapidly and intravenous arginine and sodium benzoate are available, no dialysis or exchange procedure may be necessary. We have been successful in lowering blood ammonia rapidly by aggressive use of intravenous arginine alone, and Brusilow *et al.* (1984) routinely omit intravenous sodium benzoate and phenylacetate in the acute management.

The next phase of treatment is the chronic management. The use of a low-protein diet, arginine, sodium benzoate, and perhaps phenylacetate is carried out as specified above. This phase of management requires regular dietary supervision, assessment of growth and development, and regular measurement of the serum amino acid profile. The chronic phase of management usually does not represent serious problems. The next management consideration is the occurrence of acute episodes of hyperammonemia. These can occur due to inappropriate dietary or medication prescription or to parental noncompliance with the detailed regimen. There is frequent need for dietary adjustment as growth slows during the 6- to 15-month age period. More often, episodes of hyperammonemia are triggered by minor illnesses which cause decreased caloric intake and increased protein catabolism. Significant episodes are managed by use of intravenous glucose and arginine (Brusilow *et al.*, 1984). Although such episodes can be life-threatening, they are usually aborted within hours if the illness is treated early and if intravenous arginine is available. Intravenous sodium benzoate and phenyacetate and hemodialysis may be appropriate if difficulties persist. It remains to be seen whether neonatal citrullinemia patients can survive major episodes of protein catabolism as might occur with serious infectious illnesses or major trauma. Presumably, additional dietary adjustments will be required as these patients complete growth and achieve adult status.

Prognosis

The neurological outcome for patients with neonatal citrullinemia still is relatively disappointing. Long-term neurological sequelae are usual, and there is considerable correlation with the duration of coma in the neonatal period (Msall *et al.*, 1984). In our opinion, the main reason for prolonged coma is delayed diagnosis and lack of rapid availability of specific diagnostic capacity and intravenous management. The great majority of first-born citrullinemia patients within a family have IQ outcomes well below the normal range. Presumably, the outcome would be improved markedly for subsequent siblings treated from birth, but the long-term hazards and burden of the disease appropriately discourage most families from exploring this possibility.

Prenatal Diagnosis

Prenatal diagnosis for citrullinemia is more complex and treacherous than for many enzyme deficiencies. One problem is the fact that many heterozygous individuals express very low enzyme activity in cultured skin fibroblasts (Christensen *et al.*, 1980; Su *et al.*, 1982), and this may be true for cultured amniotic cells as well. The activity for heterozygotes can be in the range of 5–10% of normal. In addition, cultured amniotic epithelial cells express lower enzyme activity than do cultured amniotic fibroblastic cells (Jacoby *et al.*, 1981). Variability also is increased, because enzyme activity is lower in subconfluent cell cultures. The major hazard appears to be the demonstration of very low enzyme activity, which might be misinterpreted to represent an affected fetus when, in fact, the fetus is heterozygous or normal. One unaffected fetus was aborted in this context (Christensen *et al.*, 1980). By growing cultured amniotic fluid cells to high density and by using a sensitive radioactive assay, no difficulties or errors have been experienced in five pregnancies at risk for neonatal citrullinemia studied in our laboratory or in four cases studied by R. McInnes (personal communication). Analysis of incorporation of [^{14}C]citrulline into acid-precipitable protein by intact cultured amniotic fluid cells is probably the most reliable indicator for prenatal diagnosis (Cathelineau *et al.*, 1981a; Jacoby *et al.*, 1981; Fleisher *et al.*, 1983; Kleijer *et al.*, 1984). This analysis readily distinguishes heterozygous fibroblasts with low enzyme activity from affected cultured fibroblasts (Su *et al.*, 1982). We perform [^{14}C]citrulline/[^{3}H]leucine incorporation studies for prenatal diagnosis of citrullinemia if enzyme activity in cultured amniotic fluid cells is low. It is likely that similar methods can be established for reliable prenatal diagnosis for citrullinemia using chorionic villus biopsy (Fleisher *et al.*, 1984). Quantitation of citrulline in amniotic fluid is of considerable value in prenatal diagnosis (Fleisher *et al.*, 1983; Kamoun *et al.*, 1983; Kleijer *et al.*, 1984). This approach avoids the tissue culture problems, is rapid, and should be used routinely; but enzyme and incorporation studies remain the definitive procedures.

MOLECULAR ANALYSIS IN CITRULLINEMIA

Analysis of the structural gene for argininosuccinate synthetase and some of the data from citrullinemia patients all indicate strongly that there is a single expressed gene for the enzyme. There is a general acceptance that the enzyme represents a homotetramer with a subunit molecular weight of 46,000. Takada *et al.* (1979) separated three forms of the enzyme in the rat, but the forms varied only in the amount of bound argininosuccinate. Many laboratories have performed somatic cell hybridization studies using fibroblasts from different citrullinemia patients. Cathelineau *et al.* (1981b, 1982) did not detect complementation, while Kennaway and Curtis (1981) and McInnes *et al* (1984) did, indicating the presence of significant genetic heterogeneity in citrullinemia. Complementation only partially restores [^{14}C]citrulline incorporation, and all mutants mapped to one major complementation group (McInnes *et al.*, 1984), suggesting that the complementation was intragenic.

Analysis of DNA, RNA, and immunoreactive protein was carried out in a series of cultured skin fibroblast lines from neonatal citrullinemia patients (Su *et al.*, 1982). All of these cell lines had less than 1% of argininosuccinate synthetase activity by direct assay. Some heterogeneity within the cell lines was suggested by variation of [^{14}C]citrulline incorporation. The majority of cell lines demonstrated the absence of cross-reacting immune material using an antibody to the enzyme, but a minority of cell lines did contain cross-reacting material. One cell line contained cross-reacting immune material which migrated slightly faster on SDS–polyacrylamide gel electrophoresis. Analysis of genomic DNA by Southern blotting did not demonstrate any abnormality in the citrullinemia fibroblasts. This analysis was complicated by the presence of multiple pseudogenes, but the possibility of heterozygous or homozygous deletion of the entire gene was eliminated in all cases. Analysis of total cellular RNA from these fibroblast lines demonstrated the presence of mRNA for argininosuccinate synthetase of near the appropriate size. Subsequent analysis of RNA from cultured fibroblasts utilizing hybridization to cDNA

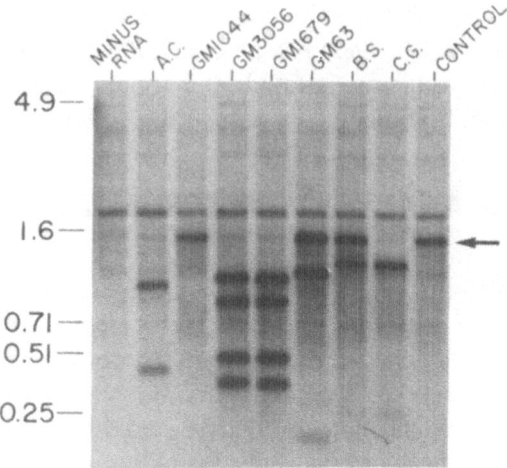

Fig. 3.   Analysis of mRNA from citrullinemia fibroblasts using S1 nuclease mapping. The mRNA was hybridized to nonradioactive cDNA and digestion was carried out with S1 nuclease. Protected DNA fragments were analyzed by agarose gel electrophoresis and Southern blotting using the cDNA as radioactive probe. The arrow indicates fully protected cDNA with normal mRNA. All lanes except those marked control and minus RNA are from neonatal citrullinemia patients. Cell line A.C. contains one S1 nuclease-detectable abnormal allele and one RNA-negative allele. GM1044 contains only fully protective mRNA. Cell lines GM3056 and GM1679 were taken from the same patient and contain two different S1 nuclease-detectable abnormal alleles. Cell lines GM63 and B.S. each contain one fully protective allele and one S1 nuclease-detectable abnormal allele. Cell line C.G. contains an S1 nuclease-detectable abnormal allele, presumably in the homozygous state, since the parents are first cousins. See Fig. 4, Table IV, and text for further interpretation. [From Su *et al.* (1983), by permission.]

and S1 nuclease digestion indicated multiple classes of abnormal mRNA, as shown in Fig. 3 (Su *et al.*, 1983). In some instances, the mRNA fully protected the available cDNA, suggesting the presence of subtle defects in the mRNA. This analysis would not detect single base changes, and the fully protective abnormal mRNAs presumably contain small defects. In other instances the abnormal mRNA failed to fully protect the cDNA, and digestion of the cDNA occurred at specific sites along the length. The sites of nuclease susceptibility varied for different alleles. The abnormal mRNAs with S1-detectable defects presumably involve larger defects such as might occur with insertions, deletions, or RNA splicing abnormalities. Many patients were demonstrated to be compound heterozygotes by this analysis.

Subsequently, we have demonstrated a third class of citrullinemia

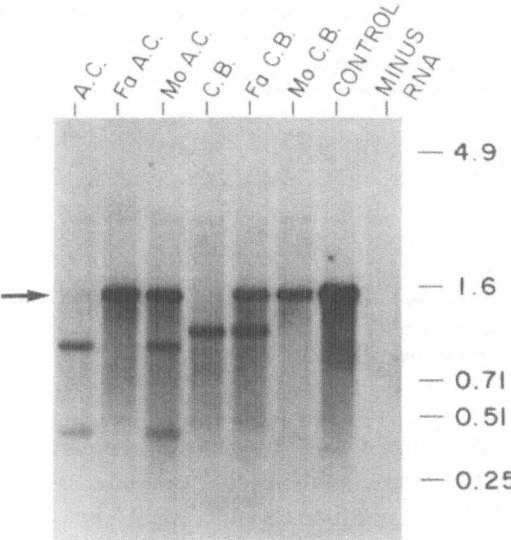

Fig. 4. Demonstration of RNA-negative allele for citrullinemia. Analysis was carried out as for Fig. 3. Two unrelated patients are designated A.C. and C.B., while parents are designated Fa for father and Mo for mother. [T.-S. Su, A.L. Beaudet, and W.E. O'Brien, (unpublished data).]

alleles, which we call RNA-negative alleles. In these instances, the genomic DNA was intact by Southern blotting analysis, but no stable mRNA was detected. This abnormality has been detected only in a compound heterozygous situation, so that documentation depends on analysis of parents and the propositus, as demonstrated in Fig. 4. We have observed two patients (A.C. and C.B. in Fig. 4) in whom there is a single class of abnormal RNA with a specific S1 nuclease-detectable defect. Analysis of the parents indicated the presence of the abnormal mRNA in one parent but not the other in each case. The data indicate that the affected children inherited one allele producing an abnormal mRNA with an S1 nuclease-detectable defect and one allele that failed to produce a stable mRNA. Southern blotting analysis, including dosage analysis and the use of intron probes, indicated that the RNA-negative allele is not a large deletion of the gene.

Our experience in analysis of citrullinemia fibroblasts is summarized in Tables IV and V. We have observed a series of alleles producing abnormal mRNAs which are distinguishable by S1 nuclease analysis, and

TABLE IV. Summary of Abnormal Alleles in Citrullinemia[a]

Cell line	Genotype	CRM	Cell line	Genotype	CRM
AC	AR	−	MV	TT or TR	+
CB	BR	−	GM1044	TT or TR	−
CG	CC	−	966	TT or TR	+
1679	DE	−	1263	TT or TR	−
KSt	BT	+	1377	TT or TR	−
BSm	CT	−	1391	TT or TR	−
GM63	FT	−			

[a] Alleles A–F have S1 nuclease-detectable abnormalities. R denotes an RNA-negative allele. T denotes a totally protective allele.

these alleles are designated A–F in Table IV. Alleles that totally protect the cDNA with S1 nuclease analysis are designated T (totally protective), and alleles that failed to produce a stable mRNA are designated R (RNA-negative). Many individuals with neonatal citrullinemia are compound heterozygotes. Many cell lines produce only a fully protective mRNA, and a TT genotype cannot be distinguished from a TR genotype. We believe that many of the fully protective alleles will represent nonsense or missense mutations or other small changes in the mRNA. Given the normal Southern blotting analysis and previous experience with thalassemia, the S1 nuclease-detectable defects in mRNA are likely to represent predominantly splicing abnormalities, although various insertions and deletions also may occur. The RNA-negative alleles may represent transcriptional defects or the occurrence of unstable mRNA. It is not surprising that cell lines producing cross-reactive immune material always contain at least one fully protective allele. Although we have not yet observed large deletions of the gene, further molecular heterogeneity is likely to be observed by study of additional patients. These studies indicate that most or all neonatal citrullinemia patients represent genetic

TABLE V. Human Mutants for Argininosuccinic Synthetase

1. Most cell lines CRM-negative
2. All Southern blots normal to date
3. S1 nuclease analysis of mRNA separates three classes of alleles:
   a. Fully protective RNA = small (?single base) changes
   b. S1-detectable abnormal RNA = large (?splicing) abnormalities
   c. RNA-negative = decreased transcription or half-life

defects at the structural locus for the enzyme, and that the various defects described above are allelic as evidenced by the data from compound heterozygotes.

MOLECULAR AND GENETIC ANALYSIS OF REGULATION

A number of distinct biological phenomena involving the argininosuccinate synthetase locus are available for investigation. These include the tissue-specific increased expression in liver and the species-specific absence and presence of enzyme activity in cultured fibroblasts from Chinese hamster and most other species, respectively. Metabolite repression of expression in tissue culture cells is a very distinct event, which should be amenable to molecular analysis. Similarly, the enzyme overproduction by Can^r cells offers a distinct form of regulation which can be studied. It remains to be determined whether there are any common regulatory mechanisms or factors involved in these somewhat diverse variations in expression.

Perhaps some lessons can be drawn from knowledge of gene regulation in lower organisms. Regulation of arginine biosynthesis in prokaryotes was reviewed by Cunin (1983). In *E. coli* the arginine biosynthetic enzymes are scattered in the genome to some extent, although all enzymes are subject to feedback regulation by arginine. The argininosuccinate synthetase locus (*arg*G) is less well studied than some of the other structural genes, although the gene has been cloned (Holowachuk and Friesen, 1982). The *arg*R locus encodes a repressor, and mutations in *arg*R are trans-recessive. The arginine pathway represents a regulon with scattered genes under the control of a common repressor. The repressor is thought to bind to conserved sequences called ARG boxes located at the 5' end of each gene. Based on *in vitro* transcription studies, free arginine is thought to be the corepressor (Cunin *et al.*, 1976). There also may be some nontranscriptional modulation of the *arg* loci, but this is unclear. The *arg* loci are noteworthy for the absence of attenuation, which is involved in the regulation of many other amino acid biosynthetic pathways. In *E. coli*, the canavanine-resistant phenotype can involve derepressed mutants (*arg*R), tRNA synthetase mutants (*arg*S), transport (*arg*P), and a separate locus (*can*), which maps near *arg*P; see Maas (1972) and Cunin (1983) for references.

Genetic regulation of arginine biosynthesis in *Saccharomyces cere-visiae* and *Neurospora crassa* was reviewed by Davis (1983). The arginine biosynthetic enzymes in yeast are dispersed in the genome and are subject to control by a complex repressor system. Three unlinked mutations define the *arg*RI, *arg*RII, and *arg*RIII loci. These loci may encode a heteromultimeric aporepressor, with arginine or arginyl tRNA as likely corepressors. The exact mechanism of regulation is uncertain, although Messenguy and Dubois (1983) have suggested that arginine-specific regulation in yeast operates at a posttranscriptional level. The most studied mechanism for canavanine resistance in yeast involves mutation of the structural gene for the arginine permease (Whelan *et al.*, 1979). There is no evidence at present for arginine-specific regulation in *Neurospora.* Canavanine resistance occurs in *Neurospora* due to expression of an enzyme that cleaves canavanine and is controlled by the *cnr* locus (Perkins *et al.*, 1982). Canavanine resistance also occurs due to mutation at the *pmb* locus, which encodes the permease for basic amino acids. All of these microorganisms are known to have genetic mechanisms for general regulation of amino acid biosynthesis, and these genetically distinct general and specific controls provide precedent for multiple levels of regulation.

The nature of Can^r human cell lines is unclear. In all instances, cells are found to be stable when grown in nonselective tissue culture media, and they are not subject to repression by arginine (Jacoby, 1978; Su *et al.*, 1981*a*). It is uncertain whether these stable cell variants represent mutants with a change in the nucleotide sequence, or whether these represent some stable epigenetic event, such as an alteration in DNA methylation or in chromatin structure. There is no detailed published analysis of the effect of mutagens or 5-azacytidine on the frequency of isolation of Can^r cells. In preliminary experiments, we have been unable to demonstrate any increase in frequency of occurrence of Can^r cells after treatment with 5-azacytidine or ethylmethane sulfonate, but these negative results cannot be considered conclusive. Although arginyl-tRNA synthetase was reported to be normal in Can^r cells (Jacoby, 1978), detailed comparison of the tRNA synthetase activity with both arginine and canavanine as substrates has not been reported. Analysis of arginine and canavanine transport has not been reported for human Can$_r$ cells.

Analysis of Can^r cells using cloned human cDNA indicated that the amount of hybridizable mRNA correlated well with the increased enzyme activity in Can^r cells, as cited above. The relative amount of hybridizable mRNA also correlated well with enzyme activity when wild-type cells were grown in citrulline as compared to arginine medium. Analysis of genomic DNA from Can^r cells indicated that gene amplification is not the mechanism for enzyme overproduction (Su *et al.*, 1981*b*). Alternative splicing of the mRNA for argininosuccinate synthetase has been detected, as discussed above (Fig. 1). Although some increased abundance of mRNA containing an additional 5' untranslated exon was detected in Can^r cells (Freytag *et al.*, 1984*b*), detailed analysis has not been completed to clarify any possible biological significance of this variation. In unpublished studies (S. O. Freytag, T.-S. Su, A. L. Beaudet, and W. E. O'-Brien), we have attempted to determine if enzyme overproduction in Can^r cells involves a *cis*-acting or *trans*-acting mechanism. Can^r lymphoblasts were isolated from an individual heterozygous for a mutation in the argininosuccinate synthetase gene with production of mRNA with an S1 nuclease-detectable defect. Analysis with S1 nuclease indicated that the Can^r lymphoblasts overproduced both normal and mutant mRNA, indicating a *trans*-acting mechanism for enzyme overproduction.

If one assumes that *trans*-acting factors regulate the expression of argininosuccinate synthetase, a variety of models can be proposed regarding the known regulatory events. If a positive-acting element exists, Can^r cells might represent a gain or increase in the expression of this positive-acting factor. This positive-acting factor could induce its own synthesis to provide a stable mechanism for enzyme overproduction. Alternatively, one might assume that enzyme overproduction involves expression of a negative-acting regulatory element. Loss or reduced expression of this negative factor could result in increased expression of argininosuccinate synthetase. A *trans*-acting repressor also could be regulated in some way by arginine, arginyl-tRNA, or other arginine-related molecules. Loss of expression of such a repressor could explain the simultaneous enzyme overproduction and loss of metabolite repression. The report of a possible regulatory form of citrullinemia could be related to genetic alterations in such hypothetical *trans*-acting factors. Similarly, differences in expression between Chinese hamster cells and other tissue culture cells could be explained by the presence or absence of *trans*-acting regulatory factors.

GENE TRANSFER USING THE ARGININOSUCCINATE SYNTHETASE LOCUS

Since Chinese hamster cells do not express argininosuccinate synthetase, tissue culture medium with citrulline substituted for arginine can be used to select for enzyme expression in these cells. This has facilitated various gene transfer studies. The feasibility of such studies was made clear by somatic cell hybridization studies, where retention of human chromosome 9 correlated with the presence of argininosuccinate synthetase activity in Chinese hamster–human hybrids (Carritt *et al.*, 1977). Chromosome-mediated gene transfer was used to transfer the human gene into Chinese hamster cells (Hudson *et al.*, 1980). The human enzyme was distinguished from hamster enzyme using isoelectric focusing. DNA-mediated gene transfer was carried out using the calcium phosphate precipitation method and human DNA isolated from Can^r cells (Su *et al.*, 1984*b*). These studies demonstrated the transfer of the single human expressed gene into the Chinese hamster cells. Very large DNA fragments (>80 kb) were transferred, and the detection of the expected genomic DNA fragments served to confirm the identity and structure of the human expressed gene. DNA-mediated gene transfer also has been carried out using the human cDNA linked to the SV40 promoter or to the promoter from Rous sarcoma virus (Partridge *et al.*, 1984). Future gene transfer studies should be helpful in analyzing regulation for this locus and may have potential relevance for gene therapy.

FUTURE DIRECTIONS

While citrullinemia is a relatively rare disorder, it remains desirable to to reduce or eliminate the burden of this disease. Improvements in the prevention and treatment of citrullinemia are likely to have implications for other inborn errors of metabolism. It is unlikely that population-wide heterozygote screening will offer a feasible, cost-effective avenue for prevention of citrullinemia or most other inborn errors of metabolism. Even if heterozygote testing using enzyme assays could be carried out inexpensively, the great potential for heterogeneity among nondisease alleles as well as disease alleles could cause high levels of false positives and false negatives in heterozygote screening programs. Assuming that first affected children will continue to be born into families, successful care for this disease will require detection prior to the occurrence of any irreversible brain injury. This would seem feasible using some form of selective neonatal screening for hyperammonemia. A device for measuring blood ammonia at the bedside using small volumes of blood is commercially available (Tada *et al.*, 1982). The use of such a device to screen for blood ammonia elevations in any infant with the most minor symptoms in the first week or two of life could represent an effective method for diagnosing neonatal citrullinemia and other forms of neonatal hyperammonemia prior to the occurrence of irreversible damage. Talbot *et al.* (1982*a,b*) described a method for newborn screening using dried filter specimens, but infants with neonatal citrullinemia would suffer brain damage prior to availability of the result, unless filters were processed much more rapidly than is conventional. The filter method holds great promise for detection of late onset citrullinemia, late onset argininosuccinic aciduria, argininemia, and various forms of ornithinemia, all diseases where time favors the potential for highly effective dietary therapy. A remaining problem is the limited availability of centers where rapid, definitive diagnosis and treatment are possible.

Once early diagnosis is established, methods for dietary and drug therapy are relatively adequate at the present time. These methods provide a temporizing form of therapy, and patients can be maintained in a state of good growth and development for months and years. Some more definitive long-term therapy is still required, since patients remain at risk for serious, life-threatening episodes of hyperammonemia. This therapy could come in the form of new drugs or in refinements in the use of existing drugs. For instance, it is possible that more aggressive use of higher doses of sodium benzoate and arginine will prove entirely adequate for management of acute episodes of catabolism. Availability of an intravenous arginine preparation with less acid load than the hydrochloride form is desirable. Liver transplantation presumably would be completely adequate to correct the metabolic abnormalities in citrullinemia. At present, the risks of liver transplantation are judged to exceed the risks of continued dietary therapy, but improved results with liver transplantation could change that perspective.

A recent development is the possibility of gene therapy using cloned DNA. Current gene therapy efforts are focused on the use of retroviruses to derive pseudovirion preparations which can efficiently infect human cells and allow for the integration and expression of a foreign gene (Williams *et al.*, 1984; Miller *et al.*, 1984; Weatherall, 1984). Although this general approach seems attractive, new methodologies are likely to evolve rapidly. We believe that citrullinemia represents an attractive model disorder for attempts at gene therapy. The enzyme in question is a homotetramer located in the cytoplasm with no known unusual requirements for cofactors or posttranslational processing. While it would seem optimal to deliver a therapeutic DNA fragment to hepatocytes, it is possible that enzyme produced in a tissue such as bone marrow would be effective in controlling the metabolic imbalance. Very high concentrations of citrulline in the blood suggest that peripheral tissues might be able to metabolize this substrate. Enzyme deficiencies involving circulating metabolites provide a particularly opportune circumstance for attempts at gene therapy. Achievement of even modest expression of enzyme activity might be quite beneficial. Excessive enzyme activity is unlikely to be harmful in many situations. Existing experience with dietary and drug therapy indicate that it is not essential to deliver enzyme activity to all tissues in the body, but some proportion of cells could accomplish the necessary metabolic processes. An animal model system would be useful for studying some of these questions. While two dogs with citrullinemia were described (Strombeck *et al.*, 1975), we have been unable to locate heterozygous or homozygous animals from that report.

Citrullinemia and other urea cycle disorders may prove to be excellent model systems for delivery of genetic material to live cells. One approach might be to perform a partial hepatectomy and transfect primary hepatocytes in tissue culture. There is a suggestion that such cells could be reimplanted in the liver (Sutherland *et al.*, 1980). Alternatively, pseudoviruses might be targeted to hepatocytes through a cell-specific receptor. The asialoglycoprotein receptor is one candidate, which is well characterized (Ashwell and Harford, 1982) and cloned (Holland *et al.*, 1984). Perhaps the ligand for this receptor could be incorporated into pseudoviruses using chemical or recombinant DNA techniques. Delivery of genetic material to hepatocytes would have implications for many important genetic diseases, such as α_1-antitrypsin deficiency, clotting factor deficiencies, and many inborn errors of metabolism.

Proposals for gene therapy have elicited considerable ethical discussion. It is important to distinguish therapeutic attempts that manipulate somatic cells from any attempt to manipulate the germ-like DNA. For example, experiments that remove bone marrow cells or hepatocytes for insertion of foreign DNA followed by replacement into the body would not seem controversial and do not broach any novel ethical considerations. So long as the germ line remains unaffected, such attempts can be evaluated strictly on the potential risks and benefits to affected patients. Incidental risk to the germ line might be acceptable, since there is precedent for accepting such risks in cancer chemotherapy. The major risk to the patient is likely to be tumorigenesis due to insertional mutagenesis

(Brinster *et al.*, 1984). The overall risk–benefit ratio will depend in large part on the prognosis for individual diseases, and more lethal disorders provide greater justification for therapeutic attempts. The long-term prognosis for citrullinemia might be considered somewhat uncertain in this regard. The feasibility of altering the germ line to correct genetic defects is exemplified by experiments introducing growth hormone genes into deficient mice (Hammer *et al.*, 1984). However, this approach is not relevant to the human situation. While experiments to manipulate somatic cells seem easily justifiable in the instance of certain untreatable disorders, attempts to manipulate the germ line are unlikely to be justifiable in the near future.

Future directions for analysis of regulation for argininosuccinate synthetase are likely to focus on gene transfer experiments. It should be possible to transfer portions of the argininosuccinate synthetase structural gene into various tissue culture cell lines. This approach should allow for confirmation of the action of any *trans*-acting factors on incoming DNA sequences. Such experiments can utilize the gene itself or can utilize recombinant DNA constructions linking regulatory DNA sequences to reporter genes, such as the chloramphenicol acetyltransferase gene and others. Using DNA-mediated transfer, it should be possible to identify *cis*-acting regulatory sequences that are essential for the regulatory phenomena of arginine repression and enzyme overproduction in Can^r cells. Using DNA-mediated gene transfer into cultured hepatoma cells, it may be possible to identify *cis*-acting sequences that allow for increased expression in hepatocytes. Recombinant DNA constructions can be introduced into mouse embryos to evaluate tissue-specific regulation. Given the availability of tissue culture selection systems, it also might be possible to try to recover DNA fragments that encode *trans*-acting regulatory factors. DNA-mediated gene transfer followed by selection of a particular tissue culture phenotype has allowed for the cloning of oncogenes, enzymes, and surface antigens. Using these strategies, it might be possible to try to clone a DNA sequence that activates the expression of the Chinese hamster gene or transfers the phenotype of enzyme overproduction. Identification of genes that specifically regulate argininosuccinate synthetase in a *trans*-acting manner is a major goal of current research.

ACKNOWLEDGMENTS. We thank Lynn Loewenstein for preparation of the manuscript. Roderick McInnes provided valuable review of the manuscript. This work was supported by research and fellowship grants from the National Institutes of Health.

REFERENCES

Aebi, H., 1976, Coordinated changes in enzymes of the ornithine cycle and response to dietary conditions, in: *The Urea Cycle* (S. Grisolia, R. Báguena, and F. Mayor, eds.), pp. 275–299, Wiley, New York.

Amos, J. A., Fleming, B. C., Gusella, J. F., and Jacoby, L. B., 1984, Relative argininosuccinate synthetase mRNA levels and gene copy number in canavanine-resistant lymphoblasts, *Biochim. Biophys. Acta* **782**:247–253.

Ashwell, G., and Harford, J., 1982, Carbohydrate-specific receptors of the liver, *Annu. Rev. Biochem.* **51**:531–554.

Bachmann, B. J., and Low, K. B., 1980, Linkage map of *Escherichia coli* K-12, Edition 6, *Microbiol. Rev.* **44**:1–56.

Batshaw, M. L., 1984, Hyperammonemia, *Curr. Probl. Pediatr.* **14**(11):1–69.

Batshaw, M. L., and Brusilow, S. W., 1978, Asymptomatic hyperammonemia in low birthweight infants, *Pediatr. Res.* **12**:221–224.

Batshaw, M. L., and Brusilow, S. W., 1980, Treatment of hyperammonemic coma caused by inborn errors of urea synthesis, *J. Pediatr.* **97**:893–900.

Batshaw, M., Brusilow, S., and Walser, M., 1975, Treatment of carbamyl phosphate synthetase deficiency with keto analogues of essential amino acids, *N. Engl. J. Med.* **292**:1085–1090.

Batshaw, M. L., Painter, M. J., Sproul, G. T., Schafer, I. A., Thomas, G. H., and Brusilow, S., 1981*a*, Therapy of urea cycle enzymopathies: Three case studies, *Johns Hopkins Med. J.* **148**:34–40.

Batshaw, M. L., Thomas, G. H., and Brusilow, S. W., 1981*b*, New approaches to the diagnosis and treatment of inborn errors of urea synthesis, *Pediatrics* **68**:290–297.

Batshaw, M. L., Brusilow, S., Waber, L, Blom, W., Brubakk, A. M., Burton, B. K., Cann, H. M., Kerr, D., Mamunes, P., Matalon, R., Myerberg, D., and Schafer, I. A., 1982, Treatment of inborn errors of urea synthesis. Activation of alternative pathways of waste nitrogen synthesis and excretion, *N. Engl. J. Med.* **306**:1387–1392.

Beaudet, A. L., Su, T.-S., and O'Brien, W. E., 1982, Dispersion of argininosuccinate synthetase-like human genes to multiple autosomes and the X chromosome, *Cell* **30**:287–293.

Bock, H.-G. O., Su, T.-S., O'Brien, W. E., and Beaudet, A. L., 1983, Sequence for human argininosuccinate synthetase cDNA, *Nucleic Acids Res.* **11**:6505–6512.

Borsook, H., and Dubnoff, J. W., 1941, The conversion of citrulline to arginine in kidney, *J. Biol. Chem.* **141**:717–738.

Brinster, R. L., Chen, H. Y., Messing, A., van Dyke, T., Levine, A. J., and Palmiter, R. D., 1984, Transgenic mice harboring SV40 T-antigen genes develop characteristic brain tumors, *Cell* **37**:367–379.

Brusilow, S., 1984, Inborn errors of ureagenesis; Results of therapy in 44 patients, *Pediatr. Res.* **18**:220A.

Brusilow, S., Valle, D. L., and Batshaw, M., 1979, New pathways of nitrogen excretion in inborn errors of urea synthesis, *Lancet* **ii**:452–454.

Brusilow, S., Tinker, J., and Batshaw, M. L., 1980, Amino acid acylation: A mechanism of nitrogen excretion in inborn errors of urea synthesis, *Science* **207**:659–661.

Brusilow, S. W., Danney, M., Waber, L. J., Batshaw, M., Burton, B., Levitsky, L., Roth, K., McKeethren, C., and Ward, J., 1984, Treatment of episodic hyperammonemia in children with inborn errors of urea synthesis, *N. Engl. J. Med.* **310**:1630–1634.

Carlock, L. R., Skarecky D., Dana S. L., and Wasmuth J. J., 1985, Deletion mapping of human chromosome 5 using chromosome specific DNA probes, *Am. J. Hum. Genet.* **37**:839–852.

Carritt, B., and Povey, S., 1979, Regional assignments of the loci AK_3, $ACON_S$ and ASS on human chromosome 9, *Cytogenet. Cell Genet.* **23**:171–181.

Carritt, B., Goldfarb, P. S. G., Hooper, M. L., and Slack, C., 1977, Chromosome assignment of a human gene for argininosuccinate synthetase expression in Chinese hamster × human somatic cell hybrids, *Exp. Cell Res.* **106**:71–78.

Cathelineau, L., Pham Dinh, D., Boué, J., Saudubray, J. M., Farriaux, J. P., and Kamoun, P., 1981*a*, Improved method for the antenatal diagnosis of citrullinemia, *Clin. Chim. Acta* **116**:111–115.

Cathelineau, L., Pham Dinh, D., Briand, P., and Kamoun, P., 1981*b*, Studies on complementation in argininosuccinate synthetase and argininosuccinate lyase deficiencies in human fibroblasts, *Hum. Genet.* **57**:282–284.

Cathelineau, L., Pham Dinh, D., Briand, P., and Kamoun, P., 1982, Complementation in argininosuccinate synthetase and argininosuccinate lyase deficiencies in human fibroblasts, *Adv. Exp. Med. Biol.* **153**:101–110.

Christensen, E., Brandt, N. J., Philip, J., and Kennaway, N. G., 1980, Citrullinaemia: The possibility of prenatal diagnosis, *J. Inherited Metab. Dis.* **3**:73–75.

Cohen, P. P., and Hayano, M., 1946, Urea synthesis by liver homogenates, *J. Biol. Chem.* **166**:251–259.

Cunin, R., 1983, Regulation of arginine biosynthesis in prokaryotes, in: *Amino Acids: Biosynthesis and Genetic Regulation* (K. M. Herrmann and R. L. Somerville, eds.), pp. 53–79, Addison-Wesley, Reading, Massachusetts.

Cunin, R., Kelker, N., Boyen, A., Yang, H.-L., Zubay, g., Glansdorff, N., and Maas, W. K., 1976, Involvement of arginine in *in vitro* repression of transcription of arginine genes C, B and H in *Escherichia coli* K 12, *Biochem. Biophys. Res. Commun.* **69**:377–382.

Daiger, S. P., and Hoffman, N. S., 1983, Comparison of Y chromosome DNA sequences between humans and chimpanzees, *Genetics* **104**:s20.

Daiger, S. P., Wildin, R. S., and Su, T.-S., 1982, Sequences on the human Y chromosome homologous to the autosomal gene for argininosuccinate synthetase, *Nature* **298**:682–684.

Daiger, S. P., Hoffman, N. S., Wildin, R. S., and Su, T.-S., 1984, Multiple, independent restriction site polymorphisms in human DNA detected with a cDNA probe to argininosuccinate synthetase (AS), *Am. J. Hum. Genet.* **36**:736–749.

Danks, D. M., Tippett, P., and Zentner, G., 1974, Severe neonatal citrullinaemia, *Arch. Dis. Child.* **49**:579–581.

Davis, R. H., 1983, Arginine synthesis in eukaryotes, in: *Amino Acids, Biosynthesis and Genetic Regulation* (K. M. Herrmann and R. L. Somerville, eds.), pp. 81–102, Addison-Wesley, Reading, Massachusetts.

Donn, S. M., and Banagale, R. C., 1984, Neonatal hyperammonemia, *Pediat. Rev.* **5**:203–208.

Donn, S. M., Swartz, R. D., and Thoene, J. G., 1979, Comparison of exchange transfusion, peritoneal dialysis and hemodialysis for the treatment of hyperammonemia in an anuric newborn infant, *J. Pediatr.* **95**:67–70.

Fleisher, L. D., Harris, C. J., Mitchell, D. A., and Nadler, H. L., 1983, Citrullinemia: Prenatal diagnosis of an affected fetus, *Am. J. Hum. Genet.* **35**:85–90.

Fleisher, L., Mitchell, D., Koppitch, F., Mariona, F., Evans, M., Goodman, S., and Nadler, H., 1984, Chorionic villous samples (CVS) for the prenatal diagnosis of amino acidopathies, *Am. J. Hum. Genet.* **36**:188S.

Freytag, S. O., Bock, H.-G. O., Beaudet, A. L., and O'Brien, W. E., 1984a, Molecular structures of human argininosuccinate synthetase pseudogenes, *J. Biol. Chem.* **259**:3160–3166.

Freytag, S. O., Beaudet,A. L., Bock, H.-G. O., and O'Brien, W. E., 1984b, Molecular structure of the human argininosuccinate synthetase gene: Occurence of alternative mRNA splicing, *Mol. Cell. Biol.* **4**:1978–1984.

Gebhardt, R., and Mecke, D., 1979, Permissive effect of dexamthasone on glucagon induction of urea-cycle enzymes in perifused primary monolayer cultures of rat hepatocytes, *Eur. J. Biochem.* **97**:29–35.

Grisolia, S., Báguena, R., and Mayor, F. (eds.), 1976, *The'Urea Cycle* Wiley, New York.

Haggerty, D. F., Spector, E. B., Lynch, M., Kern, R., Frank, L. B., and Cederbaum, S. D., 1982, Regulation by glucocorticoids of arginase and argininosuccinate synthetase in cultured rat hepatoma cells, *J. Biol. Chem.* **257**:2246–2253.

Hammer, R. E., Palmiter, R. D., and Brinster, R. L., 1984, Partial correction of murine hereditary growth disorder by germ-line incorporation of a new gene, *Nature* **311**:65–67.

Holland, E. C., Leung, J. O., and Drickamer, K., 1984, Rat liver asialoglycoprotein receptor lacks a cleavable NH_2-terminal signal sequence, *Proc. Natl. Acad. Sci. USA* **81**:7338–7342.

Holowachuk, E. W., and Friesen, J. D., 1982, Isolation of a recombinant lambda phage carrying *nus*A and surrounding region of the *Escherichia coli* K-12 chromosome, *Mol. Gen. Genet.* **187**:248–253.

Hudson, L. D., Erbe, R. W., and Jacoby, L. B., 1980, Expression of the human argininosuccinate synthetase gene in hamster transferents, *Proc. Natl. Acad. Sci. USA* **77**:4234–4238.

Irr, J. D., and Jacoby, L. B., 1978, Control of argininosuccinate synthetase by arginine in human lymphoblasts, *Somat. Cell Genet.* **4**:111–124.

Jacoby, L. B., 1974, Adaptation of cultured human lymphoblasts to growth in citrulline, *Exp. Cell Res.* **84**:167–174.

Jacoby, L. B., 1978, Canavanine-resistant variants of human lymphoblasts, *Somat. Cell Genet.* **4**:221–231.

Jacoby, L. B., Shih, V. E., Struckmeyer, C., Niermeijer, M. F., and Boué, J., 1981, Variation in argininosuccinate synthetase activity in amniotic fluid cell cultures: Implications for prenatal diagnosis of citrullinemia, *Clin. Chim. Acta* **116**:1–7.

Jinno, Y., Nomiyama, S., Wakasugi, S., Shimada, K., and Matsuda, I., 1984, Isolation and characterization of phage clones carrying the human argininosuccinate synthetase-like genes, *J. Inherited Metab. Dis.* **7**:133–134.

Kamoun, P., Parvy, P. H., Pham Dinh, D., Boué, J., and Cathelineau, L., 1983, Citrulline in amniotic fluid and the prenatal diagnosis of citrullinemia, *Prenatal Diagnosis* **3**:53–56.

Kato, H., Oyamada, I., Mizutani-Funahashi, M., and Nakagawa, H., 1976, New radioisotopic assays of argininosuccinate synthetase and argininosuccinase, *J. Biochem.* **79**:945–953.

Kennaway, N. G., and Curtis, H. C., 1981, Complementation analysis in fibroblasts from eight patients with clinically different forms of citrullinaemia, *J. Inherited Metab. Dis.* **4**:23.

Kimball, M. E., and Jacoby, L. B., 1980, Purification and properties of argininosuccinate synthetase from normal and canavanine-resistant human lymphoblasts, *Biochemistry* 19:705–709.

Kleijer, W. J., Blom, W., Huijmans, J. G. M., Mooyman, M. C. T., Berger, R., and Niermeijer, M. F., 1984, Prenatal diagnosis of citrullinemia: Elevated levels of citrulline in the amniotic fluid in the three affected pregnancies, *Prenatal Diagnosis* 4:113–118.

Krebs, H. A., 1952, Urea synthesis, in: *The Enzymes* (J. B. Sumner and K. Mÿrback, eds.), pp. 866–885, Academic Press, New York.

Krebs, H.A., 1976, The discovery of the ornithine cycle, in: *The Urea Cycle* (S. Grisolia, R. Baguena, and F. Mayor, eds.), pp. 1–12, Wiley, New York.

Lin, R. C., Snodgrass, P. J., and Rabier, D., 1982, Induction of urea cycle enzymes by glucagon and dexamethasone in monolayer cultures of adult rat hepatocytes, *J. Biol. Chem.* 257:5061–5067.

Lockridge, O., Spector, E. B., and Bloom, A. D., 1977, Argininosuccinate synthetase activity in cultured human lymphocytes, *Biochem. Genet.* 15:395–407.

Lowenthal, A., Mori, A., and Marescau, B., 1982, Urea cycle diseases, *Adv. Exp. Med. Biol.* 153:1–528.

Maas, W. K., 1972, Mapping of genes involved in the synthesis of spermidine in *Escherichia coli, Mol. Gen. Genet.* 119:1–9.

McInnes, R., Plavsic, N., and Chilton, S., 1984, Intragenic complementation in argininosuccinic acid synthetase (ASAS) deficiency, *Am. J. Hum. Genet.* 36:15S.

McLean, P., and Gurney, M. W., 1963, Effect of adrenalectomy and of growth hormone on enzymes concerned with urea synthesis in rat liver, *Biochem. J.* 87:9–104.

McMurray, W. C., Mohyuddin, F., Rossiter, R. M., Rathbun, J. C., Valentine, G. H., Koegler, S. J., and Zarfas, D.E., 1962, Citrullinuria. A new amino-aciduria associated with mental retardation, *Lancet* i:138.

Messenguy, F., and Dubois, E., 1983, Participation of transcriptional and posttranscriptional regulatory mechanisms in the control of arginine metabolism in yeast, *Mol. Gen. Genet.* 189:148–156.

Miller, A. D., Ong, E. S., Rosenfeld, M. G., Verma, I. M., and Evans, R. M., 1984, Infectious and selectable retrovirus containing an inducible rat growth hormone minigene, *Science* 225:993–998.

Morris, J. G., and Rogers, Q. R., 1978, Ammonia intoxication in the near-adult cat as a result of a dietary deficiency of arginine, *Science* 199:431–432.

Mortimer, R. K., and Schild, D., 1980, Genetic map of *Saccharomyces cerevisiae, Microbiol. Rev.* 44:519–571.

Msall, M., Batshaw, M. L., Suss, R., Brusilow, S. W., and Mellits, E. D., 1984, Neurologic outcome in children with inborn errors of urea synthesis, *N. Engl. J. Med.* 310:1500–1505.

Naylor, S. L., Busby, L. L., and Klebe, R. J., 1976, Biochemical selection systems for mammalian cells: The essential amino acids, *Somat. Cell Genet.* 2:93–111.

Nuzum, C. T., and Snodgrass, P. J., 1971, Urea cycle enzyme adaptation to dietary protein in primates, *Science* 172:1042–1043.

Nuzum, C. T., and Snodgrass, P. J., 1976, Multiple assays of the five urea-cycle enzymes in human liver homogenates, in: *The Urea Cycle* (S. Grisolia, R. Báguena, and F. Mayor, eds.), pp. 325–349, Wiley, New York.

O'Brien, W. E., 1976, A continuous spectrophotometric assay for argininosuccinate synthetase based on pyrophosphate formation, *Anal. Biochem.* 76:423–430.

O'Brien, W. E., 1979, Isolation and characterization of argininosuccinate synthetase from human liver, *Biochemistry* 18:5353–5356.

Partridge, C. A., Beaudet, A. L., and O'Brien, W. E., 1984, Expression of human argininosuccinate synthetase cDNA in Chinese hamster cells, *Am. J. Hum. Genet.* 36:150S.

Perkins, D. D., Radford, A., Newmeyer, D., and Björkman, M., 1982, Chromosomal loci of *Neurospora crassa*, *Microbiol. Rev.* **46**:426–570.

Rabier, D., Briand, P., Petit, F., Parvy, P., Kamoun, P., and Cathelineau, L., 1982, Acute effects of glucagon on citrulline biosynthesis, *Biochem. J.* **206**:627–631.

Räihä, N. C. R., 1976, Developmental changes of urea-cycle enzymes in mammalian liver, in: *The Urea Cycle* (S. Grisolia, R. Báguena, and F. Mayor, eds.), pp. 261–274, Wiley, New York.

Ratner, S., 1947, The enzymatic mechanism of arginine formation from citrulline, *J. Biol. Chem.* **170**:761–762.

Ratner, S., 1954, Urea synthesis and metabolism of arginine and citrulline, *Adv. Enzymol.* **15**:319–387.

Ratner, S., 1976, Enzymes of arginine and urea synthesis, in: *The Urea Cycle* (S. Grisolia, R. Baguena, and F. Mayor, eds.), pp. 181–219, Wiley, New York.

Ratner, S., 1982, Argininosuccinate synthetase of bovine liver: Chemical and physical properties, *Proc. Natl. Acad. Sci. USA* **79**:5197–5199.

Ratner, S., 1983, A radiochemical assay for argininosuccinate synthetase with [U-^{14}C]aspartate, *Anal. Biochem.* **135**:479–488.

Raushel, F. M., and Seiglie, J., 1983, Kinetic mechanism of argininosuccinate synthetase, *Arch. Biochem. Biophys.* **225**:979–985.

Rochovansky, O., and Ratner, S., 1967, Biosynthesis of urea: Further studies of argininosuccinate synthetase: Substrate affinity and mechanism of action,*J. Biol. Chem.* **242**:3839–3849.

Rochovansky, O., Kodowaki, H., and Ratner, S., 1977, Biosynthesis of urea: Molecular and regulatory properties of crystalline argininosuccinate synthetase, *J. Biol. Chem.* **252**:5287–5294.

Saheki, T., Kusumi, T., Takada, S., and Katsunuma, T., 1975, Crystallization and some properties of argininosuccinate synthase from rat liver, *FEBS Lett.* **58**:314–317.

Saheki, T., Ueda, A., Hosoya, M., Kusumi, K., Takada, S., Tsuda, M., and Katsunuma, T., 1981, Qualitative and quantitative abnormalities of argininosuccinate synthetase in citrullinemia, *Clin. Chim. Acta* **109**:325–335.

Saheki, T., Ueda, A., Iizima, K., Yamada, N., Kobayashi, K., Takahashi, K., and Katsunuma, T., 1982a, Argininosuccinate synthetase activity in cultured skin fibroblasts of citrullinemic patients, *Clin. Chim. Acta* **118**:93–97.

Saheki, T., Ueda, A., Hosoya, M., Sase, M., Nakano, K., and Katsunuma, T., 1982b, Enzymatic analysis of citrullinemia (12 cases) in Japan, *Adv. Exp. Med. Biol.* **153**:63–76.

Saheki, T., Sase, M., Nakano, K., Azuma, F., and Katsunuma, T., 1983a, Some properties of argininosuccinate synthetase purified from human liver and a comparison with the rat liver enzyme, *J. Biochem.* **93**:1531–1537.

Saheki, T., Yagi, Y., Sase, M., Nakano, K., and Sato, E., 1983b, Immunohistochemical localization of argininosuccinate synthetase in the liver of control and citrullinemic patients, *Biomed. Res.* **4**:235–238.

Schimke, R. T., 1962a, Adaptive characteristics of urea cycle enzymes in the rat, *J. Biol. Chem.* **237**:459–468.

Schimke, R. T., 1962b, Differential effects of fasting and protein-free diets on levels of urea cycle enzymes in rat liver, *J. Biol. Chem.* **237**:1921–1924.

Schimke, R. T., 1963, Studies on factors affecting the levels of urea cycle enzymes in rat liver, *J. Biol. Chem.* **238**:1012–1018.

Schimke, R. T., 1964, Enzymes of arginine metabolism in mammalian cell culture, *J. Biol. Chem.* **239**:136–145.

Shih, V. E., and Efron, M. L., 1972, Urea cycle disorders, in: *The Metabolic Basis of Inherited Disease* (J. B. Stanbury, J. B. Wyngaarden, and D. S. Fredrickson, eds.), pp. 370–392, McGraw-Hill, New York.

Snodgrass, P. J., Lin, R. C., Müller, W. A., and Aoki, T. T., 1978, *J. Biol. Chem.* **253:**2748–2753.

Stewart, P. M., Batshaw, M., Valle, D., and Walser, M., 1981, Effects of arginine-free meals on ureagenesis in cats, *Am. J. Physiol.* **241:**E310–E315.

Strombeck, D. R., Meyer, D. J., and Freedland, R. A., 1975, Hyperammonemia due to a urea cycle enzyme deficiency in two dogs, *J. Am. Vet. Med. Assoc.* **166:**1109–1111.

Su, T.-S., Beaudet, A. L., and O'Brien, W. E., 1981a, Increased translatable messenger ribonucleic acid for argininosuccinate synthetase in canavanine-resistant human cells, *Biochemistry* **20:**2956–2960.

Su, T.-S., Bock, H.-G. O., O'Brien, W. E., and Beaudet, A. L., 1981b, Cloning of cDNA for argininosuccinate synthetase mRNA and study of enzyme overproduction in a human cell line, *J. Biol. Chem.* **256:**11826–11831.

Su, T.-S., Bock, H.-G. O., Beaudet, A. L., and O'Brien, W. E., 1982, Molecular analysis of argininosuccinate synthetase deficiency in human fibroblasts, *J. Clin. Invest.* **70:**1334–1339.

Su, T.-S., Beaudet, A. L., and O'Brien, W. E., 1983, Abnormal mRNA for argininosuccinate synthetase in citrullinaemia, *Nature* **301:**533–534.

Su, T.-S., Nussbaum, R. L., Airhart, S., Ledbetter, D. H., Mohandas, T., O'Brien, W. E., and Beaudet, A. L., 1984a, Human chromosomal assignments for 14 argininosuccinate synthetase pseudogenes: Cloned DNAs as reagents for cytogenetic analysis, *Am. J. Hum. Genet.* **36:**954–964.

Su, T.-S., O'Brien, W. E., and Beaudet, A. L., 1984b, Genomic DNA-mediated gene transfer for argininosuccinate synthetase, *Somat. Cell. Mol. Genet.* **10:**601–606.

Sun, N. C., Sun, C. R. Y., Tennant, R. W., and Hsie, A. W., 1979, Selective growth of some rodent epithelial cells in a medium containing citrulline, *Proc. Natl. Acad. Sci. USA* **76:**1819–1823.

Sutherland, D. E. R., Hong, C., and Najarian, J. S., 1980, Cellular transplantation for enzymatic and metabolic deficiencies, *Birth Defects: Orig. Artic. Ser.* **16:**207–217.

Tada, K., Tateda, H., and Metoki, K., 1982, A new method for screening of hyperammonemia, *Adv. Exp. Med. Biol.* **153:**19–27.

Takada, S., Kusumi, T., Saheki, T., Tsuda, M., and Katsunuma, T., 1979, Studies of rat liver argininosuccinate synthetase, *J. Biochem.* **86:**1353–1359.

Talbot, H. W., Naylor, E. W., and Guthrie, R., 1982a, Neonatal urine screening for metabolic disease with auxotrophic strains of *Bacillus subtilis, Clin. Chim. Acta* **119:**345–349.

Talbot, H. W., Sumlin, A. B., Naylor, E. W., and Guthrie, R., 1982b, A neonatal screening test for argininosuccinic acid lyase deficiency and other urea cycle disorders, *Pediatrics* **70:**526–531.

Tedesco, T. A., and Mellman, W. J., 1967, Argininosuccinate synthetase activity and citrulline metabolism in cells cultured from a citrullinemic subject, *Proc. Natl. Acad. Sci. USA* **57:**829–834.

Thoene, J., Batshaw, M., Spector, E., Kulovich, S., Brusilow, S., Walser, M., and Nyhan, W., 1977, Neonatal citrullinemia: Treatment with ketoanalogues of essential amino acids, *J. Pediatr.* **90:**218–224.

Valle, D., and Simell, O., 1983, The hyperornithinemias, in: *The Metabolic Basis of Inherited Disease* (J. B. Stanbury, J. Wyngaarden, D. S. Fredrickson, J. L. Goldstein, and M. S. Brown, eds.), pp. 382–401, McGraw-Hill, New York.

Walser, M., 1983, Urea cycle disorders and other hereditary hyperammonemic syndromes, in: *The Metabolic Basis of Inherited Disease* (J. B. Stanbury, J. B. Wyngaarden, D. S. Fredrickson, J. L. Goldstein, and M. S. Brown, eds.), pp. 402–438, McGraw-Hill, New York.

Walser, M., Batshaw, M., Sherwood, G., Robinson, B., and Brusilow, S., 1977, Nitrogen metabolism in neonatal citrullinemia, *Clin. Sci. Mol. Med.* **53:**173–181.

Weatherall, D., 1984, Gene transfection, A step nearer gene therapy? *Nature* **310:**451.

Whelan, W. L., Gocke, E., and Manney, T. R., 1979, the *can*1 locus of *Saccharomyces cerevisiae*: Fine-structure analysis and forward mutation rates, *Genetics* **91:**35–51.

Wiegand, C., Thompson, T., Bock, G. H., Mathis, R. K., Kjellstrand, C. M., and Mauer, S. M., 1980, The management of life-threatening hyperammonemia: A comparison of several therapeutic modalities, *J. Pediatr.* **96:**142–144.

Williams, D. A., Lemischka, I. R., Nathan, D. G., and Mulligan, R. C., 1984, Introduction of new genetic material into pluripotent haematopoietic stem cells of the mouse, *Nature* **310:**476–480.

Windmueller, H. G., and Spaeth, A. E., 1981, Source and fate of circulating citrulline, *Am. J. Physiol.* **241:**E473–E480.

Wolfe, D. M., and Gatfield, P. D., 1975, Leukocyte urea cycle enzymes in hyperammonemia, *Pediatr. Res.* **9:**531–535.

Yamazaki, R. K., and Graetz, G. S. 1977, Glucagon stimulation of citrulline formation in isolated hepatic mitochondria, *Arch. Biochem. Biophys.* **178:**19–25.

Chapter 4

Molecular Genetics of the Human Major Histocompatibility Complex

Charles Auffray
Institut d'Embryologie du CNRS et du Collège de France
94130 Nogent sur Marne, France

Jack L. Strominger
Department of Biochemistry and Molecular Biology
Harvard University
Cambridge, Massachusetts 02138

INTRODUCTION

The ability to mount an immune response against foreign antigens and to regulate this response at the cellular level is an important characteristic of metazoans. This ability is mediated by cell-surface recognition systems that allow the distinction between self and nonself. A major histocompatibilty complex which encodes such molecules was first defined in mice through the discovery of a genetic control of graft rejection, and is now known to exist in all vertebrates examined. In man it is named the HLA complex, located on the short arm of chromosome 6, and it encodes three classes of molecules (Fig. 1).

The class I molecules, expressed on nucleated diploid cells, are composed of a 44,000-dalton, MHC-encoded transmembrane polypeptide associated with β_2-microglobulin, a 12,000-dalton invariant molecule encoded on chromosome 15 (Fig. 2). There are two main groups of class I molecules: the HLA-A,B,C antigens corresponding to the murine H-2K,D,L antigens (the classical transplantation antigens), and the non-HLA class I H.T antigens. The latter are poorly defined and probably represent the homologues of the murine Qa–Tla antigens, which occur as differentiation antigens of the hematopoietic lineage.

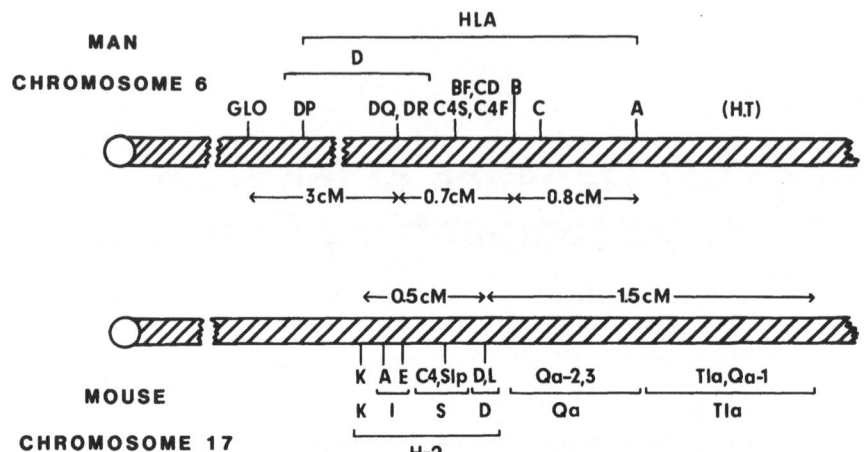

Fig. 1. Genetic map of the human and murine major histocompatibility complexes. The centromeres are indicated by circles. Genetic distances are indicated in centimorgans (cM).

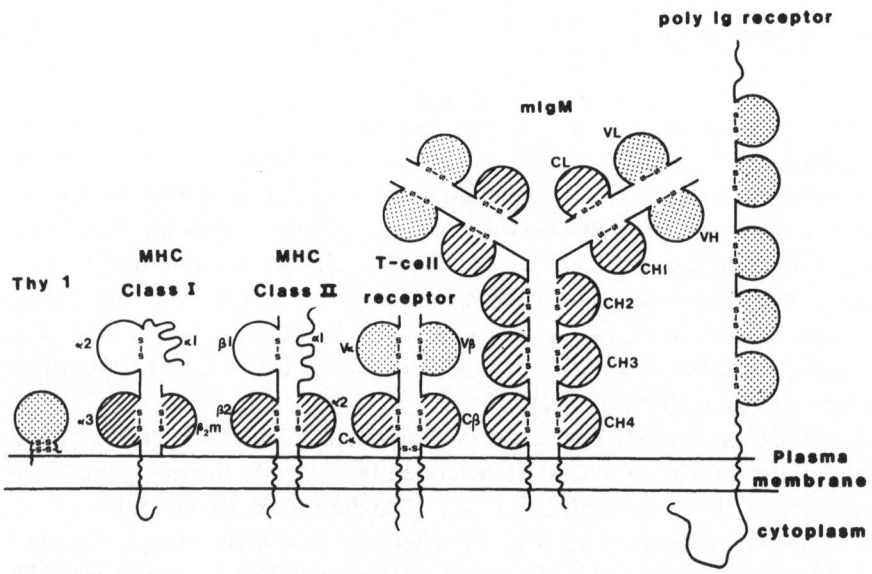

Fig. 2. Schematic representation of MHC antigens and other membrane proteins with homology to immunoglobulin constant domains (shaded) and variable domains (dotted). Redrawn from Kaufman *et al.* (1984a) with the addition of the T-cell receptor (Davis *et al.*, 1984; Mak and Yanagi, 1984) and the poly Ig receptor (Mostov *et al.*, 1984).

The class II molecules are normally expressed only by a few types of cells: B lymphocytes, and cells of the myeloid lineage, such as macrophages and dendritic cells. They also appear in certain circumstances on activated T lymphocytes and epithelial cells. They are heterodimeric integral membrane proteins consisting of a 33,000- to 34,000-dalton α chain and a 28,000- to 29,000-dalton β chain (Fig. 2), both encoded in the MHC. They transiently associate in the cytoplasm with an invariant polypeptide encoded on chromosome 5, also called Ii or γ chain [reviewed by Long (1985)]. The class II antigens encoded in the HLA-D region can be subdivided into three families, called HLA-DR, -DC (DQ), and -SB (DP). The nomenclature in parentheses indicates the new designations adopted for histocompatibility determinants after the Ninth International Histocompatibility Workshop (Bodmer *et al.*, 1984). We will use the new nomenclature HLA-DR,DQ,DP in this review, although the reader should be aware that most references cited use the old nomenclature, HLA-DR,DC,SB. HLA-DR and -DQ correspond to the murine I-E and I-A molecules, respectively, but no known homologue of HLA-DP has been found in the mouse.

The class III molecules are also involved in immunologic phenomena, since they represent components of the complement pathways. They will not be considered here, since they bear no clear relationship to the class I and II molecules aside from their genetic linkage.

Both class I and class II antigens are polymorphic molecules which function as targets for T lymphocytes that regulate the immune response. The presence of self class I antigens is a requisite for cytotoxic T lymphocytes to recognize and lyse virus-infected cells. Similarly, the class II molecules are restricting elements for regulator T lymphocytes (T helper, suppressor, and amplifier) and are encoded by the so-called immune response genes. The MHC antigens constitute an extremely polymorphic system, having at least 10–40 alleles per locus expressed in the human population. The mechanisms by which this huge polymorphism is created, propagated, and maintained are the subject of intense research and speculation. An intriguing peculiarity of certain HLA alleles is that they appear to be genetically linked to predisposition to various diseases, mainly of autoimmune nature.

Since their discovery 50 years ago, the MHC antigens have been intensively studied using serologic and cell-typing reagents. Great advances have been made in their biochemical characterization as proteins using polyclonal and monoclonal antibodies for characterization and/or purification. It is only over the last 4 years that a great deal of new information has been gained on the structure, organization, and evolution of the genes of the major histocompatibility complex, thanks to the use of the tools of molecular biology. Progress has been most impressive in the murine system [reviewed by Hood *et al.* (1982, 1983) and Steinmetz and Hood (1983)], mainly because of the availability of a large number of inbred, congenic, and recombinant strains which had been previously extensively characterized. Due to the outbred nature of the human population, studies of the HLA genes provide genetic and structural information unattainable by other means, and allow definition of new markers for which no reagents were previously available. Efforts being pursued to build a complete molecular map of the HLA complex are directed to a better understanding of the nature of HLA–disease associations. We will review here recent information acquired on the HLA class I and II genes and their use as molecular probes. Biochemical, serologic, and functional studies of HLA antigens have been reviewed recently (Ploegh *et al.*, 1981; Strominger *et al.*, 1981; Shackelford *et al.*, 1982; Kaufman *et al.*, 1984a; Lopez de Castro *et al.*, 1985; Korman *et al.*, 1985; Sanchez-Perez and Shaw, 1985).

CHARACTERIZATION OF THE HLA GENES

Isolation of the HLA (Class I and II) Genes

cDNA Cloning

Construction of cDNA Libraries.   The source of cells expressing high levels of specific proteins and their mRNAs is a key feature of cDNA cloning. In the case of the class I and II antigens, the choice of EBV-transformed lymphoblastoid B-cell lines was guided by several important considerations:

1. Al these lines are known to express five- to tenfold more of these antigens than peripheral blood lymphocytes of the individuals from whom they were derived.
2. They have been the source of material for the purification of these antigens and the subsequent determination of their primary structure.

3. They are serologically and functionally typed for most or all known HLA antigens, and some of them appear to be truly homozygous, both through typing and because they are derived from offspring of consanguineous marriages (although these criteria also have limitations; e.g., beginning with a great-grandparent, six meioses occur involving the haplotypes that result in the homozygous consanguineous cells of the offspring of a first-cousin marriage, allowing some chance for recombination, especially if the MHC contains "hot spots" for recombination).

Since the HLA class I and II antigens are transmembrane proteins, they are synthesized on membrane-bound polysomes (which therefore represent an enriched source for the corresponding mRNAs). In most cases these mRNAs have been further purified by sucrose gradient ultracentrifugation or preparative gel electrophoresis. They are assayed by cell-free translation in an mRNA-dependent rabbit reticulocyte lysate, followed by an analysis of the cell-free translation products by immunoprecipitation with specific polyclonal or monoclonal antibodies, and SDS–polyacrylamide gel electrophoresis. A difficulty in following this purification is the availability of specific antibodies able to recognize the cell-free translation products. Although this has not been a serious problem for β_2-microglobulin, it has proven to be a limiting step for the class I α chain and for both chains of the class II antigens. In these cases, most antibodies recognize the heterodimer as a complex and recognize the isolated chains poorly, if at all. Thus it has been necessary to produce antibodies specifically raised against denatured chains or to use a different translation system, such as frog oocytes. Such studies have demonstrated that the class I α chain, β_2-microglobulin, and the HLA-DR antigen chains are encoded by different mRNAs of about 1700, 900, and 1300 nucleotides, respectively. Cotranslational processing occurs in the presence of dog pancreatic microsomes, indicating the existence of a 20-24-amino acid signal peptide (Ploegh et al., 1979; Korman et al., 1980; Lee et al., 1980). cDNA libraries have been constructed using conventional methods. The mRNA purification step (10- to 40-fold), although not mandatory, has proven very useful in reducing the number of bacterial clones to be screened in order to find specific sequences, which represent as little as 0.01% of the total poly A-containing mRNA population.

Screening by Hybrid Selection of mRNA.   In this technique, DNA from pools of 5–50 recombinant cDNA clones is immobilized on nitrocellulose filters and used to purify the corresponding mRNA sequences. Thus, it relies on the preceding cell-free translation assay as a means of identifying which pool contains the desired sequence. Subsequently, clones from a positive pool are screened individually and the specific clone identified (Ploegh *et al.*, 1980; Larhammar *et al.*, 1981; Lee *et al.*, 1982*a*; Wake *et al.*, 1982*a*; Wiman *et al.*, 1982*a*; Claesson *et al.*, 1983; Strubin *et al.*, 1984; Trowsdale *et al.*, 1984*a*). This test has also been used to confirm the identity of clones isolated by other approaches (Korman *et al.*, 1982*a*). In the case of the class II antigen HLA-DR, the problem of the recognition of complexes has been circumvented by injecting the hybrid selected mRNAs for the α, β, and invariant chains into frog oocytes, in which the three chains assemble into a complex (Long *et al.*, 1982*a,b*).

Screening with Synthetic Oligonucleotides. The development of oligonucleotide synthesis has resulted in the synthesis of mixed probes corresponding to nucleotide sequences derived from the available amino acid sequences using the genetic code. In this approach, one chooses a five- to seven-amino acid sequence, which can be encoded by a limited number of nucleotide sequences since it contains amino acids encoded by only one or two codons. Then a mixture of different sequences is synthesized, one of which is a perfect match with the desired sequence. The cDNA library is then screened with this radiolabeled mixture under conditions allowing a discrimination between a perfectly matching sequence and one that differs by a single substitution. Positive clones are further characterized by DNA sequencing and/or the hybrid/selection assay. A limitation of this approach is that the probes are derived in most cases from the amino-terminal amino acid sequence, which corresponds to the 5' end of the corresponding mRNA. Therefore, only full-length clones can be detected, which in most libraries represent only a small portion of the specific clones. This technique has been used to isolate β_2-microglobulin and both class I and class II HLA-encoded proteins (Sood *et al.*, 1981; Suggs *et al.*, 1981; Stetler *et al.*, 1982). The major advantage of this technique is that a large number of clones can be screened and therefore purification steps and antibodies are not absolutely required for screening. However, it is based indirectly on these antibodies as a means of providing the basic amino acid sequence.

Immunopurification of Polysomes. The availability of antibodies that recognize the denatured HLA-DRα chain has been used to immunopurify polysomes on which the nascent polypeptide chain is being synthesized, apparently made possible through the similarity between the denatured and nascent forms. The great advantage of this technique is that mRNA can be enriched in a single step up to 3000-fold, thus providing a source for an extremely specific probe through synthesis of a complementary cDNA; alternatively, cDNA clones can be prepared directly from the immunopurified material (Korman *et al.*, 1982*a*). The lengthy process of screening is then limited to its simplest form. However, one needs to possess an RNAse-free preparation of the antibody and the technique has not been widely used.

Subsequently, cDNA clones for other class I and class II chains have been isolated by cross-hybridation with the human and mouse probes, and characterized by DNA sequencing on the basis of available amino acid sequences (Auffray *et al.*, 1982; Chang *et al.*, 1983; Long *et al.*, 1983, 1984*a*; Roux-Dosseto *et al.*, 1983*a*; Arnot *et al.*, 1984; Gustafsson *et al.*, 1984*a*, Schenning *et al.*, 1984).

In summary, cDNA clones for HLA antigens (as well as β_2-microglobulin and the HLA-DR-associated invariant chain) have been isolated and characterized through a variety of techniques, none of which can be qualified as the best one. The route to obtaining specific clones has been mostly diverse, depending on previously acquired information, reagents, or expertise.

Mapping of Genes to the HLA Region

Human genomic libraries that were available at the beginning of these studies were limited to DNA from individuals untyped for HLA antigens. Therefore the first genes isolated cannot be identified with particular alleles or loci. Although this is not a problem for invariant polypeptide chains such as β_2-microglobulin and the α chain of the HLA-DR antigen, studies of HLA polymorphism at the sequence level made the construction of libraries from HLA-typed material mandatory. This has been achieved in several laboratories using lambda phage and cosmid vectors, so that a large number of serologically defined specificities can be studied from DNA cloning experiments. With the cosmid vectors and chromosome walking techniques, clusters of tandemly organized sequences have been isolated using the various cDNA clones described above, in a similar but more limited manner to what has been achieved for the mouse MHC (see below).

A peculiarity of the HLA genes is that they belong to a multigene family of unknown size. As the number of available cDNA probes has increased, the number of corresponding genes or DNA hybridizing fragments has expanded greatly. Before a detailed analysis of a particular gene is performed, it has proven useful to ensure that it is really encoded in the HLA complex.

Three approaches to address this question have been used:

1. Southern blot analysis of DNA from mouse–human somatic cell hybrid lines that contain various sets of human chromosomes, including chromosome 6, where the HLA complex is located, and chromosome 15, bearing the β_2-microglobulin gene, has established that all sequences hybridizing to HLA probes are located on chromosome 6, whatever the probe (Lee et al., 1982a; Trowsdale et al., 1983; Spielman et al., 1984). By a similar approach, the invariant chain gene has been located on chromosome 5 (Claesson-Walsh et al., 1984).

2. Deletion mutants of larger and larger regions of the HLA complex have been produced by exposure to ethylmethane sulfonate or γ-ray irradiation of an HLA heterozygous B-cell line, with subsequent selection for the loss of specific HLA markers with corresponding antibodies. As a first step, mutants have been produced that have lost a complete HLA haplotype and are therefore hemizygous (Kavathas et al., 1980; Gladstone et al., 1982). Mutants generated subsequently have a homozygous deletion on the short arm of chromosome 6 with loss of expression of a particular HLA antigen (DeMars et al., 1983a,b, 1984). Southern blot analysis of these mutant lines has shown that there is a complete correlation between the absence of particular DNA fragments and particular serologically or functionally defined products, and has been used to map directly sequences hybridizing to cDNA probes to the short arm of chromosome 6 (Orr et al., 1982; Auffray et al., 1983a; Erlich et al., 1983a). This more precise mapping opens the possibility of ordering genes in the HLA region, a task rendered difficult by classical genetics in the absence of many recombination events localized between particular regions and the uncertainty of genetic distances based on the frequencies of these recombinations. Extensive analysis of these mutants with several restriction enzymes together with family studies have shown that many class I-like sequences map telomeric to the HLA-A locus (Orr and DeMars, 1983a,b) and are likely to represent equivalents of the murine Qa–Tla region genes.

3. DNA probes for HLA class I and DRα sequences used in in situ chromosome hybridization experiments allowed these two groups of loci to be distinguished (Morton et al., 1984). The direct visualization of se-

quences hybridizing to the short arm of chromosome 6 in this way showed that DRα at 6p21.1 is centromeric to the HLA class I sequences at 6p21.3 and agrees with the immunogenetic map (Fig. 1). The relative positions have also been confirmed by segregation in a family in which a chromosomal rearrangement has occurred with the break between these clusters (Morton *et al.*, 1984). *In situ* hybridization is a powerful tool to study chromosomal rearrangements in genetic abnormalities in man.

Multiplicity of Class I and Class II Genes

Class I Genes

The first HLA sequences isolated corresponded to HLA-B cDNA clones, which were identified by DNA sequencing and hybrid selection of mRNA. They were used as probes to isolate mouse H-2 sequences, and it is now known that there are about 32 genes on the murine chromosome 17 that share a high degree of sequence homology [for a review see Hood *et al.*, (1983)]. Southern blot and cloning experiments also provide evidence for 20–30 class I genes in the HLA complex. As for the H-2 genes, the number of class I sequences may vary from haplotype to haplotype. Individual HLA-A,B,C genes have been identified by gene transfer experiments and DNA sequencing, but it is not yet clear whether there are several of each type per haploid genome (Jordan *et al.*, 1981; Barbosa *et al.*, 1982; Le Bouteiller *et al.*, 1982; M. Malissen *et al.*, 1982*a,b*; Orr *et al.*, 1982; Bernabeu *et al.*, 1983; Lemonnier *et al.*, 1983; Orr and DeMars, 1983*a,b*).

Clusters of cosmid clones containing one or several class I genes have been isolated, but a linkage map for this region of the HLA complex is still awaited (M. Malissen *et al.*, 1982*a*).

Class II Genes

Previous studies using a panel of monoclonal and polyclonal antibodies have documented the expression of three subsets of Class II antigens on B cells, characterized by three different α chains (DRα, DQα, DPα). The β chains have been more difficult to study, particularly because of extensive polymorphism detected even after the charge microheterogeneity is resolved by treatment with neuraminidase or tunicamycin.

Thus, several studies have reported the existence of two DRβ, one DQβ, and one DPβ chains, and there is biochemical evidence for a total of seven β chains [reviewed in Kaufman *et al.* (1984*a*)].

HLA-DR Genes.   The first gene to be isolated was the DRα gene, which has been extensively characterized by several laboratories, revealing an almost complete lack of sequence variability, which agrees with observation made by biochemical and serologic techniques. There is a unique gene sequence in the human haploid genome that hybridizes strongly with it (Korman *et al.*, 1982*b*; Larhammar *et al.*, 1982*a*; Lee *et al.*, 1982*b*; Stetler *et al.*, 1982; Das *et al.*, 1983; Schamboeck *et al.*, 1983).

As for the β-chain genes belonging to the DR family, the data argue in favor of the existence of three genes per haploid genome, based on a comparison of protein and DNA sequences or restriction maps of clones obtained from the same cell line, as well as Southern blot analysis with locus-specific probes located in the 3′ untranslated region of the mRNA, which identify sequences belonging to the same family (Wake *et al.*, 1982*b*; Böhme *et al.*, 1983; Long *et al.*, 1983; Sorrentino *et al.*, 1985). The three genes are designated DRβ$_1$, DRβ$_2$, DRβ$_3$. It should be kept in mind that individual haplotypes could have more or less DRβ genes than this number, since a number of mechanisms permit gene deletion or expansion in multigene families. In fact, examination of one set of DR1–7 homozygous cell lines indicated that the DR1 cell used had only two DRβ-chain genes, while the other cells had three. Moreover the restriction enzyme patterns of DR4 and 7 cells and of DR3, 5, and w6 cells were similar, indicating a strong correlation of DRβ genes with the serologic MT2 and MT3 patterns. From studies of expressed proteins it is also apparent that the MT2 (De Préval *et al.*, 1984*a*) and MT3 (Sorrentino *et al.*, 1985) serologic specificities are the products of one of the DRβ genes. The DR serologic specificities are the products of a second DRβ gene, and in at least one haplotype the third is a pseudogene (Larhammar *et al.*, 1985).

The isolation of cosmid clones from the Priess cell line (DR4) has allowed the characterization of two parts of the HLA-DR subregion (Fig. 3): one contains the DRα gene and, 90 kb away, one DRβ gene encoding the MT3 specificity (Spies *et al.*, 1985). By comparing restriction maps of other cosmid clones containing two other DRβ-related genes with that of a DRβ pseudogene (Larhammar *et al.*, 1985), one can achieve a linkage map of the two remaining DRβ genes. Thus, one of them presumably encodes the DR4 specificity. It is interesting to note that a 2-kb sequence

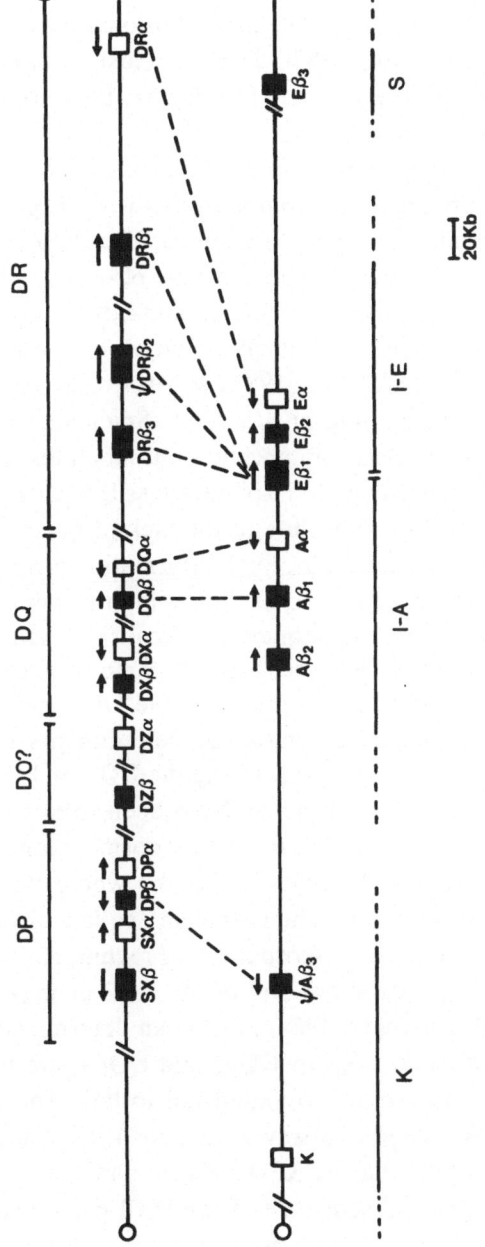

Fig. 3. Comparison of the molecular maps of the H-2I region (bottom) and the HLA-DR, DQ, and DP subregions (top). Redrawn from data taken from: H-2I region (Hood *et al.*, 1983; M. Steinmetz, personal communication); HLA-DR subregion (Spies *et al.*, 1985); HLA-DQ subregion (Okada *et al.*, 1985b); HLA-DP subregion (Trowsdale *et al.*, 1984b; Gorski *et al.*, 1984; Inoko *et al.*, 1985; Okada *et al.*, 1985b; Servenius *et al.*, 1985). The genes are indicated by boxes with an arrow indicating the direction of transcription; α genes, open box; β genes, solid box.

covering the 5' part of the gene and the signal sequence exon found in all three DRβ genes is repeated three more times between the DRα and DRβ (MT3) genes. Thus, it is possible that additional class II β genes exist in this region (Spies *et al.*, 1985). The two clusters have not been linked, but by analogy with the murine H2-I region, they are tentatively drawn in a β-β-β-α order (Fig. 3).

HLA-DQ Genes. The DQα sequence was isolated by cross-hybridization dependent on sequence homology with the DRα chain and identified using a partial amino-terminal sequence. The DQα cDNA clone hybridizes strongly to two genes on chromosome 6, one of which is the DQα gene, as shown by analysis of deletion mutants. In contrast with the DRα sequence, the DQα chain is extremely polymorphic, as much as the class II β chains (Auffray *et al.*, 1982, 1983*a,b*, 1984; Chang *et al.*, 1983; Trowsdale *et al.*, 1983; Schenning *et al.*, 1984; Spielman *et al.*, 1984; LeGall *et al.*, 1985); DXα is also polymorphic, but much less than DQα.

The DQβ cDNA clone was the first isolated class II β-chain sequence, but was not then identified as such, due to the lack of protein sequence information (Larhammar *et al.*, 1982*b*). Such information is now available from DQβ chains that are not blocked at their amino terminus (the first DQβ chain isolated could not be sequenced because it had a blocked amino terminus). It is not clear whether a DQ β-chain gene encodes any serologically defined specificity, i.e., the available DQ (also called MB or MT) antisera may recognize polymorphic determinants partially or exclusively associated with the α chain. Using the DQα and DQβ cDNA clones as probes, two α and two β genes have been isolated and characterized. They have been linked in two pairs by cosmid cloning (Fig. 3): DQα and DQβ define the DQ subregion of 48. kb where the genes are located in a tail-to-tail orientation. The complete sequences of the DQα gene (C. Auffray, J. W. Lillie, A. J. Korman, N. Fréchin, R. C. Mulligan, and J. L. Strominger, in preparation) and of the DQβ gene (Larhammar *et al.*, 1983; Boss and Strominger, 1984) have been determined. The two other genes, named DXα and DXβ or DQα$_2$ and DQβ$_2$, are linked on a 35-kb stretch of DNA and are also oriented tail to tail. Analysis of the full sequence of the DXα gene (Auffray *et al.*, 1984; C. Auffray, J. W. Lillie, A. J. Korman, N. Fréchin, R. C. Mulligan, and J. L. Strominger, in preparation) and of a partial sequence of the DXβ gene (Okada *et al.*, 1985*a*; D. Larhammar, personal communication) has not revealed any feature that would prevent their expression. Thus, it is not clear whether a DXα/β heterodimer can be expressed and whether it might correspond to any known serologically defined class II antigen.

The DX cluster might be centromeric to the DQ cluster, since the DXα gene is retained in deletion mutants typed as DR-negative, DQ-negative and which have lost the DRα gene but not the DXα gene (Auffray *et al.*, 1983*a*).

HLA-DP Genes.   The DP antigen is the last to have been identified, first by functional assays, then by biochemical analysis using specific antibodies [reviewed in Sanchez-Perez and Shaw (1985)]. DP antigens elicit allogeneic proliferative and cytotoxic responses of lymphocytes primed between donors matched at all other HLA antigens. The DP antigens constitute an allelic Mendelian segregant series, largely independent of HLA-A,B,DR types, which extends the HLA region by 1–2 cM (Fig. 1).

The identification of DPα sequences, isolated by cross-hybridization with DQα or DRα, relies on the very limited amino-terminal sequence available for DPα and is rendered difficult by the small number of positions showing amino acids different from DRα or DQα. However, factors that argue strongly in favor of this identification are correlation with loss of DP expression in deletion mutants and direct linkage with a β gene located in the DP region by genetic analysis. Sequence analysis shows that DPα is about equally distantly related to DRα and DQα. In addition to the DPα gene, there is a second gene sharing about 80% sequence homology with DPα, which has been named SXα or DPα$_2$, and which is different from all other α genes discussed so far (Auffray *et al.*, 1984; Trowsdale *et al.*, 1984*b*; Okada *et al.*, 1985*a*). Sequence analysis of the SXα gene indicates that it is a pseudogene (Boss *et al.*, 1985; Servenius *et al.*, 1985).

DPβ cDNA clones have been isolated using either mouse or other human class II β cDNA probes in cross-hybridization experiments. Their identification relies in part on a good although incomplete sequence correlation between the clones and the protein sequence of the DP antigen (due to allelic differences). It is also strongly supported by the correlation established between the DNA sequences hybridizing to these clones and the expression of particular DP antigens as shown by DNA polymorphism analysis in HLA-typed individuals, deletion mutants, and a recombinant family (Roux-Dosseto *et al.*, 1983*a*; Kappes *et al.*, 1984). There are at least two DPβ-related genes, which are linked to the DPα genes in the order SXβ-SXα-DPβ-DPα as demonstrated by cosmid cloning performed in several haplotypes (Gorski *et al.*, 1984; Trowsdale *et al.*, 1984*b*; Inoko *et al.*, 1985; Okada *et al.*, 1985*b*; Servenius *et al.*, 1985).

In addition, there is a 513-bp processed gene in one intron of the DPβ gene whose function is unknown (Trowsdale *et al.*, 1984*b*).

The genes in the DP cluster have been linked over 100 kb and they appear to be inverted in orientation when compared to other class II genes in mouse and man, i.e., they are head to head (5' to 5') rather than tail to tail (3' to 3') as are the other genes (Fig. 3). SXα and SXβ are pseudogenes in the one haplotype examined, but it is of course possible that they are intact genes in other haplotypes. The cosmid clusters have been linked in two haplotypes (DP3 and DP4). Both β-chain genes are polymorphic by restriction enzyme analysis, mainly at their 3' ends, but the remainder of the clusters are remarkably conserved. Interestingly, the amino acid polymorphism is mainly located in the β_1 domain at the 5' end, but is not reflected by a so far detected restriction enzyme polymorphism. In comparing the available DPβ sequences (DP2–4) in the β_1 domain an interesting pattern is seen in which only one of two possible sequences occurs in five regions, presumably giving rise to the immunological polymorphism (Kappes *et al.*, 1984; Okada *et al.*, 1985*b*).

Other Genes.   In addition, a gene christened DZα or DOα has been isolated as well as a corresponding cDNA (Trowsdale *et al.*, 1984*b*; Inoko *et al.*, 1985; G. Blank, personal communication), and there might be more α genes, since weakly hybridizing DNA fragments have been detected with the DQα probes. It is not yet known whether the DZα mRNA is translated and, if so, whether the putative DZα chain can associate with a class II β chain. A cDNA clone isolated using a DRβ probe in low-stringency conditions, which shows low homology to DRβ, DQβ, and DPβ but appears to be the human homologue of the $A\beta_2$ gene (E. Long, personal communication), is a good candidate for the DZβ chain. By analogy with the mouse map, this would place the DZα and β putative genes between the DP and DQ/DX regions. It is therefore possible that if a DZα/β heterodimer exists, it might correspond to the 33.1 class II antigen, which is expressed exclusively in B cells and appears to map to this region (Marti *et al.*, 1983). Further experiments should resolve this issue.

In summary, there are at least six class II α-chain genes (DRα, DQα, DXα, DPα, SXα, DZα) and eight β-chain genes (DRβ₁, DRβ₂, DRβ₃, DQβ, DXβ, DPβ, SXβ, DZβ) in the HLA-D region. Since a clear relationship has been established between three α- and four β-chain genes and the serologically or functionally defined determinants that they encode, they can be designated using the nomenclature for these determinants, that is, $DR\alpha/DR\beta_1$ and $DR\alpha/DR\beta_2$, and $DQ\alpha/DQ\beta$ and $DP\alpha/DP\beta$. We prefer to designate the other genes by their original names until they are either proven to be pseudogenes and then designated with a ψ preceding the family to which they belong, or shown to be expressed and then assigned names according to the new determinants they encode. For example if the 33.1 antigen and the $DZ\alpha$ and β genes can be correlated, they would be designated DO.

Comparison of the HLA-D region with the H-2I region (Fig. 3) reveals a similar number of known β genes (eight in man, six in mouse), but a larger number of α genes in man (six compared to two). A possible explanation of these differences is that some regions have been lost in the mouse or that subsequent to the mouse/man divergence, some loci have been duplicated in man. Alternatively, some of the mouse genes might have diverged too much to be detected with available probes. Although it is currently believed that most of the genes have been identified, it should be kept in mind that other isotypic families with low homology to those isolated could exist. For example, immunoglobulin heavy-chain constant-region genes have diverged enough to show no cross-hybridization.

Structure, Polymorphism, and Evolution of the HLA Genes

Gene Structure

Several of the isolated genes have been completely sequenced, revealing interesting features in their intron–exon structure (Fig. 4). There is an excellent correlation between exons and structural domains already identified at the protein level. That is, each gene has specific exons encoding the signal peptide and the transmembrane domain; the three class I extracellular domains ($\alpha 1$, $\alpha 2$, and $\alpha 3$) are encoded by separate exons, and the two class II α- and β-chain extracellular domains ($\alpha 1$, $\alpha 2$ and $\beta 1$, β_2) are also encoded by separate exons. The only exception to this rule concerns the intracytoplasmic domains of both class I and class II β chains, which are encoded by multiple short exons, whereas the class II α-chain cytoplasmic domain is encoded by the same exon as the transmembrane domain. The class II α-chain genes can be distinguished from

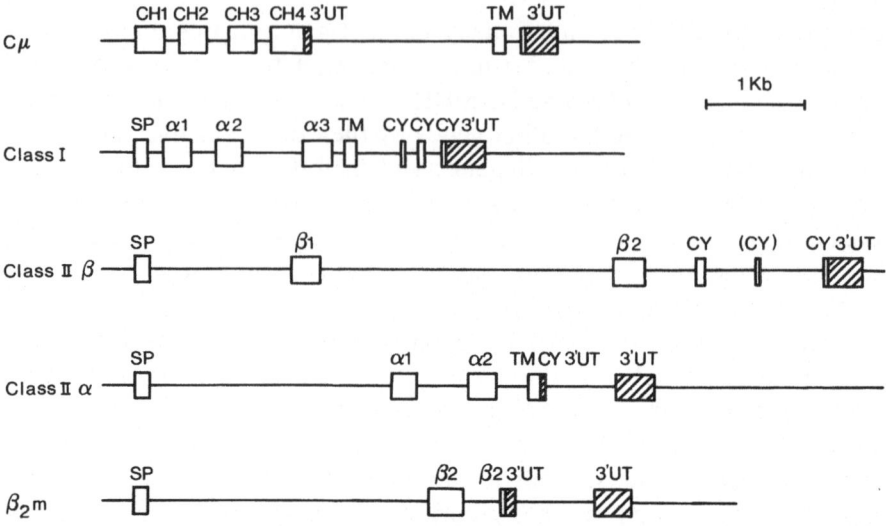

Fig. 4. Comparison of the intron–exon structure of MHC class I and class II genes with the immunoglobulin Cμ gene (Early *et al.*, 1980) and the β₂-microglobulin gene (Parnes and Seidman, 1982). The structures shown are those of class I HLA-A3 (Sodoyer *et al.*, 1984) and class II, DRα (Schamboeck *et al.*, 1983), and DQβ (Boss and Strominger, 1984). The 3′ untranslated (UT) regions are shaded; SP, signal peptide; TM, transmembrane region; CY, cytoplasmic domain (the CY exon in parentheses in the class II β gene is not functional in the DQβ gene, but is in the murine homologue Aβ).

both class I and class II β-chain genes by the structure of the 3′ untranslated region of their mRNA, which is encoded by two exons instead of one, as well as by the large length of the intron separating the signal peptide exon and the first extracellular domain. Interestingly, these two features are common to the class II α-chain genes and the β₂-microglobulin gene. Immunoglobulin genes also share many of these features, including the location of intron/exon limits between the first and second bases of a codon, providing evidence in favor of a common evolutionary origin (see below).

Genes and Pseudogenes

Since there are many more genes than known gene products, it is likely that some of them are not expressed. They might be pseudogenes or genes expressed only in certain haplotypes or tissues and/or at certain periods of development. In many instances we lack reagents that would help identify these genes, and it is possible that such reagents will be produced in the future after gene transfer experiments have succeeded. Many of the class I genes isolated fail to be expressed after transfection in mouse L cells because they are pseudogenes or because the murine fibroblast is not an appropriate recipient, or they escape detection because they encode secreted products. Two such genes have been sequenced, one having typical features of a pseudogene, namely stop codons in coding frames and altered splicing signals (Biro *et al.*, 1981). It has been argued that the second one is also a pseudogene because there is a charged residue in the transmembrane exon and a mutation of one cysteine involved in intrachain disulfide bond formation. It remains to be seen if this would be sufficient to prevent expression (M. Malissen *et al.*, 1982*b*).

The DXα and DXβ genes have no obvious feature that would prevent their expression, yet we have no evidence that they are actually expressed. The absence of transcripts of the DXα gene in B lymphocytes is not due to obvious changes in the promoter region (see below), nor to nonfunctional splicing signals. This latter possibility has been explored by cloning the DXα gene in a retroviral vector and transfection in the ψ2 packaging murine fibroblast cell line. The transfected cell lines produce recombinant retroviral genomic RNA, which can be spliced at functional sites prior to packaging in virion capsids, yielding viruses in the supernatant. The retroviral vector is engineered so that upon infection of mouse fibroblasts, the processed construct can be readily recovered as bacterial recombinant clones (Cepko *et al.*, 1984). Thus, after passage of the DXα gene through the retroviral life cycle, a "collapsed" version has been recovered. Analysis by restriction enzyme mapping and DNA sequencing has shown that it has all the features of a DXα "cDNA," the introns having been spliced out at precisely the location predicted (C. Auffray, J. W. Lillie, A. J. Korman, N. Fréchin, R. C. Mulligan, and J. L. Strominger, in preparation).

One of the isolated DRβ genes is a conventional pseudogene (Larhammar *et al.*, 1985): there are four splice junctions in which the GT/AG dinucleotides have been mutated, two stop codons in the β1 exon, and a frame shift at the end of the β2 exon caused by a 2-bp insertion. It has been proposed that inactivation of this β gene occurred by insertion of a *Kpn*I repeat upstream of the gene (Larhammar *et al.*, 1985). One of the cytoplasmic exons in the DQβ gene is not used due to a mutation of a splice junction, although the homologuos exon in the murine Aβ gene is still functional (Larhammar *et al.*, 1983; Boss and Strominger, 1984). Deletion of this part of the cytoplasmic domain does not interfere with the ability of the DQ antigen to function as a restricting element. The SXα gene has a 1-bp deletion in the α1 and transmembrane exons as well as a defect in one splice junction at the end of the α1 domain (Servenius *et al.*, 1985; Boss *et al.*, 1985). The SXβ gene has a frameshift mutation in the β2 exon followed by an in-frame stop codon 18 amino acids downstream (Okada *et al.*, 1985*b*; J. Boss, personal communication). Thus, if the SXβ gene could be expressed, the resulting polypeptide would be truncated and unlikely to be anchored in the plasma membrane. There have been no transcripts of any of these putative pseudogenes detected by Northern blot analysis or by cDNA cloning.

Immunoglobulin-like Domains

The most striking feature that emerges from the analysis of all the sequence data (protein and DNA) is the high degree of sequence homology observed between certain domains (encoded by specific exons) of class I and class II antigens with β_2-microglobulin and the constant domains of immunoglobulin heavy and light chains (Figs. 2 and 5). All these domains are members of the same family and are organized with an amino acid intrachain disulfide loop of about 60 residues. They comprise the α3 domains of class I and the α2 and β2 domains of class II antigens (Orr *et al.*, 1979; Kaufman and Strominger, 1982, 1983; Kaufman *et al.*, 1984a; Larhammar *et al.*, 1982*a,b*; Lee *et al.*, 1982*b*; Long *et al.*, 1983). Analysis of class I and class II antigens by circular dichroism has revealed a predominant β-pleated sheet structure (Lancet *et al.*, 1979; Wiman *et al.*, 1982*b*). Predictive methods show an organization of β sheets in these homologous domains similar to that of typical immunoglobulin constant domains (Novotny and Auffray, 1984; Travers *et al.*, 1984; Vega *et al.*, 1984). Moreover, if the predicted secondary structure elements are used to build a three-dimensional model of class II α2 and β2 domains, it appears that the two domains are likely to interact in a very similar manner as immunoglobulin constant domains do (Fig. 6) (J. Novotny and C. Auffray, unpublished results). A confirmation of these predictions awaits the determination of the crystal structure of HLA antigens, which is close to being solved for HLA-A2 (P. Bjorkman, J. L. Strominger, and D. Wiley, unpublished results).

```
B7α3   ADPPK-TH--VTHHPIS-DHEATLRCWALGFYPAEITLTWQR-D-G-EDQTQDTELVETRPAG-DRTFQKWAAVVV-PS---GEGQRYTCHVQHEGLPKPLTLGW
β2m    RTPKI-QV-YSRHPAENGKSNFLNCYVSGFHPSDIEVDLLK-N-G-ERIEKVEHS-DLSFSK-DWSFYLLYYTEFTPT----EKDEYACRVNHVTLSQPKIVKW

DRα2   VPPEV-TV-LTNSPVELREPNVLICFIDKFTPPVVNVTWLR-N-G-KPVTTGVSETVFLPRE-DHLFRKFHYLPFLPS----TEDVYDCRVEHWGLDEPLLKHW
DRβ2   VQPKV-TV-YPSKTQPLQHHNLLVCSVSGFYPGSIEVRWFL-N-GQEEKAGGVS--TGLIQD-DWTFQTLVMLETVPR----SGEVYTCQVEHPSVTSPLTVEW

DQα2   EVPEV-TV-FSKSPVTLGNPNTLICLVDNIFPPVVNITWLS-N-G-HSVTGGVSETSFLSKS-DHSFFKISYLTFLPS----ADEIYDCKVEHWGLDEPLLKHW
DQβ2   VEPTV-TI-SPSRTEALNHHLLVCSVTDFYPAQIKVRWFR-N-DQEETAGGVS--TPLIRNGDWTFQILVMLEMTPQ----RGDVWTCHVEHPSLQSPITVEW

DPα2   DPPEV-TV-FPKEPVELGQPNTLICHIDKFFPPVLNVTWL-C-N-G-ELVTEGVAESLFLPRT-DYSFHKFHMLTFVPS----AEDFYDCRVEHWGLDQPLLKHW
DPβ2   VQPRV-NV-SPSKKGPLQHHNLLVCHVTDFYPGSIQVRWFL-N-GQEETAGVVS--TNLIRNGDWTFQILVMLEMTPQ----QGDVMTCQVEHTSLDSPVTVEW

Cγ3    REPQVYTL-PPSREEMTKNQVSLTCLVKGFYPSDIAVEWES-NDG--EPENYKT--TPPVLDSDGSFLYSKLTVDKSRW-QEGNVFSCSVMHEALHNHYTQKS
Cλ     AAPSV-TL-FPPSSEELQANKATLVCLISDFYPGAVTVAWKA-D-S-SPVKAGVETTTPSKQS-NNKYAASSYLSLTPEQW-KSHKSYSCQVTHEGSTVEKTVAP
```

Fig. 5. Comparison of immunoglobulin-like domains. Amino acid sequences are aligned in order to maximize homology. Gaps are indicated by dashes. Residues common to eight or more of the ten sequences are boxed. The sequences shown are: B7α3, HLA-B7 α3 (Orr et al., 1979); β2m, human β2-microglobulin (Suggs et al., 1981); DRα2, HLA-DR α2 (Korman et al., 1982b); DRβ2, HLA-DR2 β2 (Kratzin et al., 1981); DQα2, HLA-DQ4 α2 (Auffray et al., 1982, 1984); DQβ2, HLA-DQ3, 6β2 (Larhammar et al., 1982b); DPα2, HLA-DP α2 (Auffray et al., 1984); DPβ2, HLA-DP4 β2 (Roux-Dosseto et al., 1983a); Cγ3, immunoglobulin Cγ3 (Edelman et al., 1969); Cλ, immunoglobulin Cλ (Poljak et al., 1973).

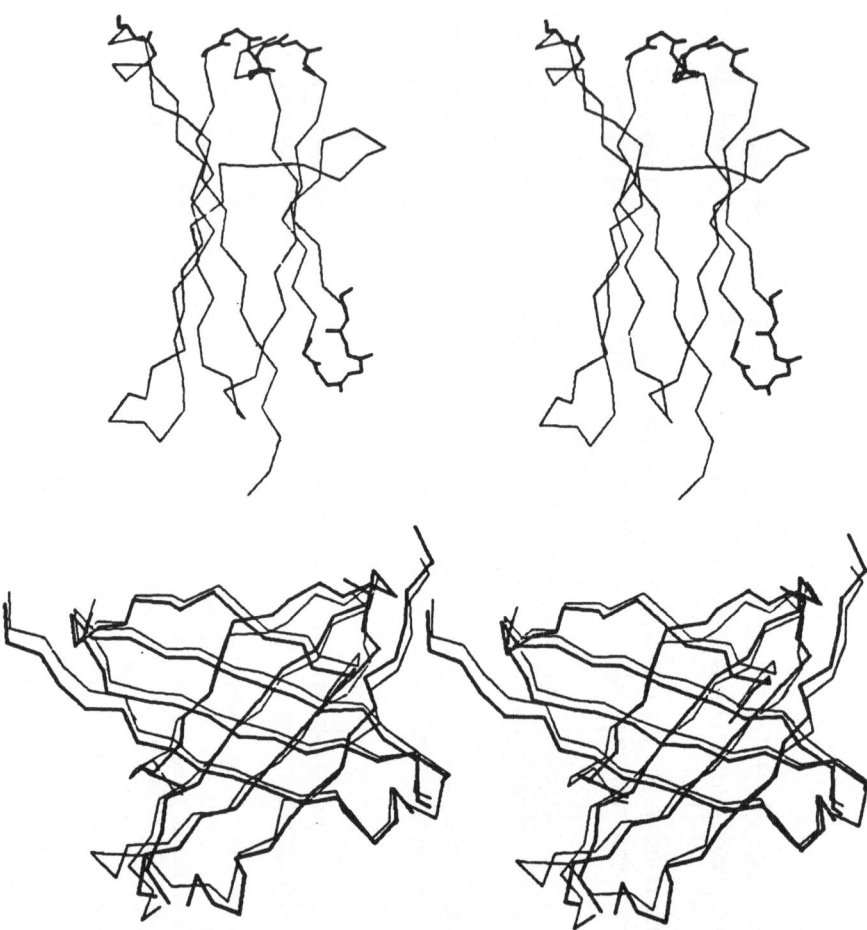

Fig. 6.   Stereodiagrams of computer-generated models of HLA-DQ antigen. Top: The β2 domain of HLA-DQβ modeled into the known 3D structure of the human immunoglobulin light-chain constant domain KOL using secondary structure predictions (Novotny and Auffray, 1984). Only the backbone of the polypeptide chain is presented. Thick lines indicate loops in KOL that have no homologue in DQβ. Bottom: The interface between the β2 (top) and α2 (bottom) domains of the HLA-DQ antigen modeled using the known CL-CH1 interface of the human immunoglobulin KOL, and energy-minimized. The two models are superimposed for comparison, with thin lines for HLA-DQ and thick lines for immunoglobulin KOL. [Figure kindly provided by Dr. J. Novotny, Harvard University, Cambridge.]

The differentiation antigen Thy-1 also belongs to the immunoglobulin superfamily (Williams and Gagnon, 1981). The poly Ig receptor (Mostov *et al.*, 1984) and the antigen-specific T-cell receptor α and β chains (Davis *et al.*, 1984; Mak and Yanagi, 1984) have been shown also to be members of the same family (Fig. 2), and new members are still being added, such as the T8 antigen (Littman *et al.*, 1985). The common structural features of these genes, which play important and various roles in the control of the immune response, strengthen the argument that they have evolved from a common ancestral gene.

Protein and DNA Sequences

A great deal of information has been accumulated in a short time both at the protein and the DNA level. Although the speed of this accumulation is likely to increase, since it should be faster to derive the protein sequence from the DNA sequence, limited protein sequences will still be necessary to identify genes with their products.

Class I Antigens. Papain-solubilized HLA class I antigens have been sequenced for two alleles at the A (A2, A28) and three at the B (B7, B40, B27) loci (Orr *et al.*, 1979; Lopez de Castro *et al.*, 1982, 1983; Ezquerra *et al.*, 1985).

Recent efforts have been made to accumulate DNA sequences from cDNA and genomic clones. As mentioned earlier, two of the sequenced genes are pseudogenes. The others correspond to genes identified by gene transfer experiments (Fig. 7): A3, Cw3, and Aw24 (Strachan *et al.*, 1984; Sodoyer *et al.*, 1984; N'Guyen *et al.*, 1985), A2 and B7 (P. A. Biro and J. Barbosa, personal communication), and cDNA clones related to A2 and B7 (Arnot *et al.*, 1984; Trowsdale *et al.*, 1984a). These studies suggests that polymorphism may be much more extensive than expected, since two A28 and two B7 sequences from homozygous (but not consanguineous) cells were in fact alleles. Although DNA sequencing is rapid, so far more sequence information has been obtained from direct protein sequencing. An important limitation of DNA sequencing is the need to isolate intact genes from libraries and then to identify these genes by immunologic methods following gene transfer expression. The use of locus-specific probes that enable distinguishing the A and B loci (Arnot *et al.*, 1984; Koller *et al.*, 1984) to screen cDNA libraries should render the accumulation of new class I sequences easier in the future.

Charles Auffray and Jack L. Strominger

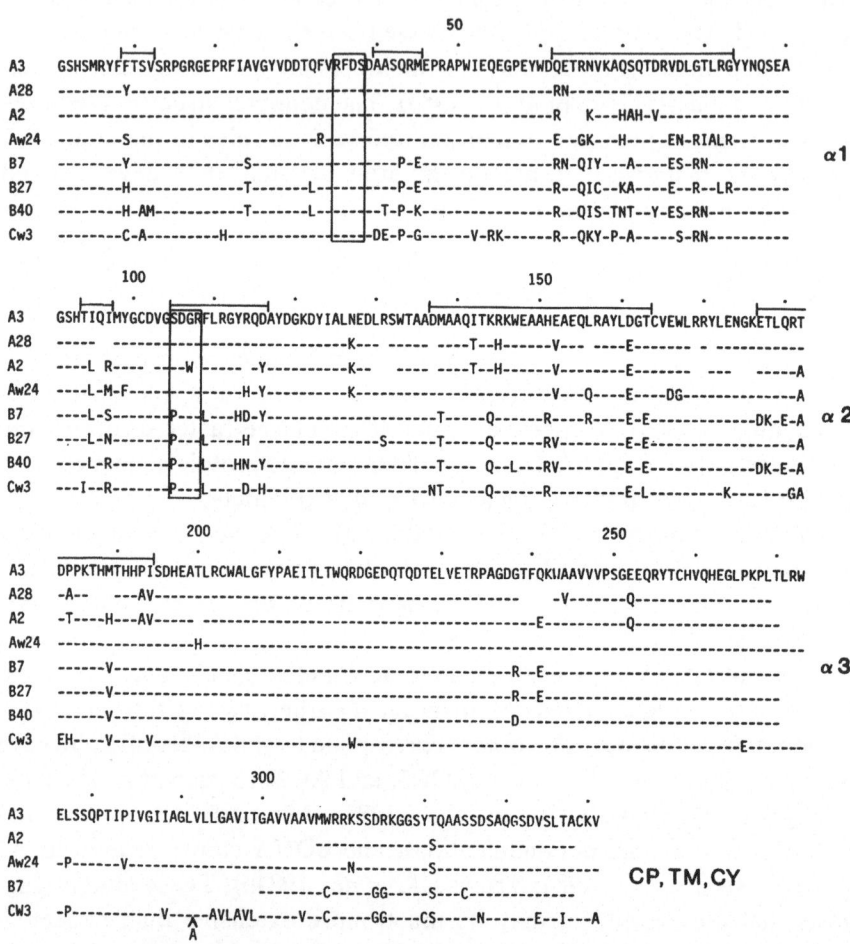

Fig. 7. The amino acid sequences of HLA-A,B,C antigens. Sequences are aligned by comparison to the HLA-A3 gene sequence (Strachan *et al.*, 1984). Identical positions are indicated by dashes. Blanks indicate residues that have not been assigned. A2 and A28 (Lopez de Castro *et al.*, 1982); Aw24 (N'Guyen *et al.*, 1985); B7 (Orr *et al.*, 1979); B27 (Ezquerra *et al.*, 1985); B40 (Lopez de Castro *et al.*, 1983); Cw3 (Sodoyer *et al.*, 1984). The polymorphic regions are indicated by bars. The two conserved sequences with homology to the fibronectin cell binding site discussed in the text are boxed.

Class II Antigens. The DRα chain has been sequenced completely by six different laboratories at the DNA level (cDNA and gene, see above) and partially by two at the protein level (Kratzin *et al.*, 1983; Knudsen *et al.*, 1985). There is an absolute correspondence between these sequences with one neutral variation (V/L) occurring in the cytoplasmic domain.

The amino acid sequence of the extracellular portion of a DR2β chain and a partial sequence of a second class II β chain found in the same homozygous cell line have been determined (Kratzin *et al.*, 1981; Götz *et al.*, 1983). These experiments have provided structural evidence for a total of seven β-chain related sequences, probably including the DQβ and DPβ related chains.

Partial and extensive sequence of the DQ-1α chain have been reported, which agree with the DNA sequence of a cDNA clone (Bono and Strominger, 1982, 1984; Götz *et al.*, 1983; Auffray *et al.*, 1984). Sequences derived from cDNA clones corresponding to the DQ-4α alleles of a DR4 and a DR7 cell line and the DQ-3α allele, as well as the genes corresponding to DQ-4α and DXα show extensive variation with the DQ-1α cDNA and genomic sequence (Auffray *et al.*, 1982, 1984; Götz *et al.*, 1983; Chang *et al.*, 1983; Schenning *et al.*, 1984). The numbering used to designate the various alleles refers to the DR haplotype on which they are encoded. Thus, DQ-4α designates the DQα chain on the DR4 haplotype.

Only limited amino acid sequence data are available for DQβ chains (Wiman *et al.*, 1982*b*; Bono and Strominger, 1984), but complete sequences corresponding probably to a DQ-1β, a DQ-3β, and a DQ-4β allele have been obtained from cDNA and genomic clones (Larhammar *et al.*, 1982*b*, 1983; Boss and Strominger, 1984; Schenning *et al.*, 1984). The DQβ sequences are polymorphic at least for DQ-1β chains on DRw6 cell lines (Shackelford *et al.*, 1983) and the extent of the DQβ polymorphism is unknown. Alternatively, some of these sequences might correspond to transcripts of the second DQβ-like gene (DXβ).

As mentioned above, amino acid sequences for the DPα and β chains are extremely limited, due to the cross-reactivity of the antibody used (Katovitch-Hurley *et al.*, 1982). The sequences of DPα, SXα, DP2, 3, and 4β and SXβ have been obtained from cDNA and genomic clones (Auffray *et al.*, 1984; Roux-Dosseto *et al.*, 1983*a*; Kappes *et al,*. 1984; Okada *et al.*, 1985*a*; Boss *et al.*, 1985).

Mechanisms for the Generation of Polymorphism

The MHC antigens represent a family of highly polymorphic molecules, that is, a large number of alleles at each locus are represented in the population. Analysis of the various sequences has provided some insight into the location of polymorphic sites and the mechanisms of their generation and propagation in the population.

The variation appears to be mostly located in the $\alpha 1$ and $\alpha 2$ domains in class I antigens (Fig. 7) and in the $\alpha 1$ and $\beta 1$ domains of class II antigens (Fig. 8), whereas the immunoglobulin-like domains are extremely conserved. For example, seven clusters of amino acid differences are apparent from comparison of putative class I alleles, the most prominent ones at positions 65–80, 105–116, and 177–194, suggesting that they correspond to alloantigenic sites. Amino acid variability plots also reveal single, highly polymorphic residues (Lopez de Castro et al., 1984). In addition, study of HLA-A2 structural variants distinguishable by cytotoxic T lymphocytes (CTL) Pious et al., 1982) indicates that discrete CTL recognition regions are located at positions 147–157 (Krangel et al., 1982, 1983a,b) and at residue 116 (Taketani et al., 1984) in precisely the same position as in the series of mouse H-$2K^b$ mutants. The HLA class I structural polymorphism is much greater than previously believed. Thus, for example, alloantibodies and CTL reagents can distinguish two and three groups of HLA-B27 subtypes, respectively [cited in Ezquerra et al., (1985)] and subdivision of A2, A3, B7, B12, and Bw44 has also been achieved using CTL reagents [reviewed in Lopez de Castro et al. (1985)].

Similar regions of hypervariability are also detected in the class II most external domains $\alpha 1$ and $\beta 1$ (Fig. 8). Only the $\alpha 1$ domain of DQα is polymorphic, with a prominent cluster of variations at positions 45–56 (Fig. 8A). It is also apparent from this comparison that the DXα gene could encode a polypeptide chain that has not diverged more than DQα alleles. As the number of sequences increases, it becomes possible to trace the history of the different alleles: DQα sequences from DR4 and DR9 cell lines (presumably DQw3) are almost identical, with the exception of one deletion and one amino acid change in $\alpha 2$ (J. Silver, personal communication), whereas they differ from DQα of a DR7 cell line by seven amino acid substitutions. In contrast, DQα from DR1 (presumably DQw1) has diverged more extensively, differing by 18 amino acids. Finally, DQα from DR3 (presumably DQw2) defines a third family of alleles. Similar observations can be made by comparing DR, DQ, and DP β chains. In particular, the three families appear as patchworks of one another, indicating the possibility that genetic exchanges have occurred repeatedly during the evolution of the families (Roux-Dosseto *et al.*, 1983*b*). Surprisingly, some of the clusters occur in the same position in the domain as in the class I antigens. In comparing the polymorphism of DQβ with that of the homologous mouse gene, I-Aβ, the regions of polymorphism in the β1 domain are not in exactly the same locations; evolution appears to have driven the polymorphism differently in the two species. It is also apparent from Fig. 8B that the same is true for the β-chain isotypes.

Another interesting observation is that in the case of class I genes and some class II genes, alleles and isotypes differ to the same extent. Analysis of the rate of accumulation of mutations at the three positions in codons indicates a strong selective pressure for the conservation of the immunoglobulin-like domain, which is best explained by the need of a particular conformation to allow interaction between the two chains. Mutations in the polymorphic domains appear to accumulate freely (Gustafsson *et al.*, 1984*b*). However, their large number and the appearance of segmental homology patterns in allelic or isotypic comparisons, that is, a cluster of mutations shared by alleles and/or isotypes, support the idea that genetic exchanges between homologous genes is in part responsible for the high degree of polymorphism observed (Auffray *et al.*, 1984). Such exchanges occurring by double unequal crossing over or gene conversion have also been proposed to affect both the class I and class II genes of the mouse MHC and immunoglobulin genes (for example, Lopez de Castro *et al.*, 1982; Hayashida and Miyata, 1983; Ollo and Rougeon, 1983; Pease *et al.*, 1983; Widera and Flavell, 1984). Thus, instead of leading to sequence homogenization, such mechanisms operating between loci or extensively diverged alleles could be used to amplify and maintain the polymorphism. The large number of potential class I (or class II) pseudogenes which are maintained could then serve as a repertoire of sequences to be used to generate new alleles at expressed loci.

Conserved Regions

The most variable domains are likely to be involved in the interaction with T-cell receptor variable regions and antigen. In contrast, there are conserved regions in the class I and class II molecules that might be relevant to specialized functions that do not require or allow variability. We have already pointed out that the immunoglobulin-like domains might

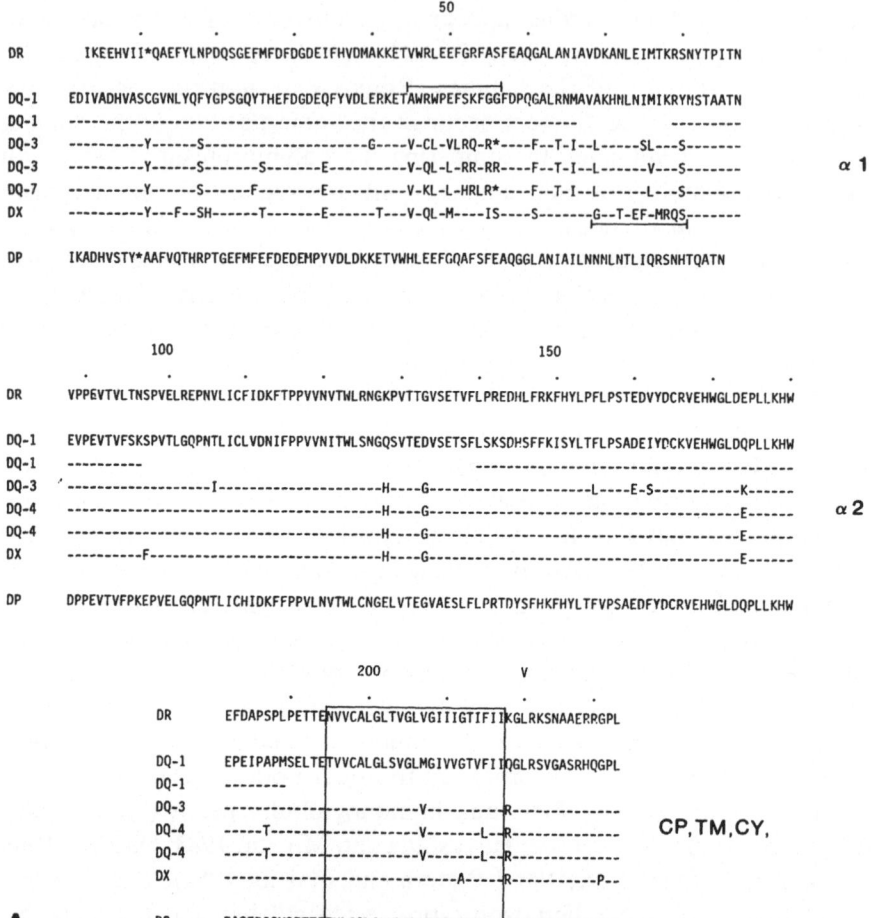

Fig. 8. The amino acid sequences of HLA class II antigens. Sequences are compared to a reference sequence for each isotype. Unassigned residues are left blank. Stars indicate gaps introduced to optimize alignments. Polymorphic regions are indicated by bars. α1, α2, β1, β2: extracellular domains; CP, TM, CY: connecting peptide, transmembrane domain, cytoplasmic domain. The transmembrane regions are boxed. (A) α chains: DRα gene and protein (Korman *et al.*, 1982*b*; Yang *et al.*, 1982). The only position found to vary in the DRα sequence is V/L at 217 (220 in the numbering system used in this figure); DQ-1α cDNA (Auffray *et al.*, 1984); DQ-1α protein (Götz *et al.*, 1983); DQ-3α cDNA (Schenning *et al.*, 1984); DQ-4α cDNA and gene (Auffray *et al.*, 1982, 1984); DQ-7α cDNA (Chang *et al.*, 1983); DXα gene (Auffray *et al.*, 1984); DPα cDNA (Auffray *et al.*, 1984). (B) β chains: DR4,6β cDNA (Long *et al.*, 1983); DR3,6β cDNA clones (Gustafsson *et al.*, 1984*b*); DR2β protein (Kratzin *et al.*, 1981; Götz *et al.*, 1983); DQ-6β cDNA (Schenning *et al.*, 1984); DQ-1β protein (Götz *et al.*, 1983); DQ-3β cDNA (Larhammar *et al.*, 1982*b*); DQ-3β gene (Boss and Strominger, 1984); DQ-4β gene (Larhammar *et al.*, 1983); DP2β cDNA (Roux-Dosseto *et al.*, 1983; Kappes *et al.*, 1984); DP3β gene (Kappes *et al.*, 1984); DP4β cDNA (Gorski *et al.*, 1984); DP4β cDNA (Gustafsson *et al.*, 1984*b*); DP4β gene (Kappes *et al.*, 1984). The tetrapeptide RFDS with homology with the fibronectin binding site (see text) is boxed.

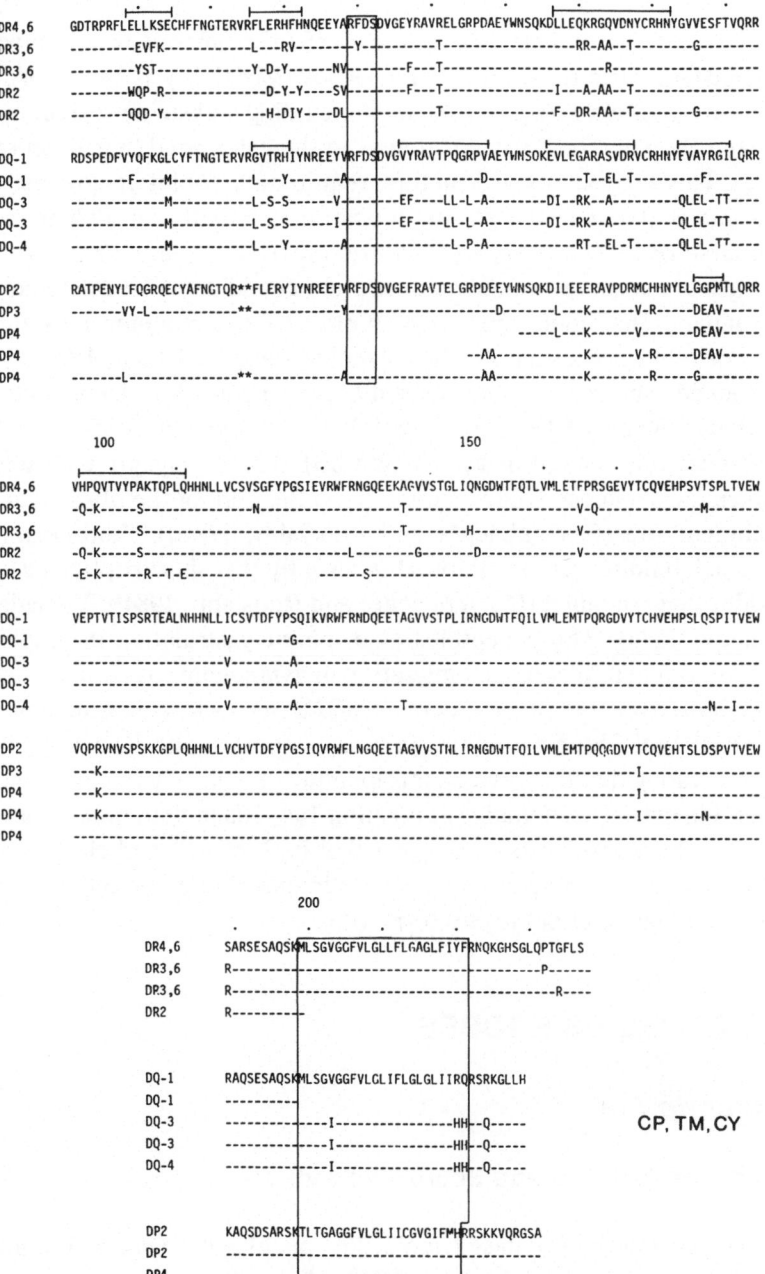

B

Fig. 8. (*continued*)

be able to interact in heterodimers in a very similar way as immunoglobulin constant regions. Another area of low variability is the transmembrane region of class II α or β chains, including a cysteine residue which has been shown to be fatty-acylated via a thioester bond (Kaufman *et al.*, 1984*b*). This suggests some structural requirement for interaction between the α and β chains in the plasma membrane, or with the γ chain during the course of biosynthesis and maturation (Kvist *et al.*, 1982). Various stretches of conserved amino acids are good candidates for monomorphic determinants that could interact with either T-cell receptor constant domains or other accessory T-cell molecules, such as T4 and T8.

Indeed, one region is conserved between class I α chains and class II β chains, namely RFDS in the first domains at positions 35–39 and 39–42, respectively (boxed in Figs. 7 and 8B). This tetrapeptide closely resembles the sequence RGDS shown to be the core of the fibronectin cell attachment site (Pierschbacher and Ruoslahti, 1984*a*). Fibronectin-mediated cell binding can be inhibited *in vitro* by this short peptide or larger peptides that contain it (Pierschbacher and Ruoslahti, 1984*b*; Yamada and Kennedy, 1984). These peptides also inhibit gastrulation in amphibian embryos and neural crest cell migration in avian embryos (Boucaut *et al.*, 1984). Moreover, the reverse peptide SGDR also shows strong inhibitory properties in a fibroblast adhesion assay (Yamada and Kennedy, 1985). It is interesting that this reverse tetrapeptide or a closely related sequence is found in class I α2 domains at position 104–108 in both mouse and man (Fig. 7). These observations suggest that both class I and class II molecules could trigger antigen-nonspecific binding of effector and target cells at the early stage of conjugate formation.

HLA GENES AS PROBES

Transcription

Differential Splicing and Secreted Products

The structure of a class I molecule specifically expressed in murine liver has been deduced from a cDNA clone. This new class I antigen appears to be secreted, lacking the normal transmembrane and cytoplasmic domains, and it has been argued that it could function as a tolerizing agent (Kress *et al.*, 1983). It is now known that it is encoded by a class I gene located in the Qa region. There is at least one more gene encoding a class I putative secreted product in this region of the mouse MHC (Lalanne *et al.*, 1985). In the human system, there is one mutant cell line that expresses a 39,000-dalton secreted class I α chain (Krangel *et al.*, 1984). Study of this line by Northern blot analysis and sequencing of cDNA clones shows that it lacks the transmembrane exon altogether (M. Krangel, personal communication). It remains to be seen if this reflects a physiological phenomenon in man also.

Several examples of alternate splicing events of class II genes have been detected by Northern blot analysis or cDNA cloning. The DRα gene can be transcribed into two mRNAs using one of two poly A addition signals located 100 bp apart (Lee *et al.*, 1982*b*; Korman *et al.*, 1982*a*). Two DQβ transcripts have been detected on Northern blots (Long *et al.*, 1982*b*; Collins *et al.*, 1984) and recent evidence indicates that this might be due to an alternate site for polyadenylation (E. Long, personal communication). In one DR4 cell line, however, cDNA clones with different 3' ends have been isolated which encode polypeptides that differ in their carboxyl terminus (J. S. Cairns, C. Dahl, and F. Bach, personal communication). A similar observation can be made when comparing several DP β-chain alleles (Fig. 8B). The cytoplasmic domain of one DP4β allele is ten amino acids longer than other DPβ chains. It is not clear whether these differences have a functional significance. The DQα gene encodes transcripts that differ in size between haplotypes: 1.1 kb in DR4, 7, and 9 (DQw3); 1.3 kb in DR1, 2, and w6 (DQw1); and 1.5 kb in DR3 (DQw2). Thus, it is possible to perform DQ typing based on mRNA length measurements (Auffray *et al.*, 1984; J. Boss, D. Piatier-Tonneau, and C. Auffray, unpublished results; Schenning *et al.*, 1984).

The unexplained observation that class II determinants are found on soluble T-helper secreted products might result from alternative splicing of the class II genes which bypass the transmembrane exon. Attempts are being made to solve this question using the corresponding exons as probes.

Regulation of Expression

Interferons α, β, and γ have been shown to modulate expression of the HLA class I antigens in various cell types. Increase of HLA-A,B,C antigens and β_2-microglobulin cell surface expression is preceded by an increase in the amount of the corresponding mRNA already detectable after 1 hr of interferon treatment (Fellous et al., 1982). There have been conflicting reports as to whether all types of interferons can also modulate the expression of class II antigens. It is now clear that only interferon γ has a pronounced effect on the level of expression, and that the level of enhancement is dependent on the basal level of transcription (although regulation at the level of mRNA stability has not been ruled out). That is, expression of class II antigens can be modulated in cells expressing them, such as B lymphocytes, but in cases where the basal expression is already high, no increase can be obtained (Basham and Merigan, 1983; Rosa et al., 1983a,b). On the other hand, in cell types that have no constitutive expression of class II antigens, such as vascular endothelial cells and dermal fibroblasts, interferon γ induces the de novo expression of class II antigens (Collins et al., 1984). In these cell lines, transcription of class I genes appears doubled by interferon γ, and there is a parallel induction of HLA-DR (both at the protein and mRNA level) and HLA-DP (detected at the mRNA level) together with the invariant chain. In contrast, HLA-DQ mRNAs and proteins are induced at a very low level. These results are very similar to those reported for promyelocytic leukemia cells and normal human monocytes or macrophages of various sources (Koeffler et al., 1984), where HLA-DR can be clearly induced without concomitant expression of HLA-DQ (protein and mRNA). Thus, it appears that the three families of HLA class II antigens can be regulated independently of each other.

The segregation of the expression of DR and DQ antigens is reminiscent of the fact that they behave as differentiation antigens in the course of maturation in the lymphoid and myeloid hematopoietic lineages. That is, in some instances expression of HLA-DR can be detected with the absence of HLA-DQ molecules on various types of leukemic cells. Expression of HLA-DQ can be restored in hairy cell leukemia cells using phorbol esters, 5-azacytidine, or sodium butyrate (Faille et al., 1985). Phorbol esters and 1,25-dihydroxy-vitamin D3 also induce the promyelocytic cell line HL60 to differentiate with characteristics of monocyte-macrophages, but only the latter induces expression of HLA-DR molecules. Since interferon γ appears to regulate expression of the class II genes at the level of transcription, it is interesting to search in the promoter region for sequences that might be involved in this regulation. By comparing DRα and I-Eα sequences upstream of the typical promoter ele-

```
                    • -110            -98                    -78        -69
Consensus α and β  CCYAGNRACNGATG                           CTGATTGGYY
       DQ-3β       --C--AG--A---G  AGGTCCTTCAGCTCCAGTG  --------TT CCTT
       DQ-4β       --T--AG--A---T  AGGTCCTTCAGCTCCAGTG  --------TT CCTT
       DXβ         --C--AGG-A---G  AGGTCCTTCAGCTCCAGTG  --------TT CCTT
       I-Aβ        --C--AG--A---G  ACAGACTTCAGGTCCAATG  --------TT CCTC

       DPβ         --T--TG-GCA--G  CTCATACAAAGCTC AGTG  TCC-----TT CTTT
       I-Eβ        A-T--CA--T---G  ATGCTGGACTCCTTTGATG  --------CT CCCA
       DRβ         A-C--CA--T---G  ATGCTATTGAACTCAGACG  -----CATT CTCC

Consensus β only                   ANRYYNYYCAGCTCCARTG             CYYY


       DQα         G-T--TA--T--GA  TGTCACCATGGGGG ATTTTT  --A-----CC AAAA
       DXα         A-TG-CA-ACA--A  TGTCACCATAGGGG ATTTTT  --------CC AAAA
       DRα         --T--CA--A---G  CGTCA TCTCAAAATATTTTT  --------CC AAAG
       I-Eα        —T--CA--A---G  TGTCAGTCT GAAACATTTTT  --------TT AAAA

Consensus α only                   TGTCANYCTNRRRRNATTTTT           AAAA
                                          A
```

•Bases upstream from the initiation of transcription of DC-3β

Fig. 9. Comparison of the upstream sequences common to the class II MHC genes. Y, Pyrimidine; R, purine; N, any nucleotide. DQ-3β (Boss and Strominger, 1984); DQ-4β (Larhammar et al., 1983); DQα, DXα, DXβ (Okada et al., 1985a); DPβ (Kappes et al., 1984); I-Eβ (Saito et al., 1983); I-Aβ and DRβ (Larhammar et al., 1985); DRα (Schamboeck et al., 1983); I-Eα (Mathis et al., 1983). [Taken from Okada et al., (1985b).]

ments corresponding to the TATA and CCAAT boxes, a region of strong homology has been detected (Mathis et al., 1983). Compilation of mouse and human class II gene sequences led to the definition of conserved elements of 14 and ten nucleotides separated by a spacer of 20 bases in α-chain genes and 19 bases in β-chain genes (Saito et al., 1983; Larhammar et al., 1985; Okada et al., 1985a). In addition to the conserved elements, there are distinguishable features of the α and β-gene spacers that suggest that this region is involved in the coordinate regulation of the expression of α- and β-chain genes (Fig. 9). They may also be involved in controlling the level of transcription and therefore of expression of the three families of class II antigens. Future experiments in which genes deleted in this area will be expressed by gene transfer will be needed to demonstrate directly the role of these sequences.

Similar experiments have been conducted in order to analyze class II negative variants of B-cell lines (Pious et al., 1980; Accolla, 1983). First, fusion of such a cell line with a normal class II-expressing cell line resulted in expression of the DR allotypes of both cells, suggesting the existence of a positive *trans*-acting regulating factor. The DR, DQ, and DP α and β genes and the invariant-chain gene are present in the DNA of these cell lines, but no α or β mRNA can be detected by Northern blot analysis, whereas the level of invariant-chain gene transcript is reduced. This suggests that these cell lines have a mutation affecting regulation of expression of the class II genes (Long *et al.*, 1984*b*). Revertants of the mutant B-cell lines that reexpress HLA-DR have been characterized. The DQ and DP antigens are not reexpressed (Levine *et al.*, 1985; R. Accolla, personal communication). The nature of the mutation is not clear, and it might well be that the class II genes are transcribed at a high level and that there is a strong requirement for an mRNA stabilizing factor whose expression needs to be turned on during differentiation and could be affected in the mutants.

A subset of severe combined immunodeficiencies, a congenital and usually lethal disease referred to as the bare lymphocyte syndrome, is characterized by failure of expression of class I and/or class II proteins. There is also no trace of corresponding mRNAs and no response to interferon γ treatment, whereas the invariant chain (protein and mRNA) appear unaffected. That this defect is due to a shutoff of transcription by an unknown mechanism is shown by the fact that there is no obvious deletion of the genes that can be reexpressed in EBV-transformed lines derived from these patients (De Préval *et al.*, 1984; Lisowska-Grospierre *et al.*, 1985).

Genetic Polymorphism and Disease Association

A major difficulty in the human system as compared to that of the mouse is the outbred nature of the population and the impossibility of conducting breeding experiments. Detailed genetic analysis has therefore relied upon family studies using serologic and functional tools. Since these two approaches recognize overlapping but nonidentical biochemical entities, it was hoped that the generation of a large panel of monoclonal antibodies would help in refining these studies. However, the complexity already obvious from serologic studies using polyclonal alloantisera has been replaced by an even greater complexity of epitopes. In many instances, cross-reactivity between various antigens has not been resolved, and in others, epitopes present on one subset of class II antigen in a given cell line have been found to be located on another subset in another cell line. Furthermore, new antigens have been defined without providing tools with a clear-cut specificity that would enable distinguishing them from the already classified antigens. Therefore the analysis of DNA polymorphisms with cloned probes provides an important complement to these studies. By Southern blot analysis of DNA from a panel of individuals typed for HLA antigens that are unrelated or members of informative families, it has been possible to establish correlations between restriction enzyme site polymorphisms and HLA specificities.

Class I Genes

Since all class I genes share a high degree of homology, a single probe detects 10–20 bands in a restriction enzyme digest of human DNA. Studies of restriction enzyme length polymorphisms (RFLP) have provided new insights into the polymorphism of the HLA region (Fig. 10). For example, among the 12–13 EcoRV fragments ranging in size between 2 and 28 kb detected with a class I probe, three are polymorphic, and one band of 8.6 kb correlates with the HLA-B8 specificity. This can be confirmed in family studies (Cann et al., 1983). In another study using various x-ray-induced deletion mutants and unrelated individuals, HLA-A1, A2, and B8 have been assigned to specific DNA fragments and 30% of the hybridizing PvuII fragments aligned (Orr and DeMars, 1983b).

In an extensive study using five restriction enzymes, 152 different fragments have been detected, 88 of which are polymorphic. Interestingly, the majority (63%) of these fragments correlate with HLA-A specificities, whereas only 13 and 5% correlate with HLA-B and C, respectively. It is possible to define clusters of polymorphic fragments that show strong association with the HLA-A1, A3, and A9, A11, and Aw19 specificities. It is noteworthy that segregation of polymorphic fragments always occurs together with HLA types, and that is there is no evidence for any polymorphic homologous gene outside of the MHC. Moreover, haplotype assignment can be performed in 99% of cases and homozygosity is easily detected. An interesting observation is that indidviduals typed as HLA-A9 seem to have fewer class I genes than normal, whereas HLA-Aw29 individuals have more genes (Cohen and Dausset, 1983; Cohen et al., 1983).

Class II Genes

Among the α-chain genes, DQα appears the most polymorphic. The DQα probe detects DNA polymorphisms of EcoRI and HindIII fragments.

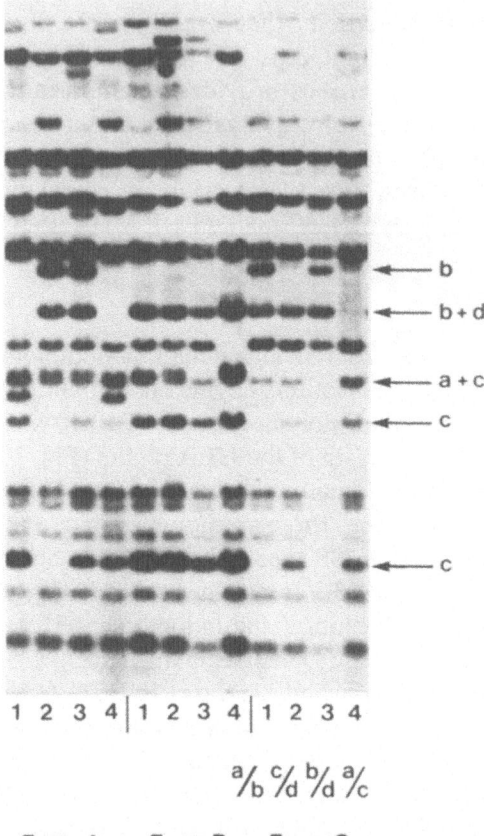

Fig. 10. Southern blot analysis of DNA from three families (A, B, C) digested with *Pvu*II
and hybridized to an HLA class I probe. In each family, lanes 1 and 2 correspond to the
parents, and lanes 3 and 4 to HLA-nonidentical children. The haplotype combinations are
indicated for family C. Arrows on the side point to polymorphic DNA fragments that can
be assigned to the indicated haplotypes in familiy C. [Figure kindly provided by D. Cohen,
Hôpital St. Louis, Paris.]

A striking result is the excellent correlation between the detected fragments and the serologically defined DR/MT linkage groups. Although it
is possible that the MT1 determinant present on DQ antigens is in part
located on the DQα chain, the MT2 and MT3 determinants are located
on DR antigens (see above). Thus, the correlation seen at the DNA level
may reflect merely a strong linkage and a subsequent cosegregation of
DR and DQ subregions in a limited number of combinations (Auffray *et*

al., 1983*b*; Trowsdale *et al.*, 1983; Spielman *et al.*, 1984). A survey of 92 haplotypes in 23 families allowed the definition of two allelic series detected with the DQα probe that segregate independently in non-DR5 or DR7 haplotypes. It appears, therefore, that recombination between loci defined by these series is infrequent in DR5 and DR7 (Le Gall *et al.*, 1985). The other α-chain genes appear to be much less polymorphic, that is, variability is detected only occasionally: *Pst*I and *Taq*I for DXα (Spielman *et al.*, 1984) and *Bgl*II for DRα (Erlich *et al.*, 1983*b*).

Ten *Eco*RI and 12 *Bam*HI fragments are detected by cross-hybridization between DRβ, DQβ, and DPβ genes. Thus, it is possible to detect patterns of *Bam*HI DNA fragments specific for the DR1, 2/w6, 3, 4, 5, 7, and 8 haplotypes with a DQβ probe, and to distinguish DR 2 and DRw6 with *Eco*RI. Further subdivision of the DQ types is accomplished with *Pst*I. Overall, the DRβ genes are the most polymorphic and the DPβ genes the least polymorphic. In another study of 88 haplotypes using six different restriction enzymes, 52 polymorphic fragments were detected with a DQβ probe. Interestingly, some clusters of polymorphic fragments correlate with DR specificities. This most probably reflects the strong linkage disequilibrium between the DQ and DR subregions of the HLA complex (see above). Therefore, these studies provide a large number of new genetic markers in this region (Owerbach *et al.*, 1983*a*; Cohen *et al.*, 1984*a*; De Préval *et al.*, 1984*b*). The Southern blot method has also been used to refine family studies, and in at least one case it has been possible to detect a new crossover in the HLA-D region using a DPβ probe (Robinson *et al.*, 1984).

Disease Association

It is of obvious interest to determine if the DNA polymorphisms can be used as more accurate markers of disease susceptibility than those available. Indeed, the DRα *Bgl*II polymorphism reproduces the DR3/4 linkage with insulin-dependent diabetes (IDDM) (Erlich *et al.*, 1984). More interesting is the finding that one of the *Bam*HI DQβ fragments (3.7 kb) is present in 30–40% of control healthy individuals (including DR4) and 0.2% of insulin-dependent diabetic patients. This negative association does not correlate with negative association of the disease with DR2, since this fragment is not found in DR2 haplotypes (Owerbach *et al.*, 1983*b*). In another study, a 2.2-kb *Eco*RI fragment detected with a DQβ probe was found to be absent in IDDM patients and present in DR2 controls or multiple sclerosis patients. Moreover, a cluster of polymorphic fragments found in DR3/4 heterozygous patients defines a group with a relative risk ten times higher than when using the serologically defined markers (Cohen *et al.*, 1984*b*).

Obviously such studies are only beginning and the question of whether HLA antigens or linked gene products are directly involved in the predisposition to disease remains open.

Function

Class I Genes

In order to identify clones containing functional class I genes, they have been introduced into mouse LTK$^-$ fibroblast cells by the calcium phosphate precipitation technique. Transfected cell lines having incorporated an HLA gene are obtained by cotransfer of the HSV TK gene and selection on HAT medium. These cell lines have been studied by immunofluorescence using a panel of monoclonal antibodies both by microscopic and flow cytometric analysis as well as by complement-mediated cytotoxicity. Thus, genes encoding the A1, A2, A3, A9, A11, Aw24, A26, B7, B14, B27, B40, Bw58, and Cw3 specificities have been identified (Barbosa *et al.*, 1982, 1984; Le Bouteiller *et al.*, 1982; Bernabeu *et al.*, 1983; Hermann *et al.*, 1983; Lemonnier *et al.*, 1983; Van de Rijn *et al.*, 1984; Yoshie *et al.*, 1984; and personal communications from J. Barbosa, D. Cohen, H. Coppens, B. Jordan, H. Orr, and P. Parham). As a result of its association with mouse β_2-microglobulin, the HLA gene product appears at the cell surface. Immunoprecipitation of the expressed polypeptide and 2D gel analysis reveal no difference from authentic HLA antigens. It is worth noting that most monomorphic or polymorphic epitopes are detectable serologically on the transfected lines. Conformational modification of the murine β_2-microglobulin upon association with the HLA chain renders it more readily labeled by iodination. In addition, it reacts with specific anti-human β_2-microglobulin antibodies. This post-association modification of antigenicity is also detected in mouse–human somatic cell hybrids. This phenomenon is seen with three out of 13 clones tested. One can speculate that class I gene products that do not associate appropriately with murine β_2-microglobulin will escape detection with the available antibodies or cytotoxic T lymphocytes. Thus, genes that fail to express in these assays are not necessarily pseudogenes (Lemonnier *et al.*, 1983).

The transfected cell lines expressing human class I products in most cases fail to be killed by specific CTLs, that is, they are resistant to both human allospecific CTLs and to murine CTLs directed against HLA antigens. This contrasts with the situation observed with cell lines transfected with murine class I genes, which are excellent targets for CTLs (Hood *et al.*, 1983). It has been suspected that association with mouse β_2-microglobulin destroys the target structure of the CTLs or that the level of expression on the target cells (5–20% of B-cell lines) might not be sufficient to reproduce physiological conditions. However, in recent studies in which the A2 and B7 genes have been transfected in murine, monkey, and human cell lines alone or in association with the human β_2-microglobulin gene, several of these possibilities have been excluded (Barbosa *et al.*, 1984; Van de Rijn *et al.*, 1984). That is, neither the expression level (no lysis is observed after enhancement of expression by interferon treatment), the possible association with mouse β_2-microglobulin (cotransfection of class I genes with the human β_2-microglobulin gene does not change the result), nor the need for species-specific cell interaction molecules on the effector CTLs explains the failure of recognition of class I human gene products expressed in mouse cells. Rather, it seems likely that species-specific "cell interaction" molecules on the target cell are required for the lytic process in addition to the class I gene product, such as ligands for LFA-1 or T8 at the adhesion step and T3 at the post-adhesion step. Indeed, recognition of HLA-A2 by CTLs on transfected cell lines can be efficiently blocked by anti-LFA-1, T8, or T3 antibodies (Van de Rijn *et al.*, 1984). Moreover, it appears that there is a lack of appropriate recognition of the transfected cell lines that fail to form conjugates with the cytotoxic cells, rather than a block of the activation of the lytic pathway [reviewed in Lopez de Castro *et al.* (1985)]. Finally, these requirements for CTL recognition are not absolute, since some cloned mouse xenogeneic CTLs can successfully kill HLA-B7 transfected lines (Hermann *et al.*, 1983). Similarly, in at least one case, a specific human CTL is able to kill an HLA-A3 variant transfected line (Cowan *et al.*, 1985). In contrast, functional expression of the HLA class I genes is readily achieved when they are introduced into human and monkey cell lines (Barbosa *et al.*, 1984; Van de Rijn *et al.*, 1984).

The regulation of the expression of the transfected genes can be studied at the level of transcription by exposing the transfected cell line to agents such as interferon. However, such experiments have to be interpreted with caution, since in one instance a truncated HLA-B7 gene gives rise to transcripts of various sizes, including a normal transcript, and the level of transcription is enhanced by interferon in a fashion similar to the physiological situation. This probably occurs through linkage of the integrated DNA with sequences providing signals for transcription initiation that are susceptible to interferon (Yoshie *et al.*, 1984).

Class II Genes

Transfection experiments have also been conducted with cloned class II genes. Since nothing was known of the possible role of the class II-associated invariant or γ chain, in one study the invariant-chain gene was contransfected in mouse fibrobasts with the DRα and DRβ genes together with the HSV TK gene as selectable marker. As the result of cotransfection of the four genes, cell lines have been isolated that stably express the HLA-DR antigen at the cell surface as shown by cellular binding radioimmunoassay, immunofluorescence, and immunoprecipitation of iodinated cell surface molecules. There is a large variation in the level of expression between cell lines, which can be as high as B-cell controls. The invariant-chain gene is not essential for successful expression, probably because the mouse L cell used itself synthesizes a significant level of the murine invariant chain (Rabourdin-Combe and Mach, 1983). By studying these transfected cell lines with a panel of monoclonal antibodies, it has been shown that the DRβ gene used encodes the BR3 (MT2) specificity and is one of the three closely related DR β-chain genes (De Préval *et al.*, 1984*a*).

Expression of the genes in the DP cosmids has been obtained in both mouse LTK⁻ cells and in a mouse macrophage line (Fig. 11). (Austin *et al.*, 1985; Okada *et al.*, 1985*a*; D. Levy and J. Strominger, unpublished results). The gene products were specifically reactive with monoclonal antibodies that react with DP molecules alone (B7/21-FA) or in addition to DR and DQ molecules (Tü39 and MHM4), but unreactive with those recognizing only DR and/or DQ molecules. The reactivity with MHM4 is puzzling, since this antibody reacts with deletion mutants that lack the DPα and DPβ genes [cited in Sanchez-Perez and Shaw (1985)], and also because the DP transfectants described in one of these studies failed to react with it (Austin *et al.*, 1985). Expression occurred in both cell lines without introduction of a γ-chain gene, but in immunoprecipitates, a γ

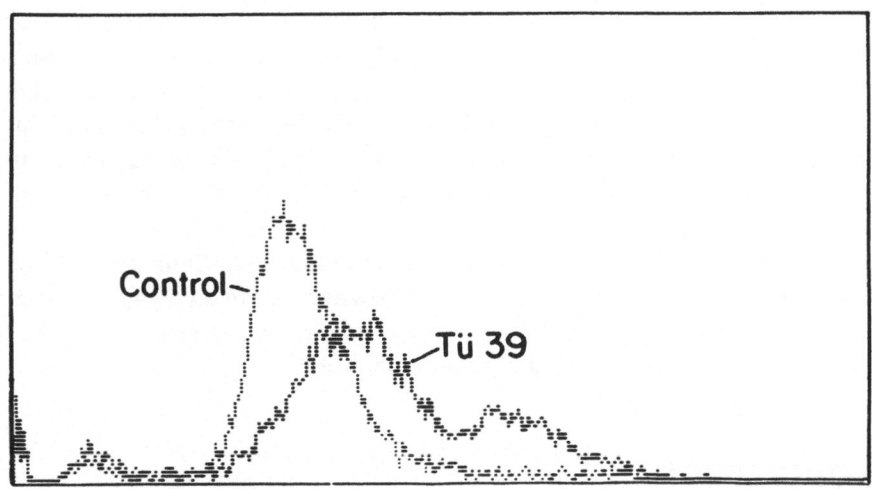

Fig. 11. Expression of the DP antigen in a mouse macrophage line by gene transfer. A cosmid clone containing the DPα, DPβ, SXα, and neomycin genes was transfected into the mouse macrophage line P3M. Expression is detected with the fluorescence-activated cell sorter after staining with the Tü39 monoclonal antibody. [From Okada *et al.*, (1985*b*).]

chain was evident, presumably derived from the host cell. In one of these studies (Austin *et al.*, 1985), the L-cell transfectants were shown to express functional DP molecules, that is, they were able to stimulate proliferation of an influenza neuraminidase-specific, DP-restricted CTL clone. Moreover, this stimulation was blocked by anti-DP antibodies. These results are very similar to those obtained previously in the murine system, showing that antigen presentation can be performed by cell types different from B lymphocytes or macrophages. It is therefore possible that the ligands for T-cell surface antigens such as T4 and LFA-1 either are not obligatory or are also present on murine fibroblasts. This in turn might depend of the nature of the antigen recognized, since murine L cells transfected with murine class II genes are able to present KLH but not ovalbumin to CTL clones specific for these antigens. (B. Malissen *et al.*, 1984).

Cosmid clones containing the DQα and DQβ genes have also been successfully transfected into murine fibroblasts and expression of DQ molecules detected at the cell surface (J. Cooper and J. Barbosa, personal communication). As for the DR genes, functional expression of these molecules in terms of antigen presentation is yet to be demonstrated.

A promising approach to functional studies of class II antigens deals with the introduction of full-length cDNA clones for the α and β chains (with or without the invariant chain) into expression vectors. Thus, using highly transmissible retroviral vectors (which have the potential of infecting a great variety of cell types), expression of DR α-, β-, and γ-chain cDNA clones has been achieved in mouse fibroblasts, with levels of expression comparable to the normal level observed in B cells (Korman et al., 1985; A. Korman, personal communication). Similarly, cDNA clones for various α and β chains placed downstream of an SV40 promoter lead to high levels of transient expression when cotransfected in monkey Cos-1 cells (E. Long, personal communication).

CONCLUSION

We now have access to a great deal of structural information on the HLA genes and their products. Thus, it is now possible to get an idea of the nature of the polymorphism, which will become more precise as the amount of information increases. The structural information will serve as a basis for the construction of new genes by exon exchanges or by site-directed mutagenesis, which can be studied by gene transfer experiments and reveal structure–function relationships. In fact, we know very little of the molecular mechanisms that allow the HLA antigens to function as restricting elements. That is, we have no precise idea of how they interact with antigen and T-lymphocyte receptors. With the recent isolation of the T-cell receptor genes, hopefully it will be possible to reconstruct completely and manipulate the recognition system that is so important for the regulation of the whole immune system. The complexity of the T-cell recognition unit, which contains a number of polypeptides in addition to the two chains of the T-cell receptor itself, makes this a difficult but extremely interesting goal. Finally, more work is needed to establish good correlations between the serology, genetics, and biochemistry of the HLA region and the new DNA probes in order to better understand the nature of HLA–disease associations. This remains one of the most challenging problems for the future.

ACKNOWLEDGMENTS. We thank A. Bonvallot, E. Bourson, L. Obert, S. Roy, and S. Tissot for secretarial assistance. We are grateful to members of our laboratories for useful discussions and for sharing unpublished results and ideas. We thank Drs. R. Accolla, F. Bach, W. Bodmer, D. Cohen, H. Coppens, J. Dausset, L. Hood, B. Jordan, P. Kourilsky, D. Larhammar, E. Long, B. Mach, H. Orr, P. Parham, P. Peterson, M. Steinmetz, S. Shaw, J. P. Thiéry, and K. Yamada for communication of their results prior to publication. Finally, we acknowledge Drs. D. Cohen and J. Novotny, who contributed illustrations for this review. This work was supported by grants from CNRS to C. A. and from NIH to J.L.S.

REFERENCES

Accolla, R. S., 1983, Human B cell variants immunoselected against a single Ia antigen subset have lost expression of several Ia antigen subsets, *J. Exp. Med.* **157**:1053–1058.

Arnot, D.,, Lillie, J. W., Auffray, C., Kappes, D., and Strominger, J. L., 1984, Inter-locus and intra-allelic polymorphism of HLA class I antigen mRNA, *Immunogenetics* **20**:237–252.

Auffray, C., Korman, A. J., Roux-Dosseto, M., Bono, R., and Strominger, J. L., 1982, cDNA clone for the heavy chain of human B cell alloantigen DC1: Strong sequence homology to the HLA-DR heavy chain, *Proc. Natl. Acad. Sci. USA* **79**:6337–6341.

Auffray, C., Kuo, J., DeMars, R., and Strominger, J. L., 1983a, A minimum of four human class II α chain genes are encoded in the HLA region of chromosome 6, *Nature* **304**:174–177.

Auffray, C., Ben-Nun, A., Roux-Dosseto, M., Germain, R. N., Seidman, J. G., and Strominger, J. L., 1983b, Polymorphism and complexity of the human DC and murine I-A α chain genes, *EMBO J.* **2**:121–124.

Auffray, C., Lillie, J. W., Arnot, D., Grossberger, D., Kappes, D., and Strominger, J. L., 1984, Isotypic and allotypic variation of the class II human histocompatibility antigen α chain genes, *Nature* **308**:327–333.

Austin, P., Trowsdale, J., Rudd, C., Bodmer, W., Feldmann, M., and Lamb, J., 1985, Functional expression of HLA-DP genes transfected into mouse fibroblasts, *Nature* **313**:61–64.

Barbosa, J. A., Karmack, M. E., Biro, P. A., Weissman, S. M., and Ruddle, F. H., 1982, Identification of human genomic clones coding the major histocompatibility antigens HLA-A2 and HLA-B7 by DNA-mediated gene transfer, *Proc. Natl. Acad. Sci. USA* **79**:6327–6331.

Barbosa, J. A., Mentzer, S. J., Minawada, G., Strominger, J. L., Burakoff, S. J., and Biro, P. A., 1984, Differential recognition of HLA-A2 and B7 antigens by cloned cytotoxic T lymphocytes following gene transfer into human, monkey and mouse cells, *Proc. Natl. Acad. Sci. USA* **81**:7549–7553.

Basham, T. Y., and Merigan, T. C., 1983, Recombinant interferon γ increases HLA-DR synthesis and expression, *J. Immunol.* **130**:1492–1497.

Bernabeu, C., Finlay, D., Van de Rijn, M., Maziarz, R. T., Biro, P. A., Spits, H., de Vries, J., and Terhorst, C. P., 1983, Expression of the major histocompatibility antigens HLA-A2 and HLA-B7 by DNA mediated gene transfer, *J. Immunol.* **131**:2032–2037.

Biro, P. A., Pereira, D., Sood, A. K., de Martinville, B., Francke, U., and Weissman, S.

M., 1981, The structure of the human major histocompatibility complex, *UCLA Symp. Mol. Cell. Biol.* **20**:315.

Bodmer, W. F., Albert, E., Bodmer, J. G., Dausset, J., Kissmeyer-Nielsen, Mayr, W. F., Payne, J. J., Van Rood, J. J., Trnka, Z., and Walford, R. L., 1984, Nomenclature for factors of the HLA system, *Immunogenetics* **20**:593–601.

Böhme, J., Owerbach, D., Denaro, M., Lernmark, A., Peterson, P. A., and Rask, L., 1983, Human class II major histocompatibility antigen β chains are derived from at least three loci, *Nature* **301**:82–84.

Bono, M. R., and Strominger, J. L., 1982, Direct evidence of homology between human DC-1 antigen and murine I-A molecules, *Nature* **299**:836–838.

Bono, M. R., and Strominger, J. L., 1984, NH_2-terminal sequence of the α and β chains of human DC-1 antigen isolated from JY cell line: Homology with murine I-A molecules, *Immunogenetics* **18**:453–459.

Boss, J. M., and Strominger, J. L., 1984, Cloning and sequence analysis of the human major histocompatibility complex gene DC-3β, *Proc. Natl. Acad. Sci. USA* **81**:5199–5203.

Boss, J. M., Mengler, R., Okada, K., Auffray, L., and Strominger, J. L., 1985, Sequence analysis of the human major histocompatibility gene SXα *Mol. Cell Biol.* (in press).

Boucaut, J. C., Darribère, T., Poole, T. J., Aoyama, H., Yamada, K. M., and Thiéry, J. P., 1984, Biologically active synthetic peptides as probes of embryonic development: A competitive peptide inhibitor of fibronectin function inhibits gastrulation in amphibian embryos and neural crest cell migration in avian embryos, *J. Cell. Biol.* **99**: 1822–1830.

Cann, H. M., Ascanio, L., Paul, P., Marcadet, A., Dausset, J., and Cohen, D., 1983, Polymorphic restriction endonuclease fragment segregates and correlates with the gene for HLA-B8, *Proc. Natl. Acad. Sci. USA* **80**:1665–1668.

Cepko, C. L., Roberts, B. E., and Mulligan, R. C., 1984, Construction and applications of a highly transmissible murine retrovirus shuttle vector, *Cell* **37**:1053–1062.

Chang, H. C., Moriuchi, T., and Silver, J., 1983, The heavy chain of the human B-cell alloantigen, HLA-DS, has a variable N-terminal region and a constant immunoglobulin-like region, *Nature* **305**:813–815.

Claesson, L., Larhammar, D., Rask, L., and Peterson, P. A., 1983, cDNA clone for the human invariant γ chain of class II antigens and its implications for the protein structure, *Proc. Natl. Acad. Sci. USA* **80**:7395–7399.

Claesson-Walsh, L., Barker, P. E., Larhammar, D., Rask, L., Ruddle, F. H., and Peterson, P. A., 1984, The gene encoding the human class II antigen-associated γ chain is located on chromosome 5, *Immunogenetics* **20**:89–93.

Cohen, D., and Dausset, J., 1983, HLA gene polymorphism, in: *Progress in Immunology V* (Y. Yamamura and T. Tada eds.), pp. 1–12, Academic Press, New York.

Cohen, D., Paul, P., Font, M. P., Cohen, O., Sayagh, B., Marcadet, A., Busson, M., Mahouy, G., Cann, H. M., and Dausset, J., 1983, Analysis of HLA class I genes with restriction endonuclease fragments: Implications for polymorphism of the human major histocompatibility complex, *Proc. Natl. Acad. Sci. USA* **80**:6289–6292.

Cohen, D., Le Gall, I., Marcadet, A., Font, M. P., Lalouel, J. M., and Dausset, J., 1984a, Clusters of HLA class II β restriction fragments described allelic series, *Proc. Natl. Acad. Sci. USA* **81**:7870–7874.

Cohen, D., Cohen, O., Marcadet, A., Massart, C., Lathrop, M., Deschamps, I., Hors, J., Schuller, E., and Dausset, J., 1984b, Class II HLA-DC β chain DNA restriction fragments differentiate among HLA-DR2 individuals in insulin-dependent diabetes and multiple sclerosis, *Proc. Natl. Acad. Sci. USA* **81**:1774–1778.

Collins, T., Korman, A. J., Wake, C. T., Boss, J., Fiers, W., Ault, K. A., Gimbrone, M. A., Strominger, J. L., and Pober, J. S., 1984, Immune interferon activates multiple class

II major histocompatibility complex genes and the associated invariant chain gene in human endothelial cells and dermal fibroblasts, *Proc. Natl. Acad. Sci. USA* **81**:4971–4921.

Cowan, E. P., Biddison, W. E., Jordan, B. R., and Colligan, J. E., 1985, Molecular cloning and DNA sequence analysis of a gene encoding an HLA-A3 subtype and its functional expression in murine L. Cells, in: *Advances in Gene Technology: Molecular Biology of the Immune System* (J. Wayne, I. W. Streilein, F. Ahmad, S. Black, B. Blomberg, and R. W. Voellmy, eds.), ICSU Short Reports Vol. 2, pp. 131–132, Cambridge University Press, Cambridge.

Das, J. K., Lawrence, S. K., and Weissman, S. M., 1983, Structure and nucleotide sequence of the heavy chain gene of HLA-DR, *Proc. Natl. Acad. Sci. USA* **80**:3543–3547.

Davis, M. M., Chien, Y. H., Gascoigne, N. R. J., and Hedrick, S. M., 1984, A murine T cell receptor gene complex: Isolation, structure and rearrangement, *Immunol. Rev.* **81**:235–258.

DeMars, R., Chang, C. C., and Rudersdorf, R., 1983a, Dissection of the D region of the human major histocompatibility complex by means of induced mutations in a lymphoblastoid cell line, *Hum. Immunol.* **8**:123–139.

DeMars, R., Chang, C. C., Marrari, M., Duquesnoy, R. J., Morren, H., Segall, M., and Bach, F. H., 1983b, Dissociation in expression of MB1/MT1 and DR1 alloantigens in mutants of a lymphoblastoid cell line, *J. Immunol.* **131**:1318.

DeMars, R., Chang, C. C., Shaw, S., Reitnauer, P. J., and Sondel, P. M., 1984, Homozygous deletions that simultaneously eliminate expression of class I and class II antigens of EBV transformed B lymphoblastoid cells, *Hum. Immunol.* **11**:77–97.

De Préval, C., Rabourdin-Combe, C., Gorski, J., and Mach, B., 1984a, Expression of a single HLA-DR antigen on DNA transfected mouse cells: Analysis by a panel of monoclonal antibodies, in: *Human MHC Class II Antigens: Genetics, Structure and Function* (C. M. Steel, ed), pp. 207–221, Wiley, New York.

De Préval, C., Gorski, J., and Mach, B., 1984b, Molecular complexity of the HLA-DR, -DC and -SB genes and genotypic split of HLA-DR serological specificities by DNA typing, in: *Histocompatibility Testing 1984*, (E. D. Albert, M. T. Baur, and W. R. Mayr, eds), pp. 569–572, Springer-Verlag, Berlin.

Early, P., Rogers, J., Davis, M., Calame, K., Bond, M., Wall, R., and Hood, L., 1980, Two mRNAs can be produced from a single immunoglobulin μ gene by alternative RNA processing pathways, *Cell* **20**:313–319.

Edelman, G., Cunningham, B. A., Gall, W. E., Gottlieb, P. D., Rutishauser, U., and Waxdal, M. J., 1969, The covalent structure of an entire γG immunoglobulin molecule, *Proc. Natl. Acad. Sci. USA* **63**:78–85.

Erlich, H., and Stetler, D., 1984, HLA class II DNA polymorphism: Markers for genetic predisposition to insulin-dependent diabetes, *Banbury Report*.

Erlich, H. A., Stetler, D., Saiki, R., Gladstone, P., and Pious, D., 1983a, Mapping of the genes encoding the HLA-DR α chain and the HLA-related antigens to a chromosome 6 deletion using genomic blotting, *Proc. Natl. Acad. Sci. USA* **80**:2300–2304.

Erlich, H., Stetler, D., and Grumet, C., 1983b, Restriction fragment length polymorphism analysis of HLA-typed families using cloned HLA probes, in: *Banbury Report 14: Recombinant DNA Applications to Human Diseases*, pp. 327–334, Cold Spring Laboratory, Cold Spring Harbor, New York.

Ezquerra, A., Bragado, R., Vega, M. A., Strominger, J. L., Woody, J. N., and Lopez de Castro, J. A., 1985, Primary structure of papain-solubilized human histocompatibility antigen HLA-B27, *Biochemistry*, **24**:1733–1741.

Faille, A., Turmel, P., and Charron, D. J., 1985, Differential expression of HLA-DR and

HLA-DC/DS molecules in a patient with hairy cell leukemia: Restoration of HLA-DC/
DS expression by 12-O tetradecanoyl phorbol 13 acetate, 5-azacytidine and sodium
butyrate, *Blood* **64**:33–37.

Fellous, M., Nir, V., Wallach, D., Merlin, G., Rubinstein, M., and Revel, M., 1982, Interferon dependent induction of mRNA for the major histocompatibility antigens in
human fibroblasts and lymphoblastoid cells, *Proc. Natl. Acad. Sci. USA* **79**:3082–3086.

Gladstone, P., Fueresg, L., and Pious, D., 1982, Gene dosage and gene expression in the
HLA region: Evidence from deletion variants, *Proc. Natl. Acad. Sci. USA* **79**:1235–
1239.

Gorski, J., Rollini, P., Long, E. O., and Mach, B., 1984, Molecular organization of the HLA-
SB region of the major histocompatibility complex and evidence for two SB β chain
genes, *Proc. Natl. Acad. Sci. USA* **81**:3934–3938.

Götz, H., Kratzin, H., Thinnes, F. P., Yang, C. Y., Kruse, T., Pauly, E., Kölbel, S., Egert,
G., Wernet, P., and Hilschmann, N. 1983, Primary structure of human class II histocompatibility antigens, *Hoppe-Seyler's Z. Physiol. Chem.* **364**:749–755.

Gustafsson, K., Emmoth, E., Widmark, E., Böhme, J., Peterson, P. A., and Rask, L.,
1984a, Isolation of a cDNA clone coding for an SB β chain, *Nature* **309**:76–78.

Gustafsson, K., Wiman, K., Emmoth, E., Larhammar, D., Böhme, J., Hyldig-Nielsen, J.,
Ronne, H., Peterson, P. A., and Rask, L., 1984b, Mutations and selection in the generation of class II histocompatibility antigen polymorphism, *EMBO J.* **3**:1655–1661.

Hayashida, J., and Miyata, T., 1983, Unusual evolutionary conservation and frequent DNA
segment exchange in class I genes of the major histocompatibility complex, *Proc. Natl.
Acad. Sci. USA* **80**:2671–2675.

Hermann, A., Parham, P., Weissman, S. M., and Engelhard, V., 1983, Recognition by
xenogeneic cytotoxic T lymphocytes of cells expressing HLA-A2 or HLA-B7 after
DNA-mediated gene transfer, *Proc. Natl. Acad. Sci. USA* **80**:5056–5060.

Hood, L., Steinmetz, M., and Goodenow, R., 1982, Genes of the major histocompatibility
complex, *Cell* **28**:685–687.

Hood, L., Steinmetz, M., and Malissen, B., 1983, Genes of the major histocompatibility
complex of the mouse, *Annu. Rev. Immunol.* **1**:529–568.

Inoko, H., Ando, A., Kimura, M., Ogata, S., and Tsuji, K., 1985, Isolation and characterization of the cDNA clones and genomic clones of the HLA class II antigens. *Proceedings of the Twentieth Japan Transplantation Society Symposiun*, Tokai Shuppan,
Tokyo (in press).

Jordan, B. R., Brégégère, F., and Kourilsky, P., 1981, Human HLA gene segment isolated
by hybridization with mouse H-2 cDNA probes, *Nature* **290**:521–523.

Kappes, D. J., Arnot, D., Okada, K., and Strominger, J. L., 1984, Structure and polymorphism of the HLA class II SB light chain genes, *EMBO J.* **3**:2985–2993.

Katovitch-Hurley, C., Shaw, S., Nadler, L., Schlossman, S., and Capra, J. D., 1982, Alpha
and beta chains of SB and DR antigens are structurally distinct, *J. Exp. Med.* **156**:1557–
1562.

Kaufman, J. F., and Strominger, J. L., 1982, HLA-DR light chain has a polymorphic N
terminal region and a conserved immunoglobulin like C terminal region, *Nature*
297:694–697.

Kaufman, J. F., and Strominger, J. L., 1983, The extracellular region of light chains from
human and murine MHC class II antigens consist of two domains, *J. Immunol.* **130**:808–
817.

Kaufman, J. F., Auffray, C., Korman, A. J., Shackelford, D. A., and Strominger, J. L.,
1984a, The class II molecules of the human and murine major histocompatibility complex, *Cell* **36**:1–13.

Kaufman, J. F., Krangel, M. S., and Strominger, J. L., 1984b, Cysteines in the transmembrane region of MHC antigens are fatty acylated via thioester bonds, *J. Biol. Chem.* **259**:7230–7238.

Kavathas, P., Bach, F. H., and DeMars, R., 1980, Gamma-ray-induced loss of expression of HLA and glyoxylase I alleles in lymphoblastoid cells, *Proc. Natl. Acad. Sci. USA* **77**:4251–4255.

Knudsen, P., McClean, J., and Strominger, J. L., 1985, A monoclonal antibody that recognizes the α chain of the HLA-DR antigens, *J. Immunol.* (in press).

Koeffler, H. P., Ranyard, J., Yelton, L., Billing, R., and Bohman, R., 1984, γ-Interferon induces expression of the HLA-D antigens on normal and leukemic human myeloid cells, *Proc. Natl. Acad. Sci. USA* **81**:4080–4084.

Koller, B. H., Sidwell, B., DeMars, R., and Orr, H. T., 1984, Isolation of HLA locus-specific DNA probes from the 3′ untranslated regions, *Proc. Natl. Acad. Sci. USA* **81**:5175–5178.

Korman, A. J., Ploegh, H. L., Kaufman, J. F., Owen, M. J., and Strominger, J. L., 1980, Cell-free synthesis and processing of the heavy and light chains of HLA-DR antigens. *J. Exp. Med.* **152**:65s–82s.

Korman, A. J., Knudsen, P. J., Kaufman, J. F., and Strominger, J. L., 1982a, cDNA clones for the heavy chain of HLA-DR antigens obtained after immunopurification of polysomes by monoclonal antibody, *Proc. Natl. Acad. Sci. USA* **79**:1844–1848.

Korman, A. J., Auffray, C., Schamboeck, A., and Strominger, J. L., 1982b, The amino acid sequence and gene organization of the heavy chain of the HLA-DR antigen: Homology to immunoglobulins, *Proc. Natl. Acad. Sci. USA* **79**:6013–6017.

Korman, A. J., Boss, J. M., Spies, T., Sorrentino, R., Okada, K., and Strominger, J. L., 1985, Genetic complexity and expression of human class II histocompatibility antigens, *Immunol. Rev.* **85**:45–86.

Krangel, M. S., Taketani, S., Biddison, W. E., Strong, D. M., and Strominger, J. L., 1982, Comparative structural analysis of HLA-A2 antigens distinguishable by cytotoxic T lymphocytes: Variants M7 and DR1, *Biochemistry* **21**:6313–6321.

Krangel, M. S., Biddison, W. E., and Strominger, J. L., 1983a, Comparative structural analysis of HLA-A2 antigens distinguishable by cytotoxic T lymphocytes: Variant DK1, evidence for a discrete CTL recognition region, *J. Immunol.* **130**:1856–1862.

Krangel, M. S., Taketani, S., Pious, D., and Strominger, J. L., 1983b, HLA-A2 mutants immunoselected *in vitro*: Definition of residues contributing to an HLA-A2-specific serological determinant, *J. Exp. Med.* **157**:324–336.

Krangel, M., Pious, D., and Strominger, J. L., 1984, Characterization of a B lymphoblastoid cell line mutant which secretes HLA-A2, *J. Immunol.* **132**:2984–2991.

Kratzin, H., Yang, C. Y., Götz, H., Pauly, E., Kölbel, S., Egert, G., Thinnes, F. P., Wernet, P., Altevogt, P., and Hilschmann, N., 1981, Primary structure of human class II histocompatibility antigens, *Hoppe-Seyler's Z. Physiol. Chem.* **363**:1665–1669.

Kratzin, H., Yang, C. Y., Götz, H., Thinnes, F. P., Kruse, T., Egert, G., Pauly, E., Kölbel, S., Wernet, P., and Hilschmann, N., 1983, Heterogeneity of class II histocompatibility antigens isolated from a human lymphoblastoid B cell line homozygous at the HLA loci, *Hum. Immunol.* **8**:65–73.

Kress, M., Cosman, D., Khoury, G., and Jay, G., 1983, Secretion of a transplantation-related antigen, *Cell* **34**:189–196.

Kvist, S., Wiman, K., Claesson, L., Peterson, P. A., and Dobberstein, B., 1982, Membrane insertion and oligomeric assembly of HLA-DR histocompatibility antigens, *Cell* **29**:61–69.

Lalanne, J. L., Transy, C., Guerin, S., Darche, S., Meulien, P., and Kourilsky, P., 1985,

Expression of class I genes in the major histocompatibility complex: Identification of eight distinct mRNAS in DBA/2 mouse liver, *Cell* **41**:469–478.

Lancet, D., Parham, P., and Strominger, J. L., 1979, Heavy chain of HLA-A and HLA-B antigens is conformationally labile: A possible role for β2-microglobulin, *Proc. Natl. Acad. Sci. USA* **76**:3844–3848.

Larhammar, D., Wiman, K., Schenning, L., Claesson, L., Gustafsson, K., Peterson, P. A., and Rask, L., 1981, Evolutionary relationship between HLA-DR antigen β chains, HLA-A,B,C antigen subunits and immunoglobulin chains, *Scand. J. Immunol.* **14**:617–622.

Larhammar, D., Gustafsson, K., Claesson, L., Bill, P., Wiman, K., Schenning, L., Sundelin, J., Widmark, E., Peterson, P. A., and Rask, L., 1982*a*, Alpha chain of HLA-DR transplantation antigen is a member of the same protein superfamily as the immunoglobulins, *Cell* **30**:153–161.

Larhammar, D., Schenning, L., Gustafsson, K., Wiman, K., Claesson, L., Rask, L., and Peterson, P. A., 1982*b*, Complete amino acid sequence of an HLA-DR antigen-like β chain as predicted from the nucleotide sequence: Similarities with immunoglobulins and HLA-A, -B and -C antigens, *Proc. Natl. Acad. Sci. USA* **79**:3687–3691.

Larhammar, D., Hyldig-Nielsen, J. J., Servenius, B., Anderson, G., Rask, L., and Peterson, P. A., 1983, Exon–intron organization and complete nucleotide sequence of a human major histocompatibility antigen DCβ gene, *Proc. Natl. Acad. Sci. USA* **80**:7313–7317.

Larhammar, D., Servenius, B., Rask, L., and Peterson, P. A., 1985, Characterization of an HLA-DR β pseudogene, *Proc. Natl. Acad. Sci. USA,* **82**:1475–1479.

Le Bouteiller, P., Foa, C., Malissen, M., Golstein, P., Galindo, T. R., Mischal, Z., Caillol, D., and Lemonnier, F. A., 1982, Expression of human histocompatibility antigens on the surface of murine cells transformed by cosmid clones containing HLA genes, *Exp. Cell. Res.* **141**:473–478.

Lee, J. S., Trowsdale, J., and Bodmer, W. F., 1980, Synthesis of HLA antigens from membrane-associated messenger RNA, *J. Exp. Med.* **152**:3s–10s.

Lee, J. S., Trowsdale, J., and Bodmer, W. F., 1982*a*, cDNA clones coding for the heavy chain of human HLA-DR antigen, *Proc. Natl. Acad. Sci. USA* **79**:545–549.

Lee, J. S., Trowsdale, J., Travers, P. J., Carey, J., Grosveld, F., Jenkins, J., and Bodmer, W. F., 1982*b*, Sequence of an HLA-DR α chain cDNA clone and intron–exon organization of the corresponding gene, *Nature* **299**:750–752.

Le Gall, I., Marcadet, A., Font, M. P., Auffray, C., Strominger, J. L., Lalouel, J. M., Dausset, J., and Cohen, D., 1985, Exuberant restriction fragment length polymorphism associated with the DQα-chain gene and the DXα-chain gene. *Proc. Natl. Acad. Sci. USA* **82**:5433–5436.

Lemonnier, F. A., Le Bouteiller, P. P., Malissen, B., Golstein, P., Mallisen, M., Mishal, Z., Caillol, D., Jordan, B. R., and Kourilsky, F. M., 1983, Transformation of murine LMTK⁻ cells with purified HLA class I genes, *J. Immunol.* **130**:1432–1438.

Levine, F., Erlich, H. A., Mach, B., and Pious, D., 1985, Transcriptional regulation of HLA class II and invariant chain genes, *J. Immunol.* **134**:637–640.

Lisowska-Grospierre, B., Charron, D. J., De Préval, C., Griscelli, C., and Mach, B., 1985, Defect of gene expression responsible for HLA-DR negative phenotype of lymphocytes from combined immunodeficiency patients, *J. Clin. Invest.* (in press).

Littman, D. R., Thomas, Y., Maddon, P. J., Chess, L., and Axel, R., 1985, The isolation and sequence of the gene encoding T8: A molecule defining functional classes of T lymphocytes, *Cell,* **40**:237–246.

Long, E. O., 1985, In search of a function for the invariant chain associated with Ia antigens, *Surv. Immunol. Res.* **4**:27–34.

Long, E. O., Gross, N., Wake, C. T., Mach, J. P., Carrel, S., Accolla, R., and Mach, B., 1982a, Translation and assembly of HLA-DR antigens in *Xenopus* oocytes injected with mRNA from a human B cell line, *EMBO J.* 1:649–654.

Long, E. O., Wake, C. T., Strubin, M., Gross, N., Accolla, R. S., Carrel, S., and Mach, B., 1982b, Isolation of distinct cDNA clones encoding HLA-DRβ chains by use of an expression assay, *Proc. Natl. Acad. Sci. USA* 79:7465–7469.

Long, E. O., Wake, C. T., Gorski, J., and Mach, B., 1983, Complete sequence of an HLA-DR β chain deduced from a cDNA clone and identification of multiple non-allelic DR β chain genes, *EMBO J.* 2:389–394.

Long, E. O., Gorski, J., and Mach, B., 1984a, Structural relationship of the SB β chain gene to HLA-D region genes and murine I region genes, *Nature* 310:233–235.

Long, E. O., Mach, B., and Accolla, R. S., 1984b, Ia-negative B cell variants reveal a coordinate regulation in the transcription of the HLA class II gene family, *Immunogenetics* 19:349–353.

Lopez de Castro, J. A., Strominger, J. L., Strong, D. M., and Orr, H. T., 1982, Structure of cross reactive human histocompatibility antigens HLA-A28 and HLA-A2: Possible implications for the generation of HLA polymorphism, *Proc. Natl. Acad. Sci. USA* 79:3813–3817.

Lopez de Castro, J. A., Bragado, R., Strong, D. M., and Strominger, J. L., 1983, Primary structure of papain solubilized human histocompatibility antigen HLA-B40 (-Bw60). An outline of alloantigenic determinants, *Biochemistry* 22:3961–3969.

Lopez de Castro, J. A., Bragado, R., Ezquerra, A., and Vega, M. A., 1984, Structural analysis of the polymorphism of HLA class I antigens, in *Histocompatibility Testing 1984* (E. D. Albert, M. T. Baur, W. R. Mayr, eds.), pp. 499–504.

Lopez de Castro, J. A., Barbosa, J. A., Krangel, M. S., Biro, P. A., and Strominger, J. L., 1985, Structural analysis of the functional sites of class I HLA antigens, *Immunol. Rev.* 85:149–168.

Mak, T. W., and Yanagi, V., 1984, Genes encoding the human T cell antigen receptor, *Immunol. Rev.* 81:221–233.

Malissen, B., Peele-Price, M., Goverman, J. M., McMillan, M., White, J., Kappler, J., Marrack, P., Pierres, A., Pierres, M., and Hood, L., 1984, Gene transfer of H-2 class II genes: Antigen presentation by mouse fibroblast and hamster B cell lines, *Cell* 36:319–327.

Malissen, M., Damotte, M., Birnbaum, D., Trucy, J., and Jordan, B. R., 1982a, HLA cosmid clones show complete, widely spaced human class I genes with occasional clusters, *Gene* 20:485–489.

Malissen, M., Malissen, B., and Jordan, B. R., 1982b, Exon/intron organization and complete nucleotide sequence of an HLA gene, *Proc Natl. Acad. Sci. USA* 79:893–897.

Marti, G. E., Kuo, M. C., Shaw, S., Chang, C. C., DeMars, R., Sogn, J. A., Coligan, J. E., and Kindt, T. J., 1983, A novel HLA-D/DR-like antigen specific for human B lymphoid cells, *J. Exp. Med.* 158:1924–1937.

Mathis, D. J., Benoist, C. D., Williams, V. E., Kanter, M. R., and McDevitt, H. O., 1983, The murine Eα immune response gene, *Cell* 32:745–754.

Morton, C. C., Kirsh, I. R., Nance, W. E., Evans, G. A., Korman, A. J., and Strominger, J. L., 1984, Orientation of loci within the human major histocompatibility complex by chromosomal *in situ* hybridization, *Proc. Natl. Acad. Sci. USA* 81:2816–2820.

Mostov, K. E., Friedlander, M., and Blobel, G., 1984, The receptor for transepithelial transport of IgA and IgM contains multiple immunoglobulin-like domains, *Nature* 308:37–43.

N'Guyen, C., Sodoyer, R., Trucy, J., Strachan, T., and Jordan, B. R., 1985, The HLA-

Aw24 gene: Sequence, surroundings and comparison with the HLA-A2 and HLA-A3 genes, *Immunogenetics* 21:479–489.

Novotny, J., and Auffray, C., 1984, A program for prediction of protein secondary structure from nucleotide sequence data: Application to histocompatibility antigens, *Nucleic Acids Res.* 12:243–255.

Okada, K., Boss, J. M., Prentice, H., Spies, T., Mengler, R., Auffray, C., Lillie, J., Grossberger, D., and Strominger, J. L., 1985a, Gene organization of the DC and DX subregions of the human major histocompatibility complex, *Proc. Natl. Acad. Sci. USA* 82:3410–3414.

Okada, K., Prentice, H., Boss, J., Levy, D., Kappes, D., Spies, T., Raghupathy, R., Auffray, C., and Strominger, J. L., 1985b, SB subregion of the human major histocompatibility complex: Gene organization, allelic polymorphism and expression in transformed cells, *EMBO J.* 4:739–748.

Ollo, R., and Rougeon, F., 1983, Gene conversion and polymorphism: Generation of mouse immunoglobulin γ2a chain alleles by differential gene conversion by γ2b chain gene, *Cell* 32:515–523.

Orr, H. T., and DeMars, R., 1983a, Class I-like HLA genes map telomeric to the HLA-A2 locus in human cells, *Nature* 302:534–536.

Orr, H. T., and DeMars, R., 1983b, Mapping of class I DNA sequences within the human major histocompatibility complex, *Immunogenetics* 18:489–502.

Orr, H. T., Lancet, D., Robb, R. J., Lopez de Castro, J. A., and Strominger, J. L., 1979, The heavy chain of human histocompatibility antigen HLA-B7 contains an immunoglobulin-like region, *Nature* 282:266–270.

Orr, H. T., Bach, F. H., Ploegh, H. L., Strominger, J. L., Kavathas, P., and DeMars, R., 1982, Use of HLA loss mutants to analyze the structure of the human major histocompatibility complex, *Nature* 296:454–456.

Owerbach, D., Lernmark, A., Rask, L., Peterson, P. A., Platz, P., and Svejgaard, A., 1983a, Detection of HLA-D/DR-related DNA polymorphism in HLA-D homozygous typing cells, *Proc. Natl. Acad. Sci. USA* 80:3758–3761.

Owerbach, D., Lernmark, A., Platz, P., Ryder, L. P., Rask, L., Peterson, P. A., and Ludvigsson, J., 1983b, HLA-D region β chain DNA endonuclease fragments differ between HLA-DR identical healthy and insulin-dependent diabetic individuals, *Nature* 303:815–817.

Parnes, J. R., and Seidman, J. G., 1982, Structure of wild-type and mutant mouse β2-microglobulin genes, *Cell* 29:661–669.

Pease, L. R., Schulze, D. H., Pfaffenbach, G. M., and Nathenson, S. G., 1983, Spontaneous H-2 mutants provide evidence that a copy mechanism analogous to gene conversion generates polymorphism in the major histocompatibility complex, *Proc. Natl. Acad. Sci USA* 80:242–246.

Pierschbacher, M. D., and Ruoslahti, E., 1984a, Cell attachment activity of fibronectin can be duplicated by small synthetic fragments of the molecules, *Nature* 309:30–33.

Pierschbacher, M. D., and Ruoslahti, E., 1984b, Variants of the cell recognition of fibronectin that retain attachment promoting activity, *Proc. Natl. Acad. Sci. USA* 81:5985–5988.

Pious, D., Martin, S., Gladstone, P., and Soderland, 1980, Linked marker analysis of spontaneous HLA variants of somatic cells, *Somat. Cell Genet.* 6:529–541.

Pious, D., Krangel, M. S., Dixon, L. L., Parham, P., and Strominger, J. L., 1982, HLA antigen structural gene mutants selected with an allospecific monoclonal antibody, *Proc. Natl. Acad. Sci. USA* 79:7832–7836.

Ploegh, H. L., Cannon, L. E., and Strominger, J. L., 1979, Cell-free translation of the mRNAs for the heavy and light chains of HLA-A and HLA-B antigens, *Proc. Natl. Acad. Sci. USA* **76**:2273–2277.

Ploegh, J. L., Orr, H. T., and Strominger, J. L., 1980, Molecular cloning of a human histocompatibility antigen cDNA fragment, *Proc. Natl. Acad. Sci. USA* **77**:6081–6085.

Ploegh, H. L., Orr, H. T., and Strominger, J. L., 1981, Major histocompatibility antigens: The human (HLA-A,-B,-C) and murine (H-2K, H-2D) class I molecules, *Cell* **24**:287–299.

Poljak, R. J., Amzel, L. M., Avey, M. P., Chen, B. L., Phizackerley, R. P., and Saul, F., 1973, Three-dimensional structure of the Fab' fragment of a human immunoglobulin at 2.8Å resolution, *Proc. Natl. Acad. Sci. USA* **75**:3305–3310.

Rabourdin-Combe, C., and Mach, B., 1983, Expression of HLA-DR antigens at the surface of mouse L cells co-transfected with cloned human genes, *Nature* **303**:670–674.

Robinson, M. A., Long, E. O., Johnson, A. H., Hartzman, R. J., Mach, B., and Kindt, T. J., 1984, Recombination within the HLA-D region: Correlation of molecular genotyping with functional data, *J. Exp. Med.* **160**:222–238.

Rosa, F., Berissi, H., Weissenbach, J., Maroteaux, L., Fellous, M., and Revel, M., 1983*a*, The β2-microglobulin mRNA in human Daudi cells has a mutated initiation codon but is still inducible by interferon, *EMBO J.* **2**:239–243.

Rosa, F., Hatat, D., Abadie, A., Wallach, D., Revel, M., and Fellous, M., 1983*b*, Differential regulation of HLA-DR mRNAs and cell surface antigens by interferon, *EMBO J.* **2**:1585–1589.

Roux-Dosseto, M., Auffray, C., Lillie, J. W., Boss, J. M. Cohen, D., De Mars, R., Mawas, C., Seidman, J. G., and Strominger, J. L., 1983*a*, Genetic mapping of a human class II antigen β chain cDNA clone to the SB region of the HLA complex, *Proc. Natl. Acad. Sci. USA* **80**:6036–6040.

Roux-Dosseto, M., Auffray, C., Lillie, J. W., Korman, A. J., and Strominger, J. L., 1983*b*, Homology matrix comparison of human and murine class II antigens, *UCLA Symp. Mol. Cell. Biol.* **8**:481–490.

Saito, H., Maki, R. A., Clayton, L. K., and Tonegawa, S., 1983, Complete primary structures of the Eβ chain and gene of the mouse major histocompatibility complex, *Proc. Natl. Acad. Sci. USA* **80**:5520–5524.

Sanchez-Perez, M., and Shaw, S., 1985, HLA-DP: Current status, in: *Human Class II Histocompatibility Antigens* (S. Ferrone, B. G. Solheim, and E. Moller, eds.), Springer-Verlag, New York, (in press).

Schamboeck, A., Korman, A. J., Kamb, A., and Strominger, J. L., 1983, Organization of the transcriptional unit of a human class II histocompatibility antigen: HLA-DR heavy chain, *Nucleic Acids Res.* **11**:8663–8675.

Schenning, L., Larhammar, D., Bill, P., Wiman, K., Jonsson, A. K., Rask, L., and Peterson, P. A., 1984, Both α and β chains of HLA-DC class II histocompatibility antigens display extensive polymorphism in their amino-terminal domains, *EMBO J.* **3**:447–452.

Servenius, B., Gustafsson, K., Widmark, E., Emmoth, E., Anderson, G., Larhammar, D., Rask, L., and Peterson, P. A., 1985, Molecular map of the human HLA-SB (HLA-DP) region and sequence of an SBα (DPα) pseudogene, *EMBO J.* **3**:3209–3214.

Shackelford, D. A., Kaufman, J. F., Korman, A. J., and Strominger, J. L., 1982, HLA-DR antigens: Structure, separation of subpopulations, gene cloning and function, *Immunol. Rev.* **66**:133–181.

Shackelford, D. A., Eibl, B., and Strominger, J. L., 1983, Structural polymorphism of the DC1 light chain from DR1, DR2 and DRw6 positive cell lines, *Immunogenetics* **18**:625–637.

Sodoyer, R., Damotte, M., Delovitch, T. L., Trucy, J., Jordan, B. R., and Strachan, T.,

1984, Complete nucleotide sequence of a gene encoding a functional human class I histocompatibility antigen (HLA-Cw3), *EMBO J.* **3**:879–885.

Sood, A. K., Pereira, D., and Weissman, S. M., 1981, Isolation and partial nucleotide sequence of a cDNA clone for human histocompatibility antigen HLA-B by use of an oligodeoxynucleotide primer, *Proc. Natl. Acad. Sci. USA* **78**:616–620.

Sorrentino, R., Lillie, J., and Strominger, J. L., 1985, Molcular characterization of MT3 antigens by two-dimensional gel electrophoresis, NH₂-terminal amino acid sequence and Southern blot, *Proc. Natl. Acad. Sci. USA,* **82**:3794–3798.

Spielman, R. S., Lee, J., Bodmer, W. F., Bodmer, J. G., and Trowsdale, J., 1984, Six HLA-D region α chain genes on human chromosome 6: Polymorphisms and associations of DCα-related sequences with DR types, *Proc. Natl. Acad. Sci. USA* **81**:3461–3465.

Spies, T., Sorrentino, R., Boss, J. M., Okada, K., and Strominger, J. L., 1985, Structural organization of the DR subregion of the human major histocompatibility complex, *Proc. Natl. Acad. Sci. USA* **82**:5165–5169.

Steinmetz, M., and Hood, L., 1983, Genes of the major histocompatibility complex in mouse and man, *Science* **222**:727–733.

Stetler, D., Das, H., Nunberg, J. H., Saiki, R., Steng-Dong, R., Mullis, K., Weissman, S., and Erlich, H. A., 1982, Isolation of a cDNA clone for the human HLA-DR antigen α chain by using a synthetic oligonucleotide as a hybridization probe, *Proc. Natl. Acad. Sci. USA* **79**:5966–5970.

Strachan, T., Sodoyer, R., Damotte, M., and Jordan, B. R., 1984, Complete nucleotide sequence of a functional class I HLA gene, HLA A3: Implications for the evolution of HLA genes, *EMBO J.* **3**:887–894.

Strominger, J. L., Engelhard, O. H., Fuks, A., Guild, B. C., Hyafil, P., Kaufman, J. F., Korman, A. J., Kostyk, T. G., Krangel, M. S., Lancet, D., Lopez de Castro, J. A., Mann, D. L., Orr, H. T., Parham, P. R., Parker, K. C., Ploegh, H. L., Pober, J. S., Robb, R. J., and Shackelford, D. A., 1981, Biochemical analysis of products of the MHC, in: *The Role of the Major Histocompatibility Complex in Immunobiology* (M. E. Dorf, ed.), pp. 115–172, Garland Press, New York.

Strubin, M., Mach, B., and Long, E. O., 1984, The complete sequence of the mRNA for the HLA-DR associated invariant chain reveals a polypeptide with an unusual transmembrane polarity, *EMBO J.* **3**:869–872.

Suggs, S., Wallace, R. B., Hirose, T., Kawashima, E. H., and Itakura, K., 1981, Use of synthetic oligonucleotides as hybridization probes: Isolation of cloned cDNA sequences for human β2-microglobulin, *Proc. Natl. Acad. Sci. USA* **78**:6613–6617.

Taketani, S., Krangel, M. S., Spits, H., de Vries, J., and Strominger, J. L., 1984, Structural analysis of an HLA-B7 antigen variant detected by cytotoxic T lymphocytes, *J. Immunol.* **133**:816–821.

Travers, P., Blimdell, T. L., Sternberg, M. J. E., and Bodmer, W. F., 1984, Structural and evolutionary analysis of HLA-D region products, *Nature* **310**:235–238.

Trowsdale, J., Lee, J., Carey, J., Grosveld, F., Bodmer, J., and Bodmer, W., 1983, Sequences related to HLA-DRα chain on human chromosome 6: Restriction enzyme polymorphism detected with DCα chain probes, *Proc. Natl. Acad. Sci. USA* **80**:1972–1976.

Trowsdale, J., Lee, J., Kelly, A., Carey, J., Jenkins, J., Travers, P., and Bodmer, W. F., 1984*a*, Isolation and sequencing of a cDNA clone for a human HLA-ABC antigen, *Mo!. Biol. Med.* **2**:53–61.

Trowsdale, J., Kelly, A., Lee, J., Carson, S., Austin, P., and Travers, P., 1984*b*, Linkage map of two HLA-SBα and two HLA-SBβ-related genes: An intron in one of the SBβ genes contains a processed pseudogene, *Cell* **38**:241–249.

Van de Rijn, M., Bernabeu, C., Royer-Pokora, B., Weiss, J., Seidman, J. G., de Vries, J., Spits, H., and Terhorst, C., 1984, Recognition of HLA-A2 by cytotoxic T lymphocytes after DNA transfer into human and murine cells, *Science* **226**:1083–1085.

Vega, M. A., Bragado, R., Ezquerra, A., and Lopez de Castro, J. A., 1984, Variability and conformation of HLA class I antigens: A predictive approach to the spatial arrangement of polymorphic regions, *Biochemistry* **23**:823–831.

Wake, C. T., Long, E. O., Strubin, M., Gross, N., Accolla, R., Carrel, S., and Mach, B., 1982a, Isolation of cDNA clones encoding HLA-DR α chains, *Proc. Natl. Acad. Sci. USA* **79**:6979–6983.

Wake, C. T., Long, E. O., and Mach, B., 1982b, Allelic polymorphism and complexity of the genes for HLA-DR β chains: Direct analysis by DNA–DNA hybridization, *Nature* **300**:372–374.

Widera, G., and Flavell, R. A., 1984, The nucleotide sequence of the murine I-Eβ[b] immune response genes: Evidence for gene conversion events in class II genes of the major histocompatibility complex, *EMBO J.* **3**:1221–1225.

Williams, A. F., and Gagnon, J., 1981, Neuronal cell Thy-1 glycoprotein: Homology with immunoglobulin, *Science* **216**:696–703.

Wiman, K., Larhammar, D., Claesson, L., Gustafsson, K., Schenning, L., Bill, P., Böhme, J., Denaro, M., Dobberstein, B., Hammerling, U., Kvist, S., Servenius, B., Sundelin, J., Peterson, P. A., and Rask, L., 1982a, Isolation and identification of a cDNA clone corresponding to an HLA-DR antigen β chain, *Proc. Natl. Acad. Sci. USA* **79**:1703–1707.

Wiman, K., Claesson, L., Rask, L., Tragardh, L., and Peterson, P. A., 1982b, Purification and partial amino acid sequence of papain solubilized class II transplantation antigens, *Biochemistry* **21**:5351–5358.

Yamada, K. M., and Kennedy, D. W., 1984, Dualistic nature of adhesive protein function: Fibronectin and its biologically active peptides can auto-inhibit fibronectin function, *J. Cell. Biol.* **99**:29–36.

Yamada, K. M., and Kennedy, D. W., 1985, Amino acid sequence specificities of an adhesive recognition signal, *J. Cell. Biochem.* (in press).

Yang, C. Y., Kratzin, H., Götz, H., Thinnes, F. P., Kruse, T., Egert, G., Pauly, E., Kölbel, S., Wernet, P., and Hilschmann, N., 1982, Primary structure of human class II histocompatibility antigens, *Hoppe-Seyler's Z. Physiol. Chem.* **363**:671–676.

Yoshie, O., Schmidt, H., Lengyel, P., Reddy, E. S. P., Morgan, W. R., and Weissman, S. M., 1984, Transcripts of human HLA gene fragments lacking the 5'-terminal region in transfected mouse cells, *Proc. Natl. Acad. Sci. USA* **81**:649–653.

Chapter 5

Genetics of Human Alcohol and Aldehyde Dehydrogenases

Moyra Smith

Department of Pediatrics
University of California at Irvine
Irvine, California 92717

INTRODUCTION

During the past 5 years considerable progress has been made in the elucidation of the biochemical genetics of human alcohol dehydrogenases (ADH) and human aldehyde dehydrogenases (ALDH). In particular, progress has been made in determining the number of gene loci coding for these enzymes and the tissue distribution of the enzymes. In addition, a number of allelic variants of specific forms of alcohol and aldehyde dehydrogenases have been described. Studies have been done on different population groups to determine the frequencies of some of these variants. The relationship of the presence of variant forms of alcohol and aldehyde dehydrogenases to altered alcohol tolerance has been investigated. Efficient procedures for purifying alcohol and aldehyde dehydrogenases have been defined. As a result, detailed studies on the kinetics of separated isozymes and amino acid sequence determinations have been possible. To date, complete amino acid sequence data have been obtained for three ADH isozymes and one ALDH isozyme, while partial amino acid sequence data have been published on a second ALDH isozyme. Antibodies to specific forms of aldehyde dehydrogenase have been used to determine the nature of the genetic variation in mitochondrial ALDH. Polyclonal and monoclonal antibodies have been used to determine the cellular distribution of the different forms of ADH and to examine the interrelationship of the different clases of ADH isozymes. Of particular interest are the recent derivations of DNA probes for the analysis of ADH and ALDH genes. In the case of class I ADH these probes have been used to examine DNA polymorphism and to begin to analyze factors that may be involved in the control of gene expression. Progress has been made in determining the chromosomal assignment of four of the ADH gene loci and three of the ALDH gene loci.

ALCOHOL DEHYDROGENASES

Definition

Alcohol dehydrogenases (EC 1.1.1.1) are enzymes that are capable of oxidizing a variety of primary, secondary, and tertiary aliphatic alcohols and a limited number of cyclic alcohols, in the presence of NAD, to generate the corresponding aldehydes.

Nomenclature of Human ADH Loci

At least five different gene loci code for human ADH. Studies by Smith et al. (1971, 1972, 1973a,b) defined three gene loci coding for three different ADH subunits, termed α coded by the ADH1 locus, β coded by the ADH2 locus, and γ, coded by the ADH3 locus. These subunits give rise to a number of different ADH isozymes, resulting from the dimerization of like and unlike subunits. Specific homodimeric isozymes (e.g., αα or ββ) exhibited similar but nonidentical properties. A different form of ADH, termed π ADH, was described by Li and Magnes (1975). Detailed studies on the properties of purified π ADH have been carried out by Bosron and coworkers (1980). This form of ADH differs significantly in its properties from the products of the three previously described ADH loci and must therefore be classified as the product of a fourth ADH locus.

Through the use of the higher molecular weight alcohols pentanol and octanol, Pares and Vallee (1981) demonstrated the occurrence in human liver of an alcohol dehydrogenase that migrates to the anode and therefore differs significantly in charge from the products of the four previously described ADH loci. The ADH isozymes with anodal mobility are termed χ ADH isozymes and are the product of a fifth ADH locus.

χ ADH isozymes differ significantly in their kinetic properties from the other forms of ADH.

Analysis of peptide profiles of purified ADH isozymes by Strydom and Vallee (1982) revealed that the three class I ADH subunits α, β, and γ had closely similar peptide profiles. However, the peptide profiles of the π and χ ADH subunits differed from each other and from the profiles of α, β, and γ. Based on the differences in homology, these authors proposed that α-, β-, and γ-containing isozymes coded by the *ADH1*, *ADH2*, and *ADH3* loci be referred to as class I ADH, while π ADH, coded by the *ADH4* locus, be referred to as class II ADH, and χ ADH isozymes, coded by the *ADH5* locus, be referred to as class III ADH.

It seems likely that as detailed studies are carried out with a broader range of alcohols and with different tissues, evidence will be obtained for the existence of additional structural gene loci coding for alcohol dehydrogenases. It seems possible, for example, that a human analogue of the recently defined rat retina-specific ADH (Julia *et al.*, 1983) will be found.

Tissue Distribution of ADH Isozymes

Class III ADH (χ ADH) is the only ADH apparently constitutively expressed, since it has been detected in all tissues examined and in white blood cells (Adinolfi *et al.*, 1984). Class I and class II ADH are primarily liver-specific isozymes; however, they are expressed in other tissues, such as kidney, gastrointestinal tract, and lung to a lesser extent. Very small amounts of class I ADH isozymes (primarily ββ) may be detected in skin cells, cultured fibroblasts, and hair roots (Goedde *et al.*, 1979b). Studies on the tissue distribution of class I ADH isozymes during different stages of development were carried out by Smith *et al.* (1971, 1972). The *ADH1* gene product, αα, is the only class I ADH isozyme detectable in fetal liver during the first trimester. Subsequently, the *ADH2* isozyme, ββ, is expressed; following birth, the *ADH3* isozyme, γγ, is detectable in liver. It is of interest to note that in nine out of 12 hepatomas examined, the α-containing ADH isozymes predominated or were the only ADH isozymes present (Fig. 1). The *ADH2* gene product, β, is the only ADH isozyme present in lung throughout life. In the upper gastrointestinal tract the *ADH3* locus is the only locus active throughout life. Studies on class II ADH (π) have concentrated primarily on liver. There is, however, evidence that isozymes with similar properties are present in other tissues, including gastrointestinal tract, kidney, and lung (Smith, 1972). To date

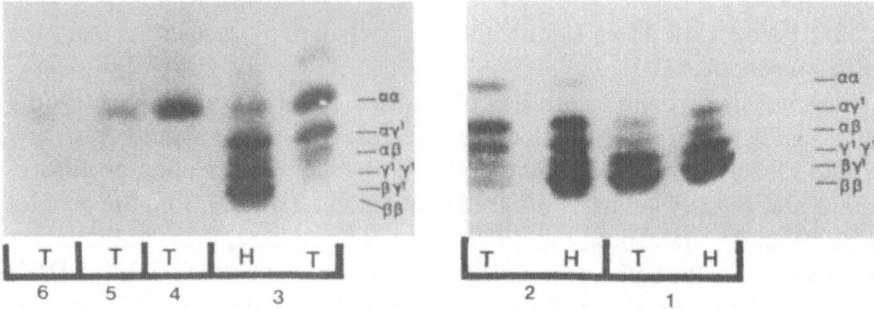

Fig. 1. ADH isozymes present in (H) host liver tissue and in (T) hepatoma tumor tissue. Tissue extracts were electrophoresed in starch gels at pH 7.7 in the presence of NAD. Note that in individual 1, a similar distribution of ADH isozymes is seen in host and tumor tissues. In cases 2 and 3, α-containing ADH isozymes predominate in the tumors. Lanes 4–6 represent ADH in tumor tissue obtained from three different adults. Note that the only ADH isozyme present is αα.

no evidence has been presented to suggest that π ADH is differentially expressed during development. The relative electrophoretic mobilities of the three classes of ADH isozymes are shown below, in Fig. 3.

Genetic Variation in ADH

Enzyme electrophoretic studies and enzyme kinetic studies have led to the identification of genetic variants at the *ADH2* and the *ADH3* gene loci.

Genetic Variation at the *ADH2* (β ADH) Gene Locus

ADH-2 Allele (β₂ Subunit). Von Wartburg and Schurch (1968), in carrying out studies on the Swiss population, discovered an atypical form of liver ADH that differed in its pH rate profile, substrate specificity, and sensitivity to metal-binding agents. These investigators defined a screening procedure to differentiate the atypical form of liver ADH from the usual form of ADH. This procedure involved assay of ADH activity at pH 8.8 and 11.0. In extracts containing the atypical ADH enzyme, the activity at pH 11 is approximately half that at pH 8.8, while in extracts containing the usual ADH, the activity at pH 11 is approximately twice that at pH 8.8.

Assays of ADH activity in 598 livers from the English population (Smith *et al.*, 1971, 1972) revealed that the atypical ADH phenotype occurred in 36 individuals. Smith *et al.* (1971, 1972) demonstrated that the atypical ADH differed from the usual ADH in its electrophoretic mobility. Studies of electrophoretic mobility and properties of ADH with the atypical pH-ratio phenotype present in liver and in lung tissue led to the conclusion that atypical ADH is due to a variant allele at the *ADH2* locus. The variant allele *ADH2-2* coded for a subunit β_2, which, when present in heterodimeric or homodimeric form, altered the electrophoretic mobility and kinetic properties of the ADH isozyme. Due to the low frequency of the atypical allele in the population described by Smith *et al.* (1972), most of the individuals in that population who displayed the atypical pH-ratio phenotype represented heterozygotes; i.e., their genotype was *ADH2* 2-1. Subsequent studies by von Wartburg and co-workers confirmed that the atypical ADH phenotype was due to a variant allele at the *ADH2* locus. The atypical allele first identified in the Swiss population is referred to as β_2 Berne (Bühler *et al.*, 1984a).

In certain Oriental populations, notably the Japanese (Fukui *et al.*, 1972; Stamatoyannopolous *et al.*, 1975; Harada *et al.*, 1978) and the Chinese (Teng *et al.*, 1979), the atypical-pH phenotype occurs in 85–90% of individuals. Studies on the atypical allele have also been carried out in Oriental individuals living in Hawaii. The atypical allele in these populations has been variously referred to as β_2Oriental or β_2Honolulu.

Recently amino acid sequence determinations have been carried out on the β_1 and β_2 subunits isolated from Swiss individuals (β_2Berne) and on β_2 subunits isolated from Oriental individuals (Buhler *et al.* 1984b; Jörnvall *et al.*, 1984). The β_2 subunit from both populations was found to be identical and to differ from the β_1 subunit in a single amino acid at position 47. The β_1 subunit has an arginine residue at this position, while the β_2 subunit has a histidine residue. This substitution can be accounted for by a single base change:

$$
\begin{array}{cc}
\text{ARG} & \text{HIS} \\
\text{CGU} & \text{CAU} \\
\text{or} & \text{or} \\
\text{CGC} & \text{CAC}
\end{array}
$$

Jörnvall *et al.* (1984) determined that the mutational change in the β_2 subunit occurs at a position that binds the pyrophosphate group of the NAD coenzyme. The authors relate this fact to the observed differences in the $\beta_2\beta_2$ and $\beta_1\beta_1$ isozymes in pH optimum and turnover number.

Indianapolis Allele (β_{Ind} Subunit). Bosron *et al.* (1979) identified a variant form of β_2 referred to as Indianapolis (β_{Ind}). Isozymes containing the β_{Ind} subunit in heterodimeric or homodimeric form have a greater cathodal mobility than the isozymes composed of β_1 subunits. Bosron *et al.* (1979a) assayed ADH activity over a broad pH range and demonstrated that specimens containing β_{Ind} isozymes showed two different pH optima for ethanol oxidation: one (higher) pH optimum at 10 and another (lower) pH optimum at 7.0. In their studies livers containing only β_1 isozymes demonstrated pH optima at 10.0–10.5, while livers of the atypical pH-ratio phenotype displayed a pH optimum at 8.5.

Subsequent studies by Bosron *et al.* (1980) on purified isozymes revealed that the β_{Ind}-containing isozymes have an altered pH optimum and an altered K_m for ethanol:

	pH optimum	K_m, mM
$\beta_1\beta_1$	10.5	1.8
$\beta_2\beta_2$	8.5	3.1
β_{Ind} homodimers and β_{Ind} heterodimers	7.0	56–74

β_{Bahai} Variant   Azevedo *et al.* (1975) examined ADH isozymes in individuals of mixed ancestry in Brazil and reported the occurrence of a β *ADH2* allele that gave rise to isozymes with greater cathodal mobility than the β_1-containing isozymes but differed from the atypical β_2-containing isozymes. It seems possible that β_{Ind} and β_{Bahai} are products of the same variant allele, which may have originated in certain African populations (see below). This variant form of β has not been encountered in European populations (Agarwal *et al.*, 1981).

Allelic Variation at the *ADH3* Locus

From electrophoretic studies on stomach and intestinal tissue from fetuses and adults and on fetal kidney tissue, where *ADH3* isozymes represent the main form of ADH, and from studies on adult livers, Smith *et al.* (1972, 1973a) determined that common genetic variation occurs at the *ADH3* locus. This variation results in the occurrence of isozymes differing in their electrophoretic mobility on starch gels containing NAD. The *ADH3*-1 allele gives rise to the γ_1 subunit, and the *ADH3*-2 allele gives rise to the γ_2 subunit. The $\gamma_1\gamma_1$ isozyme has a slower electrophoretic mobility than the $\gamma_2\gamma_2$ isozyme. Individuals heterozygous at the *ADH3* locus show a three-banded ADH pattern on electrophoresis of stomach tissues. Adinolfi and Hopkinson (1979) demonstrated that the $\gamma_1 \gamma_1$ and the $\gamma_2 \gamma_2$ isozymes differ significantly in their affinity for NAD. The $\gamma_2\gamma_2$ isozyme is significantly retarded in its mobility on starch gel when NAD is added. Further evidence of differences between $\gamma_1\gamma_1$ and $\gamma_2\gamma_2$ isozymes in coenzyme binding properties was obtained in studies on the affinity of these enzymes for Blue Sepharose (Sepharose Cibacron blud Pharmacia). Adinolfi *et al.* (1978) demonstrated that the $\gamma_2\gamma_2$ isozyme is not bound by this resin, while the $\gamma_1\gamma_1$ isozyme binds readily to Blue Sepharose and is only eluted with 5 mM NAD.

Evidence for Variant Forms of *ADH*3 with Decreased Activity. In examination of *ADH*3 isozyme patterns in kidney and intestinal samples of fetuses and in stomach samples of adults who were *ADH*3 2-1 heterozygotes, Smith (1972) noted that three different types of patterns occurred. In 76 out of 239 individuals (31%) the distribution of activity was as expected, namely $\gamma_1\gamma_1:\gamma_1\gamma_2:\gamma_2\gamma_2::1:2:1$ (Fig. 2a). In 52 out of 139 individuals (21%), the $\gamma_2\gamma_2$ isozyme was relatively more intense than the $\gamma_1\gamma_1$ isozyme and equal in intensity to the $\gamma_1\gamma_2$ isozyme. In 121 out of 239 individuals (45%) the $\gamma_2\gamma_2$ isozyme was relatively weak, while the $\gamma_1\gamma_2$ and $\gamma_1\gamma_1$ isozymes were equally intense (Fig. 2b). In a specific individual similar patterns of intensity of the *ADH*3 isozymes were noted when two different tissues were examined (stomach and kidney) from one fetus.

These findings imply that additional allelic variation may occur within the *ADH*3-1 and the *ADH*3-2 alelles, giving rise to variants with quantitatively altered activity. It is of interest to note that a similar variation has been described in *Drosophila*. Certain strains of *Drosophila* have a fast electrophoretic form of ADH, while other strains have a slow form. In addition, quantitative variation has been observed (Schwartz *et al.*, 1979). Maroni and Aulberg (1983) investigated the genetic mechanism responsible for these quantitative alterations. In the case of strains having the fast electrophoretic form, differences in activity levels were found to be due to modifier genes outside the structural ADH gene. In the case of strains having the slow electrophoretic form of ADH, activity variation was due in certain instances to changes within the structural gene that led to alterations in the primary structure and stability of the protein. Other low-activity slow variants were found to contain lower amounts of ADH mRNA, implying either differences in the rates of gene transcription or differences in rates of mRNA processing or degradation. Of particular

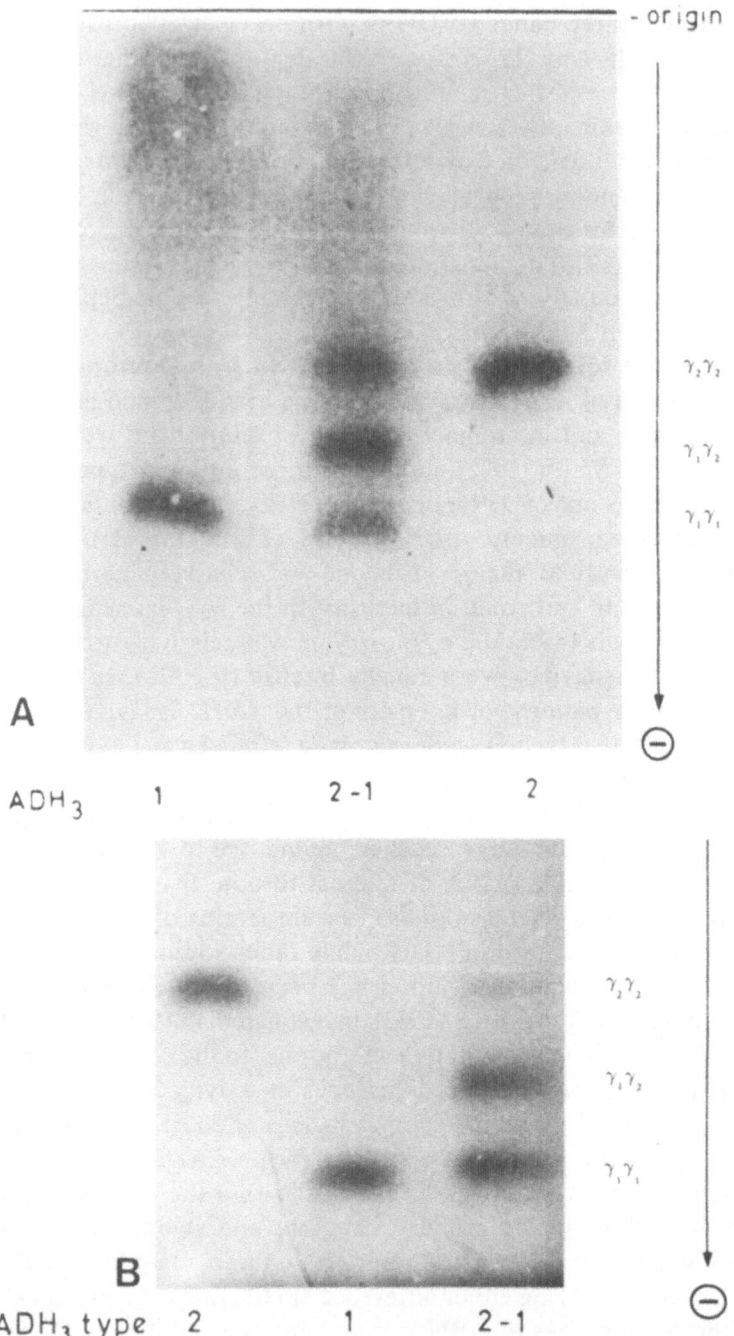

interest was the fact that one strain with slow ADH had low activity in adults and even lower activity in larvae. Maroni and Aulberg (1983) demonstrated the presence of a 5-kb insert in the 5' region of the ADH gene in this strain.

ADH1 Locus

No electrophoretic variants of *ADH*1 have been described. In the study of Smith *et al.* (1971, 1972), ADH electrophoretic studies were carried out on livers from 261 fetuses. Since αα is the predominant ADH in fetal liver, it should have been possible to detect alterations in electrophoretic mobility, but no such alterations were observed. It is possible that quantitative variation in the amount of ADH activity or kinetic differences in the αα isozymes would not have been detected in this study.

In examining electrophoretic patterns of ADH in adult livers one frequently notes that in certain individuals the αα isozyme is absent or very weak (M. Smith, unpublished observation). This finding may suggest that quantitative variations in activity occur at the *ADH*1 locus. However, since the αα ADH isozyme is relatively much less stable than the *ADH*3 gene products or the *ADH*2 gene products, it is possible that storage changes may be responsible for these quantitative variations. In a study on ADH activity in liver biopsies from alcoholic patients with liver cirrhosis, Ricciardi *et al.* (1983) noted that the αα ADH isozyme was frequently weak or absent.

Allelic variation has thus far not been documented in the class II (π) ADH genes or the class III (χ) ADH genes.

Population Frequencies of Class I ADH Allelic Variants

Frequencies of the *ADH*2-1 and the *ADH*2-2 Alleles

In studies on ADH activity in livers from 598 adults, Smith *et al.* (1972) found the atypical pH-ratio phenotype in 36 individuals (6%). Studies on the German population by Harada *et al.* (1980*a*) indicated that the

←——————————————————————————————————

Fig. 2.   The different *ADH*3 isozyme phenotypes present in samples of fetal kidney. Note the differences in two individuals with the *ADH*3 2-1 isozyme phenotype in the distribution of activity in the $\gamma_1\gamma_1$, $\gamma_1\,\gamma_2$, and $\gamma_2\gamma_2$ isozymes.

frequency of the atypical pH-ratio phenotype might be 20%. Studies on a Japanese population by Harada *et al* (1978) and on a Chinese population by Teng *et al.* (1979) demonstrated that the frequency of the atypical phenotype is 90%.

It is clear that the atypical pH-ratio phenotype is observed in individuals heterozygous or homozygous for the *ADH*2-2 allele (β_2). On starch gel electrophoresis it is difficult to distinguish the *ADH*2 2-2 from the *ADH*2 2-1 isozyme phenotype. Yin *et al.* (1984) described an agarose isoelectric focusing system that allows them to distinguish two groups among individuals with the atypical pH-ratio phenotype, namely *ADH*2 2-1 individuals and *ADH*2 2-2 individuals. Yin *et al.* (1984) also succeeded in separating the different *ADH*2 isozymes. The isolated $\beta_1\beta_1$ isozyme was found to have a pH ratio of 2.4, while the pH ratio of the $\beta_1\beta_2$ isozyme was 0.345 and that of the $\beta_2\beta_2$ isozyme was 0.3.

The atypical pH-ratio phenotype is apparently less common in blacks than in Caucasians. Bosron *et al.* (1983) described this phenotype in one of 17 American blacks, and Azevedo *et al.* (1975), studying a Brazilian population of mixed Indian, African, and European ancestry, noted that the frequency of the atypical phenotype was 2.8%.

In studies on individuals originating from the Indian subcontinent, Teng *et al.* (1979) did not detect individuals with the atypical *p*H-ratio phenotype.

Bosron *et al.* (1983*b*) determined that the frequency of the $ADH2_{Ind}$ allele is 0.16 in the American black population. Agarwal *et al.* were unable to detect individuals with the $ADH2_{Ind}$ allele in their studies on a European population.

Frequency of the *ADH*3 Alleles

In studies on the English population, Smith *et al.* (1972) found the frequency of the *ADH*3-1 allele to be 0.6 and the frequency of the *ADH*3-2 allele to be 0.4. In the Chinese and Japanese populations the frequency of the *ADH*3-1 allele is 0.91 and the frequency of the *ADH*3-2 allele is 0.09 (Teng *et al.*, 1979; Harada *et al.* 1980*a*).

It is of interest to note that in Caucasians with the atypical form of ADH (*ADH*2-2 allele), the *ADH*3-1 allele occurs with higher frequency than expected (Smith, 1972). This observation is based on studies in which the *ADH*3 isozyme phenotype was determined in tissues other than liver, so that the change in frequency is not due to inadequate typing because of the complexity of liver ADH isozyme patterns in atypical livers.

The observed and expected frequencies of the three *ADH*3 genotypes in stomach and intestinal samples from 33 individuals with liver ADH of the atypical pH-ratio phenotype are as follows:

	*ADH*3 1-1	*ADH*3 2-1	*ADH*3 2-2
Observed numbers	22	9	2
Expected numbers	12	16	5

Expected numbers were derived assuming Hardy–Weinberg equilibrium in the population and gene frequencies for *ADH*3-1 of 0.6 and for *ADH*3-2 of 0.4. One possible explanation for these discrepancies between the observed and the expected frequencies of the *ADH*3 alleles in individuals with the *ADH*2-2 allele is that linkage disequilibrium exists between the *ADH*2 and *ADH*3 alleles because the *ADH*2-2 allele was relatively recently introduced into the European population by a founder with the *ADH*3-1 genotype and that equilibrium has not yet been reached within the population. In addition, it is possible that equilibrium is being reached relatively slowly because the *ADH*2 and the *ADH*3 genes are relatively closely linked.

Studies on a mixed population by Azevedo *et al* (1975) and studies on an American black population by Bosron *et al* (1983*b*), indicate the *ADH*3-2 allele is relatively infrequent in individuals of African ancestry. The studies of Bosron *et al*. (1983*a*) indicate that in the black American population 51% of individuals are of the *ADH*3 1-1 genotype, while in the white American population the *ADH*3 1-1 genotype occurs in 21% of individuals.

In a preliminary study on the Amerindian population, Rex *et al*. (1985) examined 14 livers from a population of Indians living in northern New Mexico. Six livers were *ADH*3 2-2 (42%), four livers were *ADH*3 2-1 (28%), and two livers were *ADH*3 1-1 (14%). It will be of interest to determine whether this high frequency of the *ADH*3-2 allele continues to be observed when larger numbers of samples from the Amerindian population are examined.

Purification of Human ADH

Earlier studies on the purification of ADH exploited the fact that, in contrast to most proteins, class I ADH isozymes are positively charged

TABLE I. Order of Elution of Class
I ADH Isozymes from CM-Cellulose

Liver genotype	Elution order
ADH3 2-2, ADH2 1-1	$\gamma_2\gamma_2$
	$\alpha\gamma_2$
	$\beta_1\gamma_2$
	$\alpha\alpha$
	$\alpha\beta_1$
	$\beta_1\beta_1$
ADH3 1-1, ADH2 1-1	$\alpha\alpha$
	$\alpha\gamma_1$
	$\gamma_1\gamma_1$
	$\alpha\beta_1$, $\beta_1\gamma_1$
	$\beta_1\beta_1$

under most pH conditions. They therefore bind to the cationic exchange resin CM-cellulose and may be eluted from this resin by increasing the salt concentrations of buffers. In addition to separating ADH from other proteins, CM-cellulose is useful in separating the different ADH isozymes from each other (Blair and Vallee 1966; Smith *et al.*, 1973*a*). The homodimeric $\beta\beta$ isozymes have the greatest affinity for CM-cellulose and are therefore eluted last, at the highest salt concentration. In livers of the usual pH-ratio phenotype, the 1–1 isozyme is eluted last, while in livers of the atypical pH-ratio phenotype, the 2–2 isozyme is eluted last (Table I).

Subsequent studies have utilized variatious forms of affinity chromatography for purification of ADH. In some instances affinity of ADH for the solid matrix was based on the coenzyme binding properties of ADH; e.g., affinity chromatography of ADH on Blue Sepharose or on AMP Sepharose (Adinolfi and Hopkinson, 1978, 1979). In other cases affinity resins have been produced that incorporate ADH inhibitors. Class I ADH isozymes are specifically inhibited by pyrazole and 4-methylpyrazole. Lange and Vallee (1976) synthesized a derivative of 4-methylpyrazole which could be used to produce an affinity resin, 4(3-*N*-6 aminocaproylaminopropyl)pyrazole–Sepharose 4B, referred to as Capp-Gapp Sepharose. Class I ADH isozymes have a high affinity for this resin. Class II (π) and class III (χ) ADH are relatively uninhibited by pyrazole and have a low affinity for Capp-Gapp Sepharose. This form of affinity chromatography may therefore be used to separate the different classes of ADH isozymes.

One of the problems encountered in purifying certain forms of ADH is that certain of the isozymes are particularly labile. This is particularly true for the π ADH isozyme and the αα ADH isozyme. Stability can be increased by addition of NAD to buffer (Smith *et al.*, 1973*a,b*) or by the addition of ethanol (Bosron *et al.*, 1979).

Class III ADH isozymes are negatively charged under most *p*H conditions (Pares and Vallee, 1981). These isozymes are therefore bound by the anionic exchange resin DEAE-cellulose. Class III isozymes eluted from DEAE have been further purified by affinity chromatography on AMP Sepharose with subsequent elution with an NADH gradient (Wagner *et al.*, 1983).

Using the procedures described above, it has been possible to purify ADH isozymes. Analysis of the properties of individual isozymes has been facilitated (Vallee and Bazzone, 1983; Wagner *et al.*, 1983; Bosron *et al.*, 1983*a*). In addition, peptide mapping has been carried out (Strydom and Vallee, 1982). Amino acid sequence determinations have been obtained on β_1, β_2, and γ_1 ADH subunits (Bühler *et al.*, 1984*b*; Hempel *et al.*, 1984*b*; Jornvall *et al.*, 1984).

Kinetic Differences between ADH Isozymes

Earlier qualitative studies on the staining reactions of electrophoretically separated class I ADH isozymes (Smith *et al.*, 1973*a*) demonstrated the isozymes containing the γ ADH subunit, coded by the *ADH3* locus, differed from the other ADH isozymes in their increased activity with longer primary chain alcohols; e.g., butanol and amyl alcohol. The αα isozyme, coded by the *ADH1* locus, differed from the other class I ADH isozymes in that it showed greater activity with certain unsaturated alcohols (e.g., allyl alcohol) and certain cyclic alcohols (e.g., cyclohexanol). Recent qualitative studies demonstrate that the αα ADH isozyme, the π ADH isozyme, and the χ ADH isozyme are relatively much more active than the other ADH isozymes with the unsaturated cyclic alcohol cinnamyl alcohol.

Quantitative studies on the activity of separated ADH isozymes by Bosron *et al.* (1983*a*) revealed large differences between the isozymes in their kinetic constants for ethanol oxidation, as shown below:

Isozyme	K_m Ethanol
π	34
$\alpha\alpha$	4.2
$\gamma_1\gamma_1$	1.0
$\gamma_2\gamma_2$	0.6
$\beta_1\beta_1$	0.048
$\beta_{Ind}\beta_{Ind}$	64

Measurements by Wagner *et al.* (1983) of the activity of separated purified homo- and heterodimeric class I ADH isozymes toward a number of different substrates demonstrated that the activity of a particular heterodimer was not the mean of that observed with two homodimers.

Class I and class III ADH isozymes have been shown to be active with certain hydroxy-fatty acids, such as 16-hydroxyhexadecanoic acid and 16-hydroxydodecanoic acid (Wager *et al.* 1983). The K_m values toward these substrates were found to be 100- to 1000-fold lower than those for ethanol.

Generally the class III ADH isozyme χ has been shown to differ markedly from the other ADH isozymes in its kinetic properties. Pares and Vallee (1981) determined that short-chain (2–4 carbons) primary alcohols failed to saturate this enzyme at concentrations of 1 M, so that K_m values could not be determined. The χ isozyme has a K_m of 17 mM for hexanol and 0.8 mM for octanol. Wagner *et al.* (1983) determined that certain class I ADH isozymes had K_m values for octanol between 5 and 17 M (0.017 mM).

Determinations of the Amino Acid Sequences of ADH Isozymes

Complete amino acid sequences have been determined for the $\beta_1\beta_1$ ADH isozyme (Hempel *et al.*, 1984b), for the $\beta_2\beta_2$ isozyme from both Oriental and Swiss populations (Jornvall *et al.*, 1984; Bühler *et al.*, 1984a), and for the $\gamma_1\gamma_1$ isozyme (Buhler *et al.*, 1984b).

The polypeptide chains of the class I ADH isozymes are apparently 374 amino acids in length. In the references on amino acid sequence just cited, the length of the ADH polypeptide chain length is given as 373. This is due to the fact that two like amino acids occur in consecutive positions around position 128 and amino acid sequence analysis did not reveal this (H. Jornvall, personal communication, 1985). As described above, the β_1 and the β_2 subunits differ in a single amino acid residue at position 47. In β_1 an arginine residue is present in this position, while in β_2 a histidine residue is present. It is of interest to note that the yeast constitutive ADH also has a histidine residue present at this position (Jornvall *et al.*, 1984). The pH optimum for both the yeast constitutive ADH and the $\beta_2\beta_2$ human ADH is 8.5. Jornvall *et al.* (1984) point out that the occurrence of histidine at this position significantly alters the coenzyme interaction and the turnover number in both the yeast constitutive ADH and in the human $\beta_2\beta_2$ isozyme.

The β_1 subunit differs from the γ_1 subunit at 21 positions (Bühler *et al.*, 1984c). Of interest is the finding that 16 of the 21 differences between β_1 and γ_1 occur in the substrate-binding domain and five of the differences occur in the coenzyme-binding domain. One difference between β_1 and γ_1 occurs close to the position of the catalytic zinc atom. At position 48 serine occurs in the γ_1 subunit and in the horse E ADH, while threonine occurs in the β_1 isozyme. Differences also occur in residue 318, which lines the active site pocket: isoleucine occurs at this position in γ_1 and in the horse E ADH, while valine occurs in β_1 ADH. Bühler and coauthors postulate that these differences may account for the observed differences between $\beta_1\beta_1$ and $\gamma_1\gamma_1$ in substrate activities. Differences also occur in the amino acids present in the coenzyme binding region and it is postulated that these may account for the observed differences in the affinity of $\beta_1\beta_1$ and $\gamma_1\gamma_1$ isozymes for NAD and NADH.

Studies on the Immunologic Properties of ADH Isozymes

There is evidence that the antigenic properties of ADH isozymes differ considerably depending on whether antibodies are raised in rabbits or in mice. Furthermore, marked differences are noted in the affinities of polyclonal and monoclonal antibodies.

In the study of Adinolfi *et al.* (1978), immune sera were raised in rabbits against horse ADH and against the human $\beta_1\beta_1$ ADH. Results of these studies indicated that the immunologic activity of all of the class I ADH isozymes was identical: all class I ADH isozymes reacted with antibodies raised against horse ADH and with antibodies raised against human $\beta_1\beta_1$ isozyme. Neither of the antisera reacted with the class II ADH isozyme π. Subsequent studies by Adinolfi *et al.* (1984) indicated

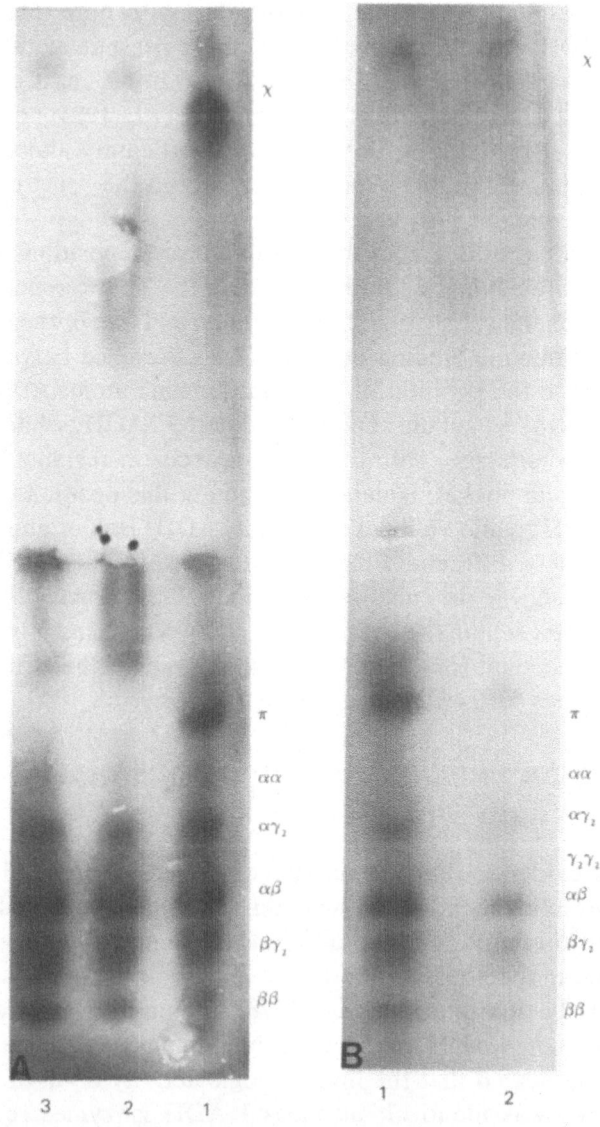

that the rabbit antisera against horse ADH and rabbit antisera against human $\beta_1\beta_1$ ADH did not react with the class III ADH isozyme. Antisera raised against the class III ADH isozyme did not cross react with human class I ADH isozymes.

Immunologic studies on ADH isozymes have also been carried out using antibodies raised in mice (Vaisanen *et al.*, 1984). Polyclonal antibodies were raised by injecting mice with horse ADH. Spleen cells from immunized mice were fused to mouse myeloma, and hybridomas were derived which produced monoclonal antibodies to horse ADH. Polyclonal antibodies were also produced by immunizing mice with the $\gamma_1\gamma_2$ isozyme isolated from intestine.

The activity of antibodies against specific ADH isozymes was determined by incubating liver extracts at 4°C overnight and then subjecting the extracts to starch gel electrophoresis.

Polyclonal antibodies raised by injecting horse ADH into mice were found to react against all forms of human ADH; i.e., class I, class II, and class III ADH isozymes (Fig. 3). One monoclonal antibody derived from spleen cells of a mouse immunized with horse ADH reacted with $\alpha\alpha$, π, and χ ADH isozymes; a second monoclonal antibody reacted with $\alpha\alpha$ and χ ADH and another reacted with π ADH.

These results suggest that there are similarities between $\alpha\alpha$, π, and χ ADH, at least as far as certain surface antigenic determinants are concerned. In this context it is of interest to note the $\alpha\alpha$, π, and χ ADH share another property in common: they are all more active with cinnamaldehyde than the other ADH isozymes (M. Smith, unpublished observations).

Differential effects of monoclonal antibodies on electrophoretic mobility and activity of specific isozymes can also be observed (Fig. 4). Using mice, it has also been possible to produce an antibody with specificity for particular class I ADH isozymes. Immunization of mice with the $\gamma_1\gamma_2$ isozyme isolated from human intestinal tissue has made it possible to raise an antibody that apparently reacts only with γ-containing ADH isozymes (Fig. 5) (Vaisanen *et al.*, 1984).

Bühler *et al.* (1983) have used antibodies against pyrazole-inhibited

←——————————————————————————————————————

Fig. 3. ADH isozymes present in extracts of (lane 1) adult liver and in extracts incubated with (A) polyclonal antibody to horse ADH or (B) monoclonal antibody to horse ADH. Note that the polyclonal antibody reacts with all class I ADH isozymes and with class II ADH, (π) and reacts weakly with class III ADH (χ). The monoclonal antibody reacts only with class II and class III ADH.

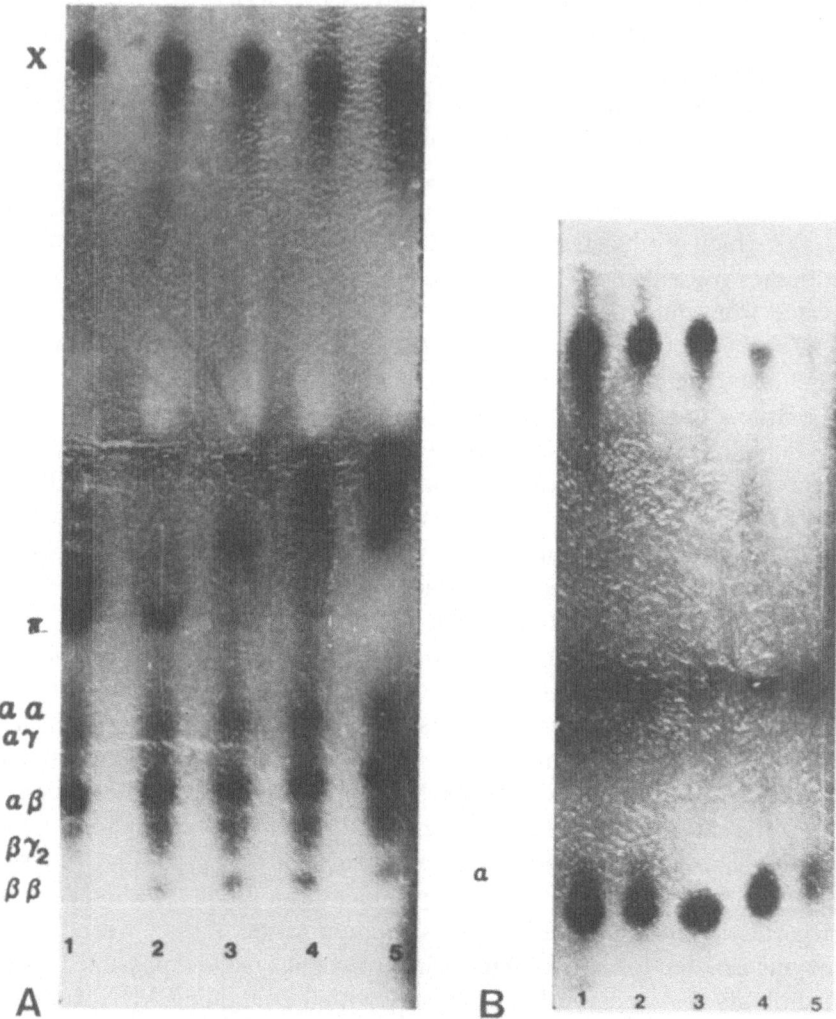

Fig. 4.   Extracts of (A) adult liver and (B) fetal liver incubated prior to electrophoresis with monoclonal antibodies (A) P3A3 and (B) P1G1. (Lane 1) Control extracts; (lanes 2–5) extracts incubated with increasing concentrations of antibody. Note that the P3A3 monoclonal antibody binds to π ADH (class II ADH) isozyme, and with increasing concentrations of antibody the electrophoretic mobility of this isozyme is progressively retarded. P3A3 does not affect the activity or mobility of the class I ADH isozymes. The P1G1 monoclonal antibody inhibits the activity of the αα and χ ADH isozymes present in extracts of fetal liver.

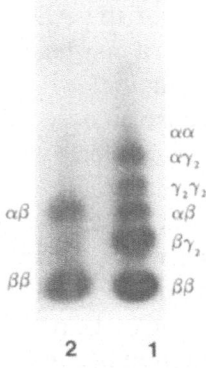

αα
αγ₂
γ₂γ₂
αβ
βγ₂
ββ

Fig. 5. ADH isozymes present in (lane 1) an extract of adult liver and (lane 2) this same extract incubated with antibody to the γ₁γ₂ ADH isozyme. Note that this antibody removes γ-containing isozymes from the extract.

(i.e., class I) ADH raised in rabbits to examine the cellular distribution of ADH in particular organs by means of histochemical techniques. These studies revealed a widespread though uneven distribution of ADH in many tissues. Von Wartburg and Bühler (1984) have stressed that it is important to note that although the overall activity of ADH in a particular tissue may be low (and therefore not readily detectable in extracts of that tissue), high concentrations may be present in particular cell types. In studies on the brain, for example, Purkinje cells in the cerebellum were found to stain strongly. Organs with abundant ADH were found to have an uneven distribution of ADH activity. In the liver, ADH was present primarily in pericentral hepatocytes; in kidney, ADH occurred primarily in the tubular epithelium; in the gastrointestinal tract, ADH was present primarily in the mucosa.

Molecular Genetic Studies on Alcohol Dehydrogenase

One of the problems in the genetic analysis of class I and class II ADH is that these isozymes are primarily tissue-specific and are not present in readily assayable quantities in accessible tissues such as white blood cells. Family studies have therefore not been carried out. In addition, it has not been possible to evaluate the role of ADH polymorphism in the generation of altered alcohol tolerance and in the susceptibility to alcoholism. These problems may be overcome by the development of DNA probes to examine ADH genes in DNA samples derived from white blood cell samples. The ADH genes are subject to developmental and tissue-specific changes in gene expression as well as to changes in expression during malignant transformation in the liver (Fig. 1) (Smith, 1972).

Through development of DNA probes and analysis of the ADH gene family at the chromosomal level and at the mRNA level, it may be possible to define certain underlying mechanisms in gene regulation.

cDNA probes for class I ADH genes have been isolated by Duester *et al.* (1984) and Ikuta and *et al.* (1984). These two groups have used different methods to derive the cDNA probes for human ADH.

Duester *et al.* (1984) used amino acid sequence data for the $\beta_1\beta_1$ ADH isozyme to identify a sequence of five amino acids, with relatively low code degeneracy, near the carboxy terminal of the polypeptide (amino acids 332–336). An oligonucleotide probe corresponding to the region was obtained. This probe consisted of a mixture of 16 different oligomers, one of which was perfectly complementary to ADH mRNA. The radiolabeled oligonucleotide probe was used to screen colonies derived from the adult human liver cDNA library of Orkin (Woods *et al.*, 1982). One clone isolated in this way, designated pADH12, was found to contain an insert of 1100 bp (base pairs). A restriction map of this clone was derived. Restriction fragments were then cloned into the M13 bacteriophage and sequenced. Analysis of the DNA sequence of the insert revealed that it contained a 593-bp 3'-untranslated region in addition to a 273-bp translated region coding for 91 amino acids. The DNA sequence of this clone predicted exactly the amino acid sequence of the 3' terminal 91 amino acids in β ADH as determined by Jornvall *et al.* (1984).

Ikuta *et al.* (1984) used antibodies against ADH and an expression library of human liver cDNA in the bacteriophage vector lambda gt11 to isolate clones. Additional screening for ADH clones was then carried out using 14mer oligonucleotide probes corresponding to a region closer to the amino terminal of the β ADH polypeptide. One of the clones isolated in this way was found to contain a 1.7-kb insert and to represent a full-length cDNA for ADH.

The pADH12 clone isolated by Duester *et al.* (1984) has been used to examine human genomic DNA (Smith *et al.*, 1984a,b; Duester *et al.*, 1985).

Analysis of Human Genomic DNA with the pADH12 cDNA Probe

When *Eco*R1-digested human DNA bound to nitrocellulose is hybridized to radiolabeled pADH12 and then washed under conditions of medium stringency (1 × SSC, 55°C for 40 min), six fragments are detected. The molecular sizes of these fragments are 10.5, 7.4, 4.2, 3.2, 2.9,

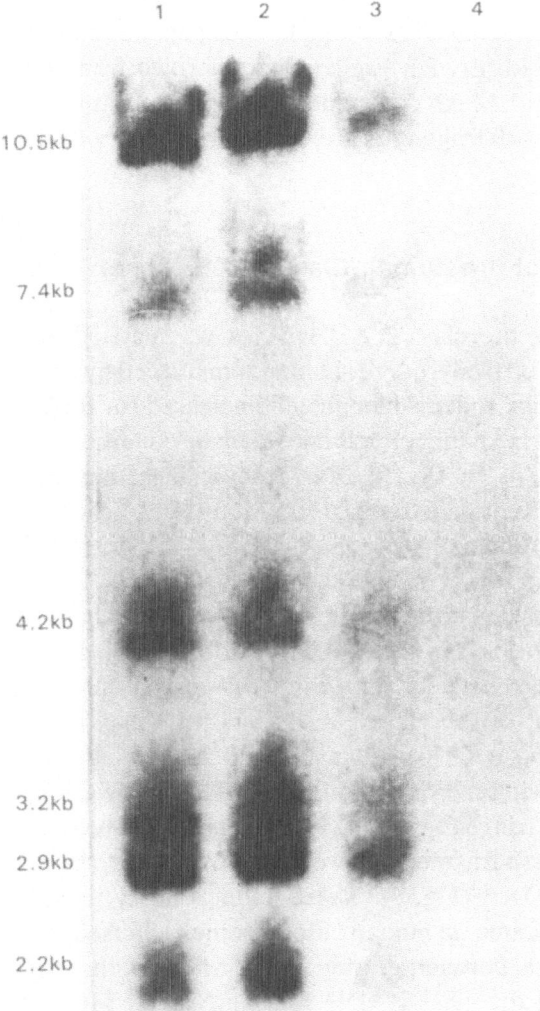

Fig. 6. Southern blot of DNA from (lanes 1 and 2) human leukocytes, (lane 4), CHO Chinese hamster cells, and (lane 3) a Chinese hamster–human somatic cell hybrid that contained chromosome 4 as the only human chromosome, DNA was digested with *Eco*R1. Filters with transferred fragments were hybridized with the pADH12 probe. Note that all DNA fragments present in the human DNA samples are also present in the hybrid DNA.

and 2.2 kb (Fig. 6). Following a high-stringency wash (0.1 × SSC, 65°C for 40 min), two fragments remain, the 10.5- and 2.9-kb fragments. These findings suggested that the pADH12 clone hybridized with the 3′ ends of the three class I ADH genes (genes coding for α, β, and γ) under conditions of low stringency, while under conditions of high stringency pADH12 hybridized only with fragments derived from the gene coding for β ADH. Subsequently the pADH12 clone was used to isolate clones of human ADH from the Maniatis library of human DNA in lambda phage. DNA sequencing and Southern blot analysis of the lambda genomic clones indicate that the 2.9- and 10.5-kb *Eco*R1 fragments are derived from the β ADH gene, while the 3.2- and 2.2-kb fragments are derived from the α ADH gene and the 4.2- and 7.4-kb fragments are derived from the γ ADH gene.

Chromosomal Assignment of the Human Class I ADH Genes

Chromosome mapping of the class I ADH genes was carried out through analysis of DNA derived from rodent–human somatic cell hybrids (Smith *et al.*, 1984a, 1985c). The rodent–human cell lines used for fusion included rat, mouse, and Chinese hamster cell lines. Under conditions of medium stringency ($1 \times$ SSC, 65°C, 4 min), DNA from Chinese hamster cells or from rat cells does not hybridize to pADH12. Mouse DNA showed a single hybridizing fragment under these conditions, but this fragment was electrophoretically separate from the human DNA fragments. Analysis of the human chromosomal constitution of 13 different rodent–human somatic cell hybrids that hybridized to the pADH12 probe revealed that the only human chromosome consistently present was human chromosome 4. Definitive assignment of the class I ADH loci to human chromosome 4 was obtained using a CHO–human hybrid containing only human chromosome 4. Following hybridization to pADH12 and washing under conditions of medium stringency, six *Eco*R1 fragments were identified in this hybrid clone. These fragments were identical in size to those observed in human genomic DNA (Fig. 6). These findings imply that all three class I ADH genes are located on human chromosome 4. Subsequent studies on somatic cell hybrids containing fragments of human chromosome 4 provide evidence that the class I ADH genes are located on the long arm of human chromosome 4 between q21 and q24 (Smith *et al.*, 1985a).

Studies on the Structure of the *ADH2* Gene

Through sequence analysis of a series of genomic clones, the coding region of the *ADH2* gene has been shown to be 15 kb in length and to be divided into nine exons by eight introns (Duester *et al.*, 1985).

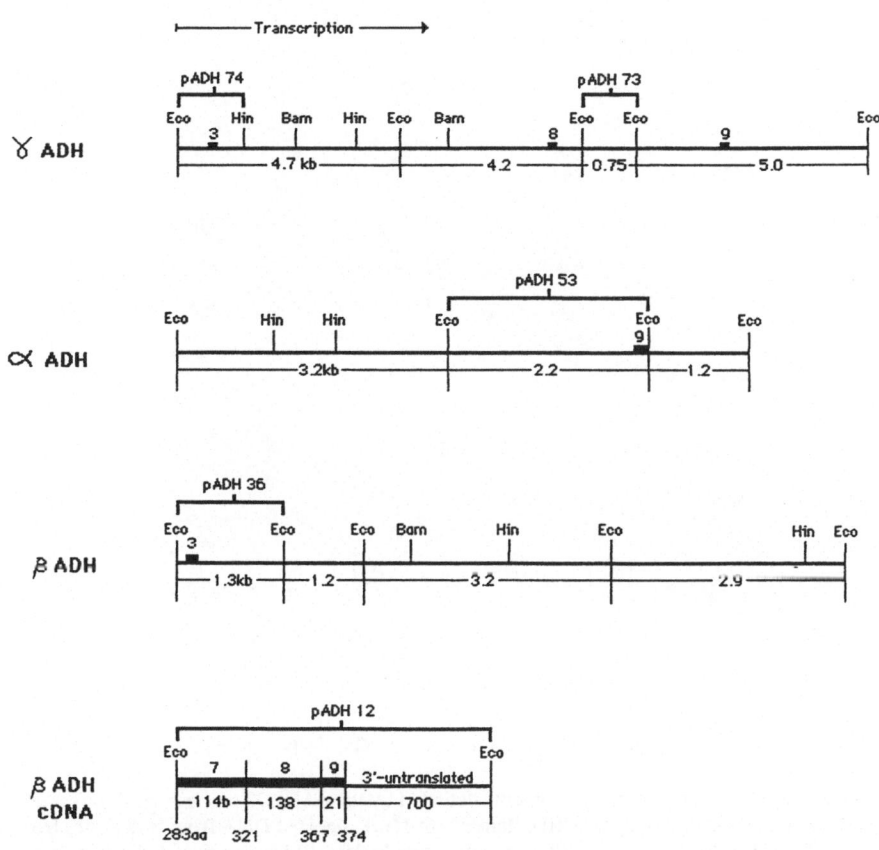

Fig. 7. Restriction maps of three ADH-containing lambda genomic clones from which probes were derived, and of one ADH cDNA clone. The regions used for deriving probes are bracketed under the name given to the probe: pADH 74 (γ), pADH73 (γ), pADH53 (α), pADH36 (β), and pADH12 (β). Exons present in regions homologous to the probe are indicated in black bars. In the pADH12 clone (β) the positions of the amino acids coded by the exon are indicated aa.

Investigation of ADH Genetic Variation Using ADH Genomic DNA Probes

Using specific probes isolated from ADH genomic clones (Fig. 7), a number of different restriction endonucleases, and DNA isolated from leukocytes obtained from more than 100 individuals, it has been possible to identify DNA polymorphisms in each of the class I ADH genes (Smith *et al.*, 1985a; 1985c). The genes of origin of specific cloned ADH genomic

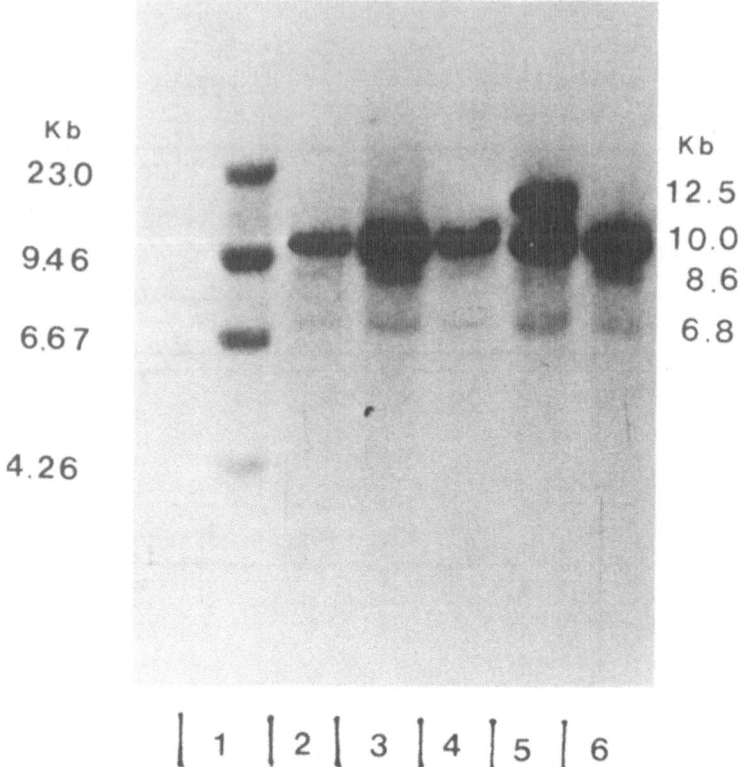

Fig. 8.   Southern blot of DNA fragments detected by the pADH73 probe (γ ADH). (Lane1)
Marker fragments (lambda (*Hind*III); (lanes 2–6) *Msp*1-digested DNA from leukocytes from
five different individuals. Note that in four individuals a 10-kb fragment hybridizes most
stringently to the probe, while in one individual 12.5- and 10-kb fragments are present.

DNA fragments used as probes was determined by DNA sequence analysis and comparison of exon sequences in specific clones with amino acid
sequence of the β ADH polypeptide (Jornvall *et al.*, 1984), the γ ADH
polypeptide (Bühler *et al.*, 1984c), and partial amino acid sequence information for the α polypeptide (von Bahr-Lindstrom *et al.*, 1985).

As might be expected from the close homology of the three class I
ADH genes, it is difficult to derive DNA probes that specifically hybridize
to a single ADH gene. However, through analysis of Southern-transferred
DNA fragments (Southern, 1975), following washes of varying stringency,
it is possible to determine which DNA fragments hybridize most stringently to a specific probe and are therefore most analogous to that probe.

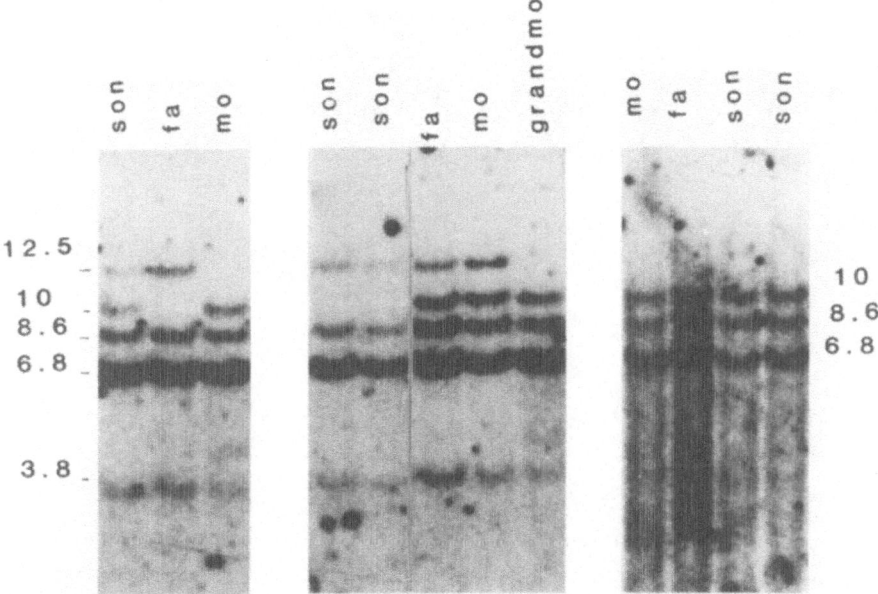

Fig. 9. Southern blot of DNA fragments detected by the pADH53 probe in individuals in three nuclear families. DNA extracted from leukocytes was digested with $Msp1$. Note polymorphism in 12.5- and 10-kb fragments. Stringency studies indicated that these fragments are not most analogous to this probe (see Fig. 8).

$Msp1$ Polymorphism at the 3′ End of the $ADH3$ Gene. This polymorphism has been demonstrated using probes pADH53 and pADH73, from the 3′ end of the $ADH1$, and the $ADH3$ genes (Figs. 7–9). The probe that hybridizes most stringently to the polymorphic DNA fragments was derived from the 3′ terminal intron in the $ADH3$ gene (γ) (Fig. 8). This probe, designated pADH73, is approximately 750 bases in length. Three groups of individuals can be identified: individuals in whom a 12-kb fragment is present, individuals having a 10-kb fragment, and individuals who have been the 12- and the 10-kb fragments. Mendelian inheritance of this polymorphism has been determined in nuclear families.

Xba Polymorphism Close to the 5′ End of the $ADH3$ Gene. Fragments involved in this polymorphism hybridize most stringently to a genomic ADH probe designated pADH74. This probe is a 1.5-kb fragment derived from a region surrounding exon 3 of the γ ADH gene. Polymorphism is due to the presence or absence of an Xba site: some indi-

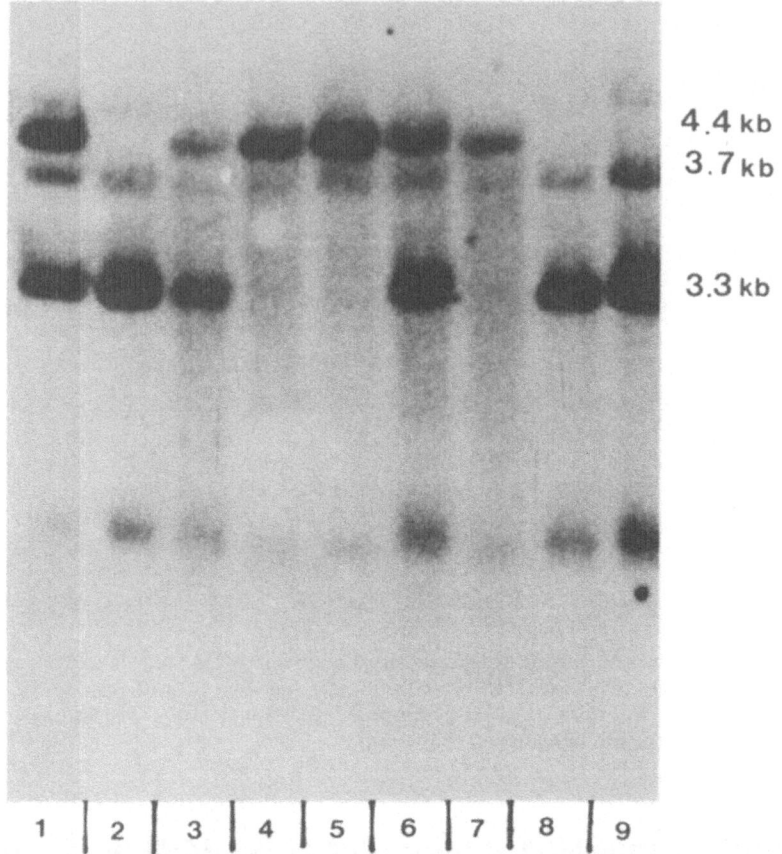

Fig. 10. Southern blot of DNA fragments detected by the pADH74 probe. DNA derived
from leukocytes from nine individuals was digested with *Xba* and then electrophoresed on
a 0.8% agarose gel. Note polymorphism in 4.4- and 3.3-kb fragments. Individuals 4 and 5
represent homozygotes for the 4.4-kb fragments; individuals 2, 8, and 9 are homozygous
for the 3.3-kb fragment; individuals 1, 3, and 6 are heterozygotes.

viduals have a 4.4-kb fragment, which hybridizes most stringently, other
individuals have a 3.3-kb fragment, while in some individuals both fragments are present (Fig. 10).

Rsa Polymorphism Close to the 5′ End of the ADH2 (β) Gene.
Fragments involved in this polymorphism hybridize most stringently to
a 1.3-kb genomic DNA probe derived from the region surrounding exon
3 in the *ADH2* gene. This probe has been designated pADH36. In some

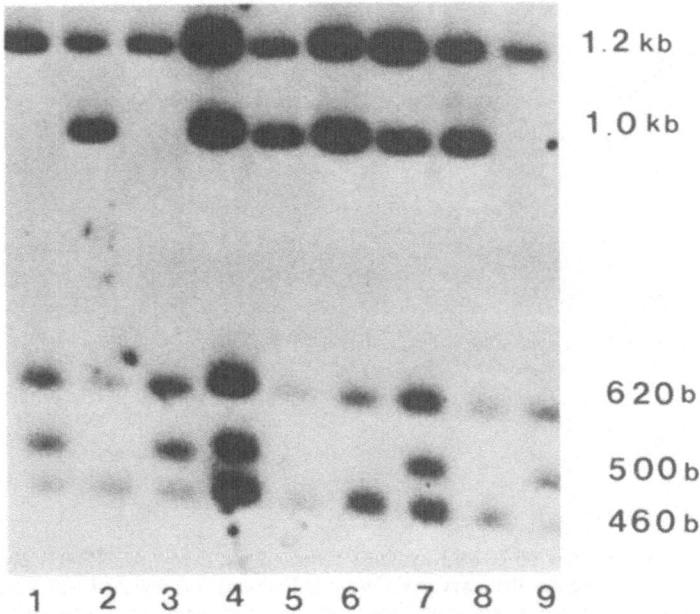

Fig. 11.   Southern blot of DNA fragments detected by the pADH36 probe (β). (Lanes 1–9) *Rsa*-digested DNA derived from leukocytes from nine different individuals. Note that in individuals 1, 3, and 9 the 1.0-kb fragment is missing and an additional 500-base fragment is present. These individuals are homozygous (+ +) for the polymorphis *Rsa* site. Individuals 4 and 7 are heterozygous for the polymorphic *Rsa* site: both 1-kb abd 500-base fragments are present.

individuals a 1-kb *Rsa* fragment hybridizes most stringently to this probe, while in other individuals the 1-kb fragment is absent and a fragment of approximately 500 bases is present (Fig. 11). Heterozygous individuals (i.e., individuals possessing both fragments) have also been identified.

There is evidence that an *Xba* polymorphism exists near the 5' end of the β ADH gene. This polymorphism may depend on the variable insertion of DNA fragments. Note that the 3.7-kb fragment present in Fig. 12 hybridizes most stringently to the pADH36 (β) probe and that there is a slight difference in the molecular weight of this fragment in different individuals.

Polymorphisms in the *ADH*1 (α) Gene.   An *Msp*1 polymorphism in the *ADH*1 gene can be demonstrated with probes derived from the

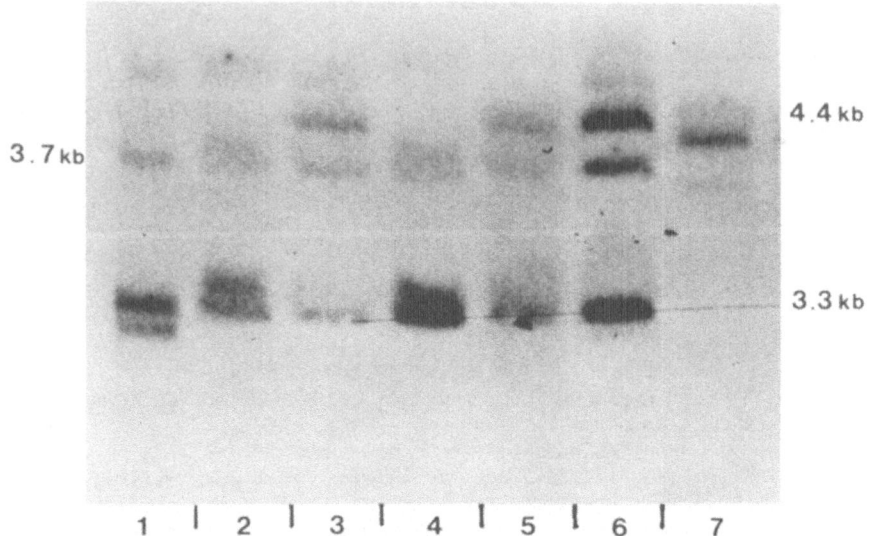

Fig. 12.   Southern blot of DNA fragments detected with the pADH74 (γ) probe. DNA extracted from leukocytes from seven different individuals was digested with *Xba* and electrophoresed on 1% agarose gels. Note that in addition to the polymorphism with respect to the 4.4- and 3.3-kb fragments, there are also small differences in fragment sizes in different individuals.

region surrounding exon 9 (i.e., the 3' untranslated region of the ADH genes. This polymorphism has been demonstrated with a genomic DNA probe derived from the α ADH gene. This probe, designated pADH53, hybridizes most stringently to a constant 6.8-kb fragment and a variable 10-kb fragment (i.e., a fragment present in some individuals but not in others). Scoring of this polymorphism may be difficult in individuals who have the polymorphic 10-kb *Msp*1 fragment derived from the *ADH*3 gene.

Studies on *Xba* digests indicate that a polymorphism exists close to the 5' end of the *ADH*1 gene and that this polymorphism may be determined by the variable insertion of DNA fragments.

Future Studies on ADH DNA Polymorphisms.   Probes are being developed to study other regions of the ADH genes. Extension of the DNA polymorphism studies to include individuals of different population groups will be of great interest. In addition, it will be of interest to determine whether specific DNA polymorphisms can be correlated with previously described ADH polymorphisms that give rise to electrophoretic and kinetic differences in ADH isozymes.

Use of ADH DNA Probes to Examine Developmental Changes in ADH Expression

Studies on ADH mRNA have been initiated (Bilanchone *et al.*, 1985; Duester *et al.*, 1985*b*). mRNA was isolated from adult and fetal liver, electrophoresed, transferred to nitrocellulose, and then hybridized with ADH-specific DNA probes [Northern blotting procedure (Maniatis *et al.*, 1982)]. Hybridization of Northern blots with the pADH12 probe (β ADH 3' cDNA probe) reveals that multiple bands are present in fetal and adult liver. In the case of total mRNA these brands range in size from 28S to 16S. In poly A mRNA these bands range in size from 23S to 16S, approximately 154 bases. In polyA mRNA from fetal liver the 20S bands predominate (Fig. 13).

When Northern blots are hybridized with pADH53, a genomic probe derived from the 3' end of the *ADH1* (α) gene, a distinct difference between the mRNA present in fetal and adult liver is noted. This difference is present in total mRNA, but is particularly noticeable in the poly A mRNA. In adult liver a number of high- and low-molecular weight bands are visible while in fetal liver only the lower molecular weight bands (16S–18S), are visible (Fig. 14).

Possible Implications of These Findings

First, fully processed mRNA species derived from the three class I ADH genes may differ in size, ranging between 16S and 18S (approximately 1540 and 1760 bases). This finding is compatible with the existence of a number of different potential polyadenylation sites within the 3' untranslated region of the ADH clone described by Duester *et al.* (1984), and with the finding of cDNA clones for β ADH that differ in length (von Bahr-Lindstrom *et al.*, 1985).

Second, results of experiments with pADH12 imply that only a subset of β ADH gene transcripts are fully processed in fetal liver. Of interest is the fact that the fetal liver used in this experiment was found to express only small quantities of β ADH, as is usual for a second-trimester fetus.

Third, results of experiments with the α ADH-specific probe ADH53 imply that in adult liver both partially processed and fully processed forms of α ADH mRNA occur. However, in fetal liver fully processed α ADH mRNA predominates. In fetal liver the αα ADH isozyme is the predominant form of ADH.

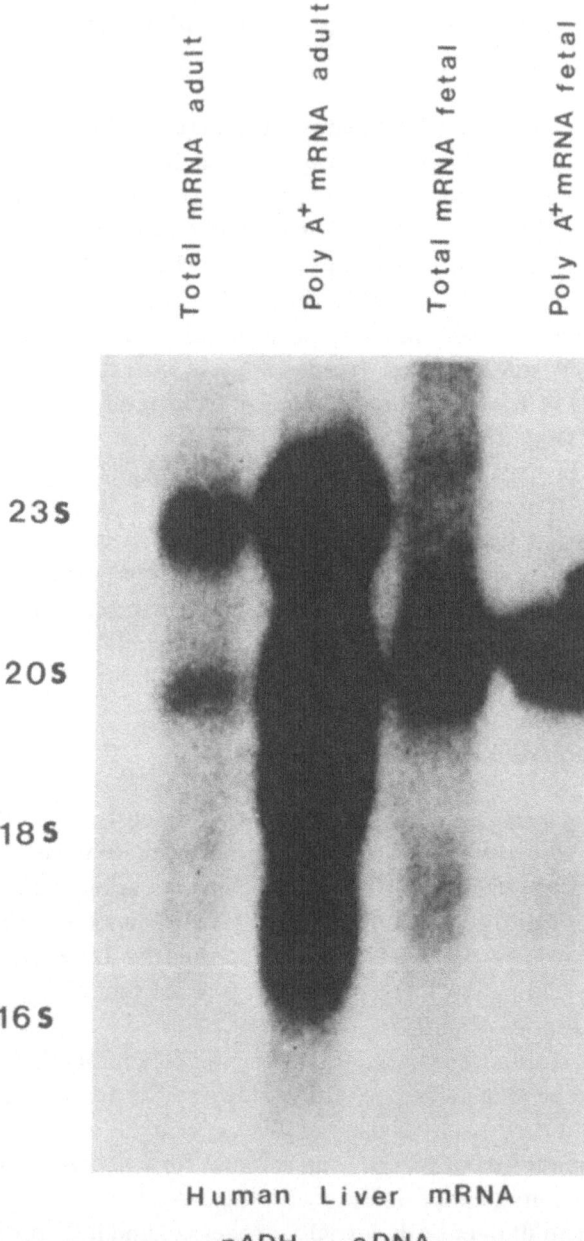

Fig. 13. Northern blot of mRNA isolated from adult and fetal liver and probed with pADH12 (β cDNA). Note that in fetal liver the probe hybridizes primarily to RNA that is approximately 20S in size.

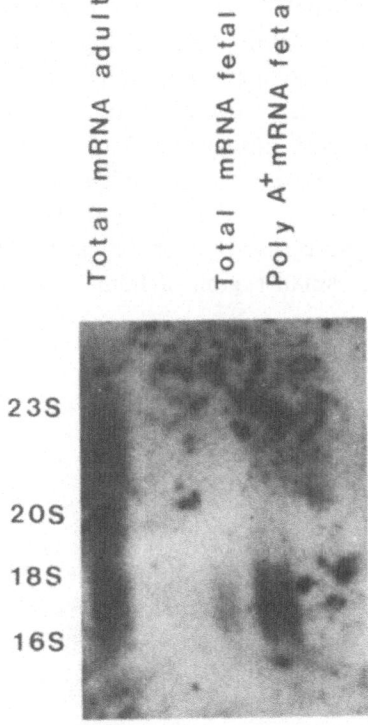

Total mRNA adult

Total mRNA fetal

Poly A⁺ mRNA fetal

23S

20S

18S

16S

Fig. 14.   Northern blot of mRNA isolated from adult liver and fetal liver probed with the pADH53 probe (α). Note that in total RNA from adult liver the probe hybridizes to mRNA that ranges in size from 23A to 16S. In fetal total mRNA and in poly A+ mRNA from fetal liver the probe hybridizes primarily to mRNA that ranges in size between 16S and 18S.

These findings therefore suggest that some of the regulation of ADH expression may take place at the level of mRNA processing.

Future Prospects

Through further expansion of these studies to include the use of other tissues in which single class I ADH genes are expressed and the use of probes specific for the 3' end of the γ ADH gene, it will be possible to determine the roles of gene transcription and RNA processing in the control of ADH gene expression.

Mapping of the Class III Gene

Human class III ADH (χ ADH) represents a constitutively expressed enzyme, which can be detected in human leukocytes and fibroblasts and in rodent–human somatic cell hybrids. Starch gel electrophoresis has been used to separate human and Chinese hamster (CHO) χ ADH. Using CHO–human leukocyte somatic cell hybrids, it has been possible to assign the gene coding for χ ADH to human chromosome 4 (Smith *et al.*, 1984*a*; 1985*b*). Additional studies on the expression of human ADH in somatic cell hybrids with derivatives of human chromosome 4 have allowed further localization of the class III ADH gene locus to the region 4q21–q24 (Carlock *et al.*, 1985). It is of interest to note that both the class I and the class III ADH loci are located in this small region of human chromosome 4.

ALDEHYDE DEHYDROGENASES

Definition

Aldehyde dehydrogenases (aldehyde:NAD oxidoreductase, EC 1.2.1.3) are enzymes that oxidize a number of different aliphatic and cyclic aldehydes in the presence of NAD to produce the corresponding keto acids.

Nomenclature of Human Aldehyde Dehydrogenase (ALDH) Loci

Current information suggests that there are four groups of ALDH isozymes. Isozymes within a particular group differ from the isozymes in other groups with respect to their electrophoretic mobility, kinetic properties, subcellular location, and tissue distribution. In some cases isozymes in different groups differ in their molecular size and subunit structure (Forte-McRobbie and Pietruszko, 1985; Santisteban *et al.*, 1985). Genetic variation occurs independently in two and possibly three of the groups of ALDH isozymes. Taken together these facts provide strong evidence that the four groups of enzymes are coded by four independent gene loci, *ALDH1*, *ALDH2*, *ALDH3*, and *ALDH4*. Further evidence for the existence of independent gene loci has come from mapping experiments: three of the human ALDH loci have been assigned chromosomally, each to a different chromosome (see below).

Current publications on human ALDH appear to conform to the nomenclature developed for the horse ALDH enzyme, where E1 represents the cytosolic ALDH and E2 represents the mitochondrial ALDH. Thus the human cytosolic enzyme is referred to as ALDH1, while the mitochondrial enzyme is referred to as ALDH2. One confusing point is that human ALDH isozymes visualized on starch gel do not follow a sequential numbering pattern according to the nomenclature. Thus, ALDH2 (mitochondrial enzyme) migrates more anodally than ALDH1 (cytosolic enzyme), while ALDH3 migrates less anodally thatn ALDH1, and ALDH4 is the least anodal isozyme. In older publications ALDH isozymes were referred to as ALDH I, II, III, and IV, where ALDH I had the greatest anodal mobility and ALDH IV the least anodal mobility (Harada *et al.*, 1980).

Particularly when isoelectric focusing is used to separate ALDH isozymes, secondary isozymes may be visualized. These apparently arise from the four isozymes described above through posttranslational modification.

Tissue Distribution of ALDH Isozymes

Studies on the tissue distribution of ALDH isozymes have been described by Harada *et al.* (1978), 1980*a,b*), G. L. Jones and Teng (1983), Pietruszko (1983), and Santisteban *et al.* (1985). Using propionaldehyde as substrate, all four ALDH isozymes can be visualized in appropriate tissues (Harada *et al.*, 1980*b*).

The mitochondrial ALDH isozyme (ALDH2) has highest activity in liver, kidney, and heart tissue. This form of ALDH is weak or absent in livers of fetuses (M. Smith, unpublished observations). The cytosolic ALDH1 isozyme is constitutively expressed and occurs in all cell types, including erythrocytes. ALDH3 isozymes occur primarily in stomach and lung, while ALDH4 isozymes are most abundant in liver and kidney.

Allelic Variation in ALDH Isozymes

Harada *et al.* (1978) in studies on livers from 40 Japanese individuals, noted that an unusual ALDH phenotype occurred in approximately half of the specimens. The most anodal ALDH isozyme (mitochondrial) was absent. Goedde *et al.* (1973*a*) proposed that the flushing reaction and symptoms of acute alcohol intoxication induced by small doses of alcohol in a high proportion of Oriental individuals was due to deficiency of the mitochondrial ALDH.

Impraim *et al.* (1982) developed antibodies to purified ALDH1 and ALDH2 isozymes by immunizing rabbits with purified preparations of these isozymes. The antibodies produced reacted with both isozymes. However, the antigenic activity of each isozyme could be separately determined following crossed immunoelectrophoresis. This consisted of starch gel electrophoresis in the first dimension followed by electrophoresis of the separated isozymes into agarose gels containing antibody. Impraim *et al.* (1982) used this technique to examine liver extracts from Japanese individuals who were apparently deficient in mitochondrial ALDH. In these extracts they were able to demonstrate enzymatically inactive but antigenically active ALDH2. On the basis of these studies, they postulated that the absence of ALDH2 in Oriental individuals was due to a structural gene mutation, which led to synthesis of an enzymatically inactive protein. Subsequently, Yoshida *et al.* (1983) extended these studies by using a combination of determinations of liver ALDH enzyme activity and quantitative determinations of liver ALDH immunologic activity to examine the genotype in individuals in the Japanese population. In studies on ten livers they were able to demonstrate that certain livers that contained ALDH2-active enzyme also contained enzymatically inactive, immunologically active material. These livers were therefore derived from individuals who were heterozygous for the normal *ALDH2* allele and the deficient *ALDH2* allele. Yoshida *et al.* (1983) reported that *ALDH2-1/ALDH2-1* (normal) homozygotes occurred with a frequency of 0.11, *ALDH2-1/ALDH2-2* heterozygotes occurred with a frequency of 0.33, and the *ALDH2-2/ALDH2-2* (deficient) homozygotes occurred with a frequency of 0.56.

Quantitative Variation in the *ALDH*1 (Cytoplasmic) Gene Product

Yoshida *et al.* (1983) detected absence of the *ALDH*1 isozyme in the liver of a Japanese individual. Nongenetic factors are also responsible for reduction in cytoplasmic ALDH activity. Cytosolic liver ALDH is reduced in individuals with alcoholic liver disease (Jenkins and Peters, 1983). Reduced cytoplasmic ALDH in erythrocytes has also been described (Agarwal *et al.*, 1983). The exact mechanism of reduction in activity under these circumstances is unknown.

Genetic Variation of ALDH3

Four percent of Europeans have been found to have a variant form of ALDH3. In these individuals a three-banded ALDH3 pattern is visible on electrophoresis (Santisteban *et al.*, 1985), suggesting heterozygosity for an *ALDH*3 allele, which results in a gene product with altered electrophoretic mobility.

Structure of ALDH Isozymes

ALDH1 and ALDH2 isozymes have been found to be tetrameric enzymes; the mitochondrial ALDH isozyme (ALDH2) has a subunit molecular weight of approximately 51,000, while the ALDH1 (cytoplasmic) ALDH isozyme has a molecular weight of approximately 53,000 (G.L. Jones and Teng, 1983). Studies by Santisteban *et al.* (1985) indicate that the ALDH3 isozyme has a molecular weight of 85,000. The occurrence of a three-banded pattern in individuals who are heterozygous at the *ALDH*3 locus suggests that ALDH3 is a dimer. Forte-McRobbie and Pietruszko (1985) purified the ALDH4 isozyme and found that it is a dimeric enzyme composed of subunits with a molecular weight of 69,000.

Properties of ALDH Isozymes

Substrate Activities

Each of the aldehyde dehydrogenases shows a broad range of activity with a number of different aliphatic aldehydes, including formaldehyde, acetaldehyde, propionaldehyde and butyraldehyde (Harada *et al.*, 1980*b*; G. L. Jones and Teng, 1983). The ALDH3 isozymes are particularly active with the cyclic aldehydes benzaldehyde and furfuraldehyde (Santisteban *et al.*, 1985).

Measurements of the K_m values of ALDH isozymes for proprionaldehyde (Harada *et al.*, 1980*b*) indicated that the mitochondrial ALDH isozyme had the lowest K_m, 3.5 μM, while the ALDH4 isozyme had the highest, 1.40 μM. In a number of publications the mitochondrial enzyme is referred to as the "low-K_m" aldehyde dehydrogenase (Greenfield and Pietruszko, 1977).

pH Optima

Harada *et al.* (1980*b*) determined that the human mitochondrial ALDH had a pH optimum of 9.7, while the other ALDH isozymes had a pH optimum of 8.8.

Coenzyme Binding

While NAD is the required cofactor for ALDH2 (mitochondrial) and ALDH4 isozymes, the ALDH1 (cytosolic) and ALDH3 isozymes can use either NAD or NADP (Santisteban *et al.*, 1985).

Inhibition Characteristics

There is a marked difference in the sensitivity of the mitochondrial and cytoplasmic ALDH isozymes to inhibition with Disulfiram (Antibuse). Characteristically, the cytoplasmic form is highly sensitive to Disulfiram inhibition (Greenfield and Pietruszko, 1977).

Stability

Studies on the stability of the ALDH isozymes indicate that benzaldehyde dehydrogenase is the least stable enzyme, while cytoplasmic ALDH is the most stable (Harada *et al.*, 1980*b*; Santisteban *et al.*, 1985).

Amino Acid Sequence Determinations of ALDH Polypeptides

Hempel *et al.* (1984*c*) have purified human cytoplasmic ALDH to homogeneity using ion exchange chromatography on CM-Sephadex and DEAE-Sephadex, followed by affinity chromatography on 5'-AMP Sepharose. The complete amino acid sequence of cytoplasmic ALDH has been determined (Hempel *et al.*, 1984*c*). Partial amino acid sequence information has also been obtained for mitochondrial ALDH (Hempel *et al.*, 1984*a*). Comparison of amino acid sequences from the two polypeptides reveals that there are short regions of similarity in the two sequences, i.e., amino acids in the regions from position 194 to 235 are highly conserved. Amino acid sequence information has been determined for a carboxyl-terminal segment of the usual form of mitochondrial ALDH and a corresponding segment derived from the functionally deficient Oriental variant of mitochondrial ALDH (Hempel *et al.*, 1984*a*). The usual and variant forms of mitochondrial ALDH have been shown to vary in a single amino acid: glutamine at position -14 in the carboxyl-terminal segment of the normal enzyme is replaced by lysine in the variant enzyme. This substitution is compatible with a single-base mutation.

Formaldehyde Dehydrogenase (FDH)

This enzyme is distinct from other forms of aldehyde dehydrogenase in that it requires reduced glutathione (GSH) as a cofactor in addition to NAD. The reaction carried out by this enzyme is

formaldehyde + GSH + NAD

$$\xrightarrow{\text{FDH}} S\text{-formylglutathgione} + \text{NADH}$$

Castle and Board (1982) have determined that FDH is present in a number of tissues, including liver, spleen, kidney, and intestine.

Meera Khan *et al.* (1984) demonstrated that FDH is also produced by human fibroblasts and by rodent–human somatic cell hybrids. They assigned the gene coding for this enzyme to human chromosome 4. Using Chinese hamster–human somatic cell hybrids containing derivatives of human chromosome 4, Hiroshige *et al.* (1985) demonstrated that this gene is located in the region 4qter–4q24.

Molecular Genetic Studies on ALDH Genes

These studies have been initiated by Yoshida and coworkers (Ikuta *et al.*, 1984; Hsu *et al.*, 1985; L. C. Hsu, T. Mohandas, and A. Yoshida, personal commnication). cDNA clones for human ALDH have been isolated by screening a human liver cDNA library cloned into the lambda gt11 expression library with antibodies to human cytoplasmic and mitochondrial ALDH. Further screening of clones was carried out using synthetic oligonucleotide probes corresponding to portions of the cytoplasmic and mitochondrial ALDH polypeptides. Using these methods, one clone for cytoplasmic ALDH and two clones for mitochondrial ALDH have been isolated. DNA sequencing of the clones was carried out. Through these studies, Hsu *et al.* (1985; and L. C. Hsu, T. Mohandas, and A.

Yoshida, personal communication) established that the degree of homology between the coding regions of ALDH1 and ALDH2 is 66%.

Chromosomal Assignment of ALDH1 and ALDH2 genes

Using DNA probes, Hsu *et al.* (1985*a,b*) assigned the ALDH1 (cytoplasmic) locus to human chromosome 12 and the ALDH2 (mitochondrial) locus to human chromosome 9. cDNA clones for ALDH2 were also isolated by Smith *et al.* 1985*d* and used to confirm the assignment of this gene to human chromosome 12.

ACKNOWLEDGMENTS. Studies in our laboratory are supported by NIAAA grant AA05781. I thank Karin Anderson for her help in preparing the figures and Dr. Virginia Bilanchone for the mRNA illustrations. I also acknowledge the excellent technical assistance of Steve Hiroshige.

REFERENCES

Adinolfi, A., and Hopkinson, D. A., 1978, Blue Sepharose chromatography of human alcohol dehydrogenase: Evidence for interlocus and interallelic differences in affinity characteristics, *Ann. Hum. Genet.* **41**:399–407.

Adinolfi, A., and Hopkinson, D. A., 1979, Affinity characteristics of human alcohol dehydrogenase (ADH) isozymes, *Ann. Hum. Genet.* **43**:109–119.

Adinolfi, A., Adinolfi, M., Hopkinson, D. A., and Harris, H., 1978, Immunological properties of the human alcohol dehydrogenase (ADH) isozymes, *J. Immunogenet.* **5**:283–296.

Adinolfi, A., Adinolfi, M., and Hopkinson, D. A., 1984, Immunological and biochemical characterization of the human alcohol dehydrogenase chi ADH isozyme, *Ann. Hum. Genet.* **48**:1–10.

Agarwal, D. P., Meier-Tackman, D., Harada, S., and Goedde, H. W., 1981, A search for the Indianapolis variant of human alcohol dehydrogenase in liver samples from Northern Germany and Japan, *Hum. Genet.* **50**:170–171.

Agarwal, D. P., Tobar-Rojas, L., Harada, S., and Goedde, H. W., 1983, Comparative study of erythrocyte aldehyde dehydrogenase in alcoholics and control subjects, *Pharmacol. Biochem. Behav.* **18**:89–95.

Azevedo, E. S., da Silva, M. C., and Tavares-Neto, J., 1975, Human alcohol dehydrogenase *ADH*1, *ADH*2, and *ADH*3 loci in a mixed population of Bahia, Brazil, *Ann. Hum. Genet.* **39**:321–327.

Bilanchone, V., Duester, G., and Smith, M., 1985, Developmental and tissue specific variation in human class I ADH mRNA, *Nucleic Acid Res.* (submitted).

Blair, A. H., and Vallee, B. L., 1966, Some catalytic properties of human liver alcohol dehydrogenase isoenzymes, *Biochemistry* **5**:2026–2034.

Bosron, W. F., Li, T. K., Dafeldecker, W. P., and Vallee, B. L., 1979a, Human liver pi alcohol dehydrogenase kinetic and molecular properties, *Biochemistry* **18**:1101–1105.

Bosron, W. F., Li, T. K., and Vallee, B. L., 1979b, Heterogeneity and new molecular forms of human liver alcohol dehydrogenase, *Biochem. Biophys. Res. Commun.* **91**:1549–1555.

Bosron, W. F., Li, T. K., and Vallee, B. L., 1980, New molecular forms of liver alcohol dehydrogenase: Isolation and characterization of ADH Indianapolis, *Proc. Natl. Acad. Sci. USA* **77**:5784–5788.

Bosron, W. F., Crabb, D. W., and Li, T. K., 1983a, Relationship between kinetics of liver alcohol dehydrogenase and alcohol metabolism, *Pharmacol. Biochem. Behav.* **18**:223–227.

Bosron, W. F., Magnes, L. J., and Li, T. K., 1983b, Human liver alcohol dehydrogenase: ADH Indianapolis results from genetic polymorphism at the *ADH2* gene locus, *Biochem. Genet.* **21**:735–744.

Bühler, R., Pestalozzi, D., Hess, M., and von Wartburg, J. P., 1983, Localization of alcohol dehydrogenase in human tissue: An immunohistochemical study, *Pharmacol. Biochem. Behav.* **18**:55–59.

Bühler, R., Hempel, J., von Wartburg, J. P., and Jornvall, H., 1984a, Atypical human alcohol dehydrogenase: the beta 2 Berne sub-unit has an amino acid exchange that is identical to the one in the beta 2 Oriental chain, *FEBS Lett.* **173**:360–366.

Bühler, R., Hempel, J., Kaiser, R., De Zalenski, C., von Wartburg, J. P., and Jornvall, H., 1984b, Human liver alcohol dheydrogenase 2: The primary structure of the gamma 1 protein chain. *Eur. J. Biochem.* **145**:447–453.

Bühler, R., Hempel, J., Kaiser, R., von Wartburg, J. P., and Vallee, B. L., 1984c, Human alcohol dehydrogenase: Structural differences between beta and gamma sub-units suggest parallel duplications in isoenzyme evolution and predominant expression of separate gene descendants in livers of different mammals, *Proc. Natl. Acad. Sci. USA* **81**:6320–6324.

Carlock, L., Hiroshige, S., and Smith, M., 1985, Assignment of the gene coding for class III ADH to human chromosome 4: 4q21–4q25, *Cytogenet. Cell Genet.*, **46**:(in press).

Castle, S. L., and Board, P. G., 1982, Electrophoretic investigation of formaldehyde dehydrogenase in human tissues, *Hum. Hered.* **32**:222–224.

Duester, G., Hatfield, G. W., Buhler, R., Hempel, J., Jornvall, H., and Smith, M., 1984, Molecular cloning and characterization of a cDNA for the beta sub-unit of human alcohol dehydrogenase, *Proc. Natl. Acad. Sci. USA* **81**:4055–4059.

Duester, G., Hatfield, G. W., and Smith, M., 1985a, Molecular genetic analysis of human alcohol dehydrogenase, *Alcohol*, **2**:53–56.

Duester, G., Smith, M., Bilanchone, V., and Hatfield, G. W., 1985b, Organization, structure and expression of the genes encoding human alpha, beta, and gamma alcohol dehydrogenase, *J. Biol. Chem.* (in press).

Forte-McRobbie, C. M., and Pietruszko, R., 1985, Purification and characterization of a high Km liver aldehyde dehydrogenase, *J. Biol. Chem.* (in press).

Fukui, M., and Wakasugi, C., 1972, Liver alcohol dehydrogenase in a Japanese population, *Jpn. J. Legal Med.* **26**:46–51.

Goedde, H. W., Harada, S., and Agarwal, D. P., 1979a, Racial differences in alcohol sensitivity: A new hypothesis, *Hum. Genet.* **51**:331–334.

Goedde, H. W., Agarwal, D. P., and Harada, S., 1979b, Alcohol metabolizing enzymes: Studies of isozymes in human biopsis and cultured fibroblasts, *Clin. Genet.* **16**:29–33.

Greenfield, N. J., and Pietruszko, R., 1977, Two aldehyde dehydrogenases from human liver. Isolation via affinity chromatography and characterization of the isozymes, *Biochim. Biophys. Acta* **483**:35–45.

Harada, S., Agarwal, D. P., and Goedde, H. W., 1978, Human liver alcohol dehydrogenase isoenzyme variations, *Hum. Genet.* **40**:215–220.

Harada, S., Misawa, S., Agarwal, D. P., and Goedde, H. W., 1980a, Liver alcohol dehydrogenase and aldehyde dehydrogenase in the Japanese: Isozyme variation and its possible role in alcohol intoxication, *Am. J. Hum. Genet.* **32**:8–15.

Harada, S., Agarwal, D., and Goedde, H. W., 1980b, electrophoretic and biochemical studies of human aldehyde dehydrogenase isozymes in various tissues, *Life Sci.* **26**:1773–1780.

Hempel, J., Kaiser, R., and Jornvall, H., 1984a, Human liver mitochondrial aldehyde dehydrogenase: A C terminal segment positions and defines the structure corresponding to the one reported to differ in the Oriental enzyme variant, *FEBS Lett.* **173**:367–373.

Hempel, J., Buhler, R., Kaiser, R., Holmquist, B., De Zalenski, C., von Wartburg, J. P., Vallee, B. L., and Jornvall, H., 1984b, Human liver alcohol dehydrogenase 1. The primary structure of the beta 1 beta 1 isoenzyme, *Eur. J. Biochem.* **145**:437–455.

Hempel, J., von Bahr-Lindstrom, H., and Jornvall, H., 1984c, Aldehyde dehydrogenase from human liver: Primary structure of the cytoplasmic isoenzyme, *Eur. J. Biochem.* **141**:21–35.

Hiroshige, S., Carlock, L., Wasmuth, J., and Smith, M., 1985, Regional assignment of human formaldehyde dehydrogenase (FDH) to the region 4q21–4q25, *Cytogenet. Cell Genet.*, **41**:(in press).

Hsu, L. C., Mohandas, T., Yoshida, A. 1985a, Chromosomal assignment of *ALDH1* and *ALDH2* genes, *Cytogenet. Cell Genet.* **41**:(in press).

Hsu, L. C., Tani, K., Fujiyoshi, T., and Yoshida, A., 1985b, Cloning of cDNA for human aldehyde dehydrogenase 1 and aldehyde dehydrogenase 2, *Proc. Nat. Acad. Sci. USA* **82**:3771–3775.

Ikuta, T., Fujiyoshi, T., Hsu, L., Kurachi, K., and Yoshida, A., 1984, Cloning of cDNAs for human alcohol and aldehyde dehydrogenase, *Am. J. Hum. Genet.* **36**:141s.

Impraim, C., Wang, G., and Yoshida, A., 1982, Structural mutation in a major human aldehyde dehydrogenase gene results in loss of enzyme activity, *Am. J. Hum. Genet.* **34**:837–841.

Jenkins, W. J., and Peters, T. J., 1983, The sub-cellular localisation of acetaldehyde dehydrogenase in human liver, *Cell Biochem. Function* **1**:37–40.

Jones, G. L., and Teng, Y.-S., 1983, A chemical and enzymological account of the multiple forms of human liver aldehyde dehydrogenase, *Biochem. Biophys. Acta* **745**:162–174.

Jörnvall, H., Hempel, J., Vallee, B. L., Bosron, W. F., and Li, T. K., 1984, Human liver alcohol dehydrogenase: Amino acid substitution in the beta 2 beta 2 Oriental enzyme explains functional properties, establishes an active site structure and parallels mutational exchanges in the yeast enzyme, *Proc. Natl. Acad. Sci. USA* **81**:3024–3028.

Julia, P., Farres, J., and Pares, X., 1983, Purification and partial characterization of a rat retina alcohol dehydrogenase active with ethanol and retinol, *Biochem. J.* **213**:547–550.

Lange, L. G. and Vallee, B. L., 1976, Double ternary complex affinity chromatography: Preparation of alcohol dehydrogenases, *Biochemistry* **15**:4681–4686.

Li, T. K., and Magnes, L. J., 1975, Identification of a distinct molecular form of alcohol dehydrogenase in human livers with high activity, *Biochem. Biophys. Res. Commun.* **63**:202–208.

Maniatis, T., Sambrook, J., and Fritsch, E., 1982, *Handbook of Molecular Cloning Techniques*, Cold Spring Harbor Laboratories, Cold Spring Harbor, New York.

Maroni, G., and Aulberg, C. C. L., 1983, Genetic control of ADH expression in *Drosophila melanogaster*, *Genetics* **105**:921–933.

Meera Khan, P., Wynen, L. M. M., Hagemeier, A., and Pearson, P., 1984, Human formaldehyde dehydrogenase (FDH) and its assignment to chromosome 4, *Cytogenet. Cell Genet.* **38**:112–115.

Pares, X., and Vallee, B. L., 1981, New human liver alcohol dehydrogenase forms with unique kinetic characteristics, *Biochem. Biophys. Res. Commun.* **98**:122–130.

Pietruszko, R., 1983, Aldehyde dehydrogenase isozymes, in: *Isozyme: Current Topics in Biological and Medical Research* (M. C. Rattazi, J. G. Scandalios, G. S. Whitt, eds.), Vol 8, pp. 195–217, Alan R. Liss, New York.

Rex, D. K., Smialek, J. E., Bosron, W. F., and Li, T. K., 1985, Alcohol and aldehyde dehydrogenase isozenzymes in a North American Indian population, *Alcohol*, in press.

Ricciardi, B. R., Saunders, J. B., William, R., and Hopkinson, D. A., 1983, Hepatic ADH and ALDH isoenzymes in different racial groups and in chronic alcoholism, *Pharmacol. Biochem. Behav.* **18**(Suppl. 1):61–65.

Santisteban, I., Povey, S., West, L. F., Parrington, J. M., and Hopkinson, D. A., 1985, Chromosome assignment, biochemical and immunological studies on a human aldehyde dehydrogenase (ALDH3), *Ann. Hum. Genet.*, **49**:87–100.

Schwartz, M., O'Donnell, J., and Sofer, W., 1979, Origin of multiple forms of alcohol dehydrogenase from *Drosophila melanogaster*, *Arch. Biochem. Biophys.* **194**:365–378.

Smith, M., 1972, Studies on the Developmental Changes and Polymorphism of Human Alcohol Dehydrogenase, Ph D Thesis, University of London.

Smith, M., Hopkinson, D. A., and Harris, H., 1971, Developmental changes and polymorphism in human alcohol dehydrogenase, *Ann. Hum. Genet.* **34**:251–271.

Smith, M., Hopkinson, D. A., and Harris, H., 1972, Alcohol dehydrogenase isozymes in stomach and liver: Evidence for activity of the *ADH3* locus, *Ann. Hum. Genet.* **35**:243–253.

Smith, M., Hopkinson, D. A., and Harris, H., 1973a, Studies on the properties of the human alcohol dehydrogenase isozymes determined by the different loci *ADH1*, *ADH2*, *ADH3*, *Ann. Hum. Genet.* **37**:49–67.

Smith, M., Hopkinson, D. A., and Harris, H., 1973b, Studies on the sub-unit structure and molecular size of the human alcohol dehydrogenase isozymes determined by the different loci *ADH1*, *ADH2*, *ADH3*, *Ann. Hum. Genet.* **36**:401–414.

Smith, M., Duester, G., Bilanchone, V., Carlock, L., and Hatfield, G. W., 1984a, Derivation of probes for molecular genetic analysis of human class I alcohol dehydrogenase (ADH), a polymorphic gene family on human chromosome 4, *Am. J. Hum. Genet.* **36**:153s.

Smith, M., Duester, G., and Hatfield, G. W., 1985a, Development of DNA probes to investigate genetic variations of human alcohol metabolizing enzymes, in: *NIDA/NIAAA Technical Review Genetic and Biological Markers of Drug Abuse and Alcoholism*, NIDA Research Monograph, Government Printing Press, Washington.

Smith, M., Duester, G., Carlock, L., and Wasmuth, J., 1985b, Assignment of alpha, beta and gamma ADH encoding genes to human chromosome 4q21–4q25, *Cytogenet. Cell Genet.* **41**:(in press).

Smith, M., Duester, G., Hiroshige, S., Anderson, K. A., and Murray, J., 1985c, DNA polymorphism in three class I ADH genes, *Am. J. Hum. Genet.* (submitted).

Smith, M. Hiroshige, S., Saxon, P., Wasmuth. J., 1985d, Assignment of the gene encoding mitochondrial aldehyde dehydrogenase (ALDH2) to chromosome 12, *Cytogenet. Cell Genet.* **41**:(in press).

Southern, E., 1975, Detecting of specific sequences among DNA fragments separated by gel electrophoresis, *J. Mol. Biol.* **98**:503–517.

Stamatoyannopoulos, G., Chen, S.-H., and Fukui, M., 1975, Liver alcohol dehydrogenase in Japanese: High frequency of atypical form and its role in alcohol sensitivity, *Am. J. Hum. Genet.* **27**:789–796.

Strydom, D. J., and Vallee, B. J., 1982, Characterization of human alcohol dehydrogenase isoenzymes by high performance liquid chromatographic peptide mapping, *Anal. Biochem.* **123**:422–429.

Teng, Y. S., Jehan, S., and Lie-Ijo, L. E., 1979, Human alcohol dehydrogenase *ADH*2 and *ADH*3 polymorphisms in ethnic Chinese and Indians of West Malaysia, *Hum. Genet.* 53:87–90.

Vaisanen, P., Bilanchone, V., and Smith, M., 1984, Development of monoclonal antibodies to determine relationships of different alcohol dehydrogenase isozymes, *Am. J. Hum. Genet.* 36:131s.

Vallee, B. L., and Bazzone, T. J., 1983, Isozymes of human liver alcohol dehydrogenase, in: *Isozymes: Current Topics in Biological and Medical Research*, Vol. 8, pp. 219–244, Liss, New York.

Von Bahr-Lindstrom, H., and Jornvall, J., 1985, Isolation of cDNA clones for class I ADH genes, *EMBO J.* (in press).

Von Bahr-Lindstrom, H., Jornvall, J., and Vallee, B. L., 1985, Amino acid sequence of human *ADH*1 (alpha) polypeptide, *EMBO J.* (in press).

Von Wartburg, J. P., and Schurch, P. M., 1968, Atypical human alcohol dehydrogenase, *Ann. N. Y. Acad. Sci.* 151:936–944.

Von Wartburg, J. P., and Bühler, R., 1984, Biology of disease alcoholism and aldehydism: New biomedical concepts, *Lab. Invest.* 50:5–15.

Wagner, F. W., Burger, A. R., and Vallee, B. L., 1983, Kinetic properties of human liver alcohol dehydrogenase: Oxidation of alcohols by class I isoenzymes, *Biochemistry* 22:1857–1863.

Woods, K. R., and Wang, K. T., 1967, *Biochim. Biophys. Acta* 133:369–370.

Woods, D. E., Markham, A. F., Ricker, R. T., Goldberger, G., Colten, H. R., 1982, Isolation of cDNA clones for the human complement protein Factor B, a Class III major histocompatibility complex gene product, *Proc. Nat. Acad. Sci.* 79:5661–5665.

Yin, S. J., Bosron, W. F., Li, T. K., Ohnishi, K., Okuda, K., Ishii, H., and Tsuchiya, M., 1984, Polymorphism of human liver alcohol dehydrogenase: Identification of *ADH*2 2-1 and *ADH*2 2-2 phenotypes in the Japanese by isoelectric focusing, *Biochem. Genet.* 22:169–180.

Yoshida, A., Wang, G., and Dave, V., 1983, Determinations of genotypes of human aldehyde dehydrogenase *ALDH*2 locus, *Am. J. Hum. Genet.* 35:1107–1116.

Addendum

CHAPTER 3: THE HUMAN ARGININOSUCCINATE SYNTHETASE LOCUS AND CITRULLINEMIA

Arthur L. Beaudet, William E. O'Brien,
Hans-Georg O. Bock, Svend O. Freytag,
and Tsung-Sheng Su

Analysis of regulation of argininosuccinate synthetase (AS) has been extended using a recombinant plasmid containing 3 kb of DNA upstream from the 5' end of the gene and 9 kb downstream including the first four exons. This fragment of the gene was linked to the bacterial chloramphenicol acetyltransferase (CAT) gene to form a CAT minigene. The CAT minigene was regulated by arginine when transfected into cultured human cells indicating the presence of *cis* regulatory sequences near the 5' end of the AS gene (Jackson *et al.*, 1985). The CAT minigene was expressed at a low level in canavanine resistant (Can^r) cells, but was derepressed when Can^r cells were subjected to arginine starvation. The results indicate that Can^r cells, which overproduce AS, are repressed with regard to arginine regulation; although the AS gene is no longer responsive to this regulation in Can^r cells.

Efforts directed at development of gene therapy for citrullinemia have resulted in construction of a retroviral vector which encodes AS activity. The human cDNA was inserted in a retroviral vector and defective viral particles were produced when the construction was introduced into ψ2 cells, a cell line developed for packaging ecotropic retrovirus (Mann *et al.*, 1983). Rodent cultured cells infected with the defective virus preparation synthesize human AS (Wood *et al.*, 1985). A rapid method for evaluating viral stocks for ability to transfer the functional AS cDNA was developed based on [^{14}C]citrulline incorporation into acid precipitable protein. Citrullinemia remains a good model disorder for evaluation of somatic gene therapy. Transfer of functional DNA sequences into bone marrow cells and into hepatocytes is being explored in animals.

REFERENCES

Jackson, M. J., Surh, L. C., Beaudet, A. L., and O'Brien, W. E., 1985, On defining the cis- and trans-acting components which regulate the human argininosuccinate synthetase (AS) locus, *Am. J. Hum. Genet.* **37**:A158.

Mann, R., Mulligan, R. C., and Baltimore, D., 1983, Construction of a retrovirus packaging mutant and its use to produce helper-free defective retrovirus. *Cell* **33**:153–159.

Wood P. A., O'Brien, W. E., and Beaudet, A. L., 1985, Development of citrullinemia as a model for gene therapy. *Am. J. Hum. Genet.* **37**:A183.

Index